T0226410

Soft Tissue Surgery

Editors

KURT K. SLADKY
CHRISTOPH MANS

VETERINARY CLINICS
OF NORTH AMERICA:
EXOTIC ANIMAL PRACTICE

www.vetexotic.theclinics.com

Consulting Editor
AGNES E. RUPLEY

January 2016 • Volume 19 • Number 1

ELSEVIER

1600 John F. Kennedy Boulevard ● Suite 1800 ● Philadelphia, Pennsylvania, 19103-2899

http://www.vetexotic.theclinics.com

VETERINARY CLINICS OF NORTH AMERICA: EXOTIC ANIMAL PRACTICE Volume 19, Number 1
January 2016 ISSN 1094-9194, ISBN-13: 978-0-323-41474-6

Editor: Patrick Manley
Developmental Editor: Meredith Clinton

Veterinary Clinics of North America: Exotic Animal Practice (ISSN 1094-9194) is published in January, May, and September by Elsevier, Inc., 360 Park Avenue South, New York, NY 10010-1710. Subscription prices are $260.00 per year for US individuals, $438.00 per year for US institutions, $100.00 per year for US students and residents, $305.00 per year for Canadian individuals, $528.00 per year for Canadian institutions, $340.00 per year for international individuals, $528.00 per year for international institutions and $165.00 per year for Canadian and foreign students/residents. To receive student/resident rate, orders must be accompanied by name of affiliated institution, date of term, and the *signature* of program/residency coordinator on institution letterhead. Orders will be billed at individual rate until proof of status is received. Foreign air speed delivery is included in all *Clinics* subscription prices. All prices are subject to change without notice. **POSTMASTER:** Send address changes to *Veterinary Clinics of North America: Exotic Animal Practice*, Elsevier Health Sciences Division, Subscription Customer Service, 3251 Riverport Lane, Maryland Heights, MO 63043. **Customer Service: Telephone: 1-800-654-2452** (U.S. and Canada); **1-314-447-8871** (outside U.S. and Canada). **Fax: 1-314-447-8029. E-mail: journalscustomerservice-usa@elsevier.com (for print support); journalsonlinesupport-usa@elsevier.com (for online support).**

Reprints. For copies of 100 or more of articles in this publication, please contact the Commercial Reprints Department, Elsevier Inc., 360 Park Avenue South, New York, New York 10010-1710. Tel.: 212-633-3874; Fax: 212-633-3820; E-mail: reprints@elsevier.com.

Veterinary Clinics of North America: Exotic Animal Practice is covered in *MEDLINE/PubMed (Index Medicus)*.

Contributors

CONSULTING EDITOR

AGNES E. RUPLEY, DVM
Diplomate, American Board of Veterinary Practitioners (Avian Practice); Director and Chief Veterinarian, All Pets Medical and Laser Surgical Center, College Station, Texas

EDITORS

KURT K. SLADKY, MS, DVM
Diplomate, American College of Zoological Medicine; Diplomate, European College of Zoological Medicine (Herpetology); Clinical Associate Professor, Department of Surgical Sciences, School of Veterinary Medicine, University of Wisconsin-Madison, Madison, Wisconsin

CHRISTOPH MANS, Dr med vet
Diplomate, American College of Zoological Medicine; Clinical Assistant Professor, Department of Surgical Sciences, School of Veterinary Medicine, University of Wisconsin-Madison, Madison, Wisconsin

AUTHORS

GEORGIA BOSSCHER, DVM
Department of Surgical Sciences, School of Veterinary Medicine, University of Wisconsin-Madison, Madison, Wisconsin

KATRIONA BRADLEY, BVMS, MRCVS
Tai Wai Small Animal and Exotic Hospital, Hong Kong, China

CASEY BUDGEON, DVM
Resident in Small Animal Surgery, Department of Surgical Sciences, School of Veterinary Medicine, University of Wisconsin-Madison, Madison, Wisconsin

ALANE KOSANOVICH CAHALANE, DVM, MA
Diplomate, American College of Veterinary Surgeons (Small Animal); Small Animal Surgeon, Co-Founder and CEO, VSH Hong Kong, Hong Kong, China

NORIN CHAI, DVM, MSc, PhD
Diplomate, ECZM (ZHM); Ménagerie du Jardin des Plantes, Muséum national d'Histoire Naturelle, Paris, France

ELSBURGH O. CLARKE III, DVM
Audubon Nature Institute, New Orleans, Louisiana

SARA A. COLOPY, DVM, PhD
Diplomate, American College of Veterinary Surgeons; Clinical Instructor, Department of Surgical Sciences, School of Veterinary Medicine, University of Wisconsin-Madison, Madison, Wisconsin

REBECCA CSOMOS, DVM, PhD
Department of Surgical Sciences, School of Veterinary Medicine, University of Wisconsin-Madison, Madison, Wisconsin

NICOLA DI GIROLAMO, DVM, MSc(EBHC)
Clinica per Animali Esotici, Centro Veterinario Specialistico, Roma, Italy

KATHRYN A. DIEHL, MS, DVM
Diplomate, American College of Veterinary Ophthalmologists; Assistant Professor, Department of Small Animal Medicine and Surgery, University of Georgia College of Veterinary Medicine, Athens, Georgia

STEPHEN J. DIVERS, BSc(Hons), BVetMed, FRCVS
DZooMed; DECZM (Herpetology); DECZM (Zoo Health Management); DACZM; Department of Small Animal Medicine and Surgery (Zoological Medicine), University of Georgia College of Veterinary Medicine, Athens, Georgia

DAVID SANCHEZ-MIGALLON GUZMAN, LV, MS
Diplomate of the European College of Zoological Medicine (Avian, Small Mammal); Diplomate of the American College of Zoological Medicine; Associate Professor of Clinical Companion Zoological Animal Medicine and Surgery, Department of Veterinary Medicine and Epidemiology, School of Veterinary Medicine University of California Davis, Davis, California

ROBERT HARDIE, DVM
Diplomate, ACVS; Diplomate, ECVS; Department of Surgical Sciences, School of Veterinary Medicine, University of Wisconsin-Madison, Madison, Wisconsin

KEVIN T. KRONER, DVM
Resident in Small Animal Surgery, Department of Surgical Sciences, School of Veterinary Medicine, University of Wisconsin-Madison, Madison, Wisconsin

CHRISTOPH MANS, Dr med vet
Diplomate, American College of Zoological Medicine; Clinical Assistant Professor, Department of Surgical Sciences, School of Veterinary Medicine, University of Wisconsin-Madison, Madison, Wisconsin

JOERG MAYER, Dr med vet, MSc
Diplomate, American Board of Veterinary Practitioners (Exotic Companion Mammal); Diplomate, European College of Zoological medicine (Small Mammal); Diplomate, American College of Zoological Medicine; Associate Professor, Zoological Medicine, University of Georgia College of Veterinary Medicine, Athens, Georgia

JO-ANN McKINNON, DVM
Diplomate, American College of Veterinary Ophthalmologists; Loudon, Tennessee

MEGAN A. MICKELSON, DVM
Resident in Small Animal Surgery, Department of Surgical Sciences, School of Veterinary Medicine, University of Wisconsin-Madison, Madison, Wisconsin

YASUTSUGU MIWA, DVM, PhD
Miwa Exotic Animal Hospital, Tokyo, Japan

MOLLY SHEPARD, DVM
Diplomate of the American College of Veterinary Anesthesia and Analgesia; Certified Canine Rehabilitation Practitioner, Certified Veterinary Medical Acupuncturist, Assistant Clinical Professor, Anesthesiology, University of Georgia College of Veterinary Medicine, Athens, Georgia; Veterinary Anesthesiologist and Physiotherapist, Chicago Veterinary Emergency & Speciality Center, Chicago, Illinois

IZIDORA SLADAKOVIC, BVSc (Hons I), MVS
Department of Small Animal Medicine and Surgery (Zoological Medicine), University of Georgia College of Veterinary Medicine, Athens, Georgia

KURT K. SLADKY, MS, DVM
Diplomate, American College of Zoological Medicine; Diplomate, European College of Zoological Medicine (Herpetology); Clinical Associate Professor, Department of Surgical Sciences, School of Veterinary Medicine, University of Wisconsin-Madison, Madison, Wisconsin

ZOLTAN SZABO, Dr med vet, GpCert(ExAP), MRCVS
Diplomate, American Board of Veterinary Practitioners (Exotic Companion Mammal Practice); Tai Wai Small Animal and Exotic Hospital, Hong Kong, China

Contents

The article focuses mainly on appropriate patient preparation for an anes-thetic episode. Special attention is given to evaluate the environmental sit-uation for optimal adjustment to reduce stress before the anesthetic event. During the anesthetic event, special attention must be paid regarding monitoring and evaluating the patient during and after the anesthetic episode.

The diversity implicit in exotic animal surgery requires a tailored approach to optimize successful outcomes. Outlined is information on patient prep-aration, instrumentation, hemostatic techniques, and magnification as it pertains to the exotic animal. Application of topical antiseptic solutions and judicious removal of pelage and feathers will decrease bacterial load during patient preparation. The use of specific barrier protection en-sures proper aseptic technique and enables optimal patient monitoring. Magnification combined with a focal light source enhances visual acuity, allowing for better use of delicate instrumentation and identification of anatomic structures.

The care of wounds in exotic animal species can be a challenging endeavor. Special considerations must be made in regard to the animal's temperament and behavior, unique anatomy and small size, and tendency toward secondary stress-related health problems. It is important to assess the entire patient with adequate systemic evaluation and consideration of proper nutrition and husbandry, which could ultimately affect wound heal-ing. This article summarizes the general phases of wound healing, factors that affect healing, and principles of wound management. Emphasis is placed on novel methods of treating wounds and species differences in wound management and healing.

Fish surgical procedures are commonplace in aquaria, zoos, laboratory fa-cilities, and pet clinical practice. To incorporate fish surgery into a clinical setting, an understanding of anatomic differences between mammals and fish, bath anesthetics, and recirculating anesthesia techniques must be developed, a system or different size systems to accommodate anesthesia and surgery of particular species of concern at an institution or practice constructed, and familiar mammalian surgical principles applied with some adaptations. Common surgical procedures in fish include coeliotomy for intracoelomic mass removal, reproductive procedures, gastrointestinal foreign body removal, radiotransmitter placement, and integumentary mass excision.

Amphibian surgery has been especially described in research. Since the last decade, interest for captive amphibians has increased, and so have the indications for surgical intervention. Clinicians should not hesitate to advocate such manipulations. Amphibian surgeries have no overwhelming obstacles. These patients heal well and tolerate blood loss more than higher vertebrates. Most procedures described in reptiles (mostly lizards) can be undertaken in most amphibians if equipment can be matched to the patients' size. In general, the most difficult aspect would be the provision of adequate anesthesia.

The surgical approach to reptiles can be challenging. Reptiles have unique physiologic, anatomic, and pathologic differences. This may result in frustrating surgical experiences; however, recent investigations provided novel, less invasive, surgical techniques. The purpose of this review was to describe the technical aspects behind soft tissue surgical techniques that have been used in reptiles, so as to provide a general guideline for veterinarians working with reptiles.

Basic surgical instrumentation for avian soft tissue surgery includes soft tissue retractors, microsurgical instrumentation, surgical loupes, and head-mounted lights. Hemostasis is fundamental during the surgical procedures. The indications, approach, and complications associated with soft tissue surgeries of the integumentary (digit constriction repair, feather cyst excision, cranial wound repair, sternal wound repair, uropygial gland excision), gastrointestinal (ingluviotomy, crop biopsy, crop burn repair, celiotomy, coelomic hernia and pseudohernia repair, proventriculotomy, ventriculotomy, enterotomy, intestinal resection and anastomosis, cloacoplasty, cloacopexy), respiratory (rhinolith removal, sinusotomy, tracheotomy, tracheal resection and anastomosis, tracheostomy, pneumonectomy) and reproductive (ovocentesis, ovariectomy, salpingohysterectomy, cesarean section, orchidectomy, vasectomy, phallectomy) systems are reviewed.

VETERINARY CLINICS OF NORTH AMERICA: EXOTIC ANIMAL PRACTICE

THE CLINICS ARE NOW AVAILABLE ONLINE!
Access your subscription at:
www.theclinics.com

Preface

Soft Tissue Surgery

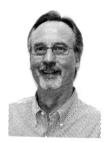 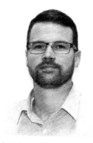

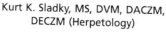

Kurt K. Sladky, MS, DVM, DACZM,   Christoph Mans, Dr med vet, DACZM
DECZM (Herpetology)

Editors

"The only weapon with which the unconscious patient can immediately retaliate upon the incompetent surgeon is hemorrhage."

—*William Stewart Halsted*

William Stewart Halsted (1852-1922), a human surgeon, was not only the founder of the medical residency training system as we know it today, but he also formulated the so-called Halsted's principles, which include gentle handling of tissue, meticulous hemostasis, preservation of blood supply, strict aseptic technique, minimum tension on tissues, accurate tissue apposition, and obliteration of dead space. These basic principles of human surgery also apply to animal patients, and adherence to these principles will greatly improve the success of surgery. While adherence to these principles is one important prerequisite for a successful outcome of a surgical procedure in exotic animals, another important consideration is the anatomic and physiologic features unique to many of these species.

Surgical techniques and equipment used in exotic animals have continued to evolve over the past 10 years, and many techniques and equipment used in human and small animal surgery have successfully been applied to exotic animal species. With these new and improved techniques, we are now able to perform surgical procedures with a less invasive approach and with less tissue trauma. Consequently, our patients will experience more rapid recoveries with less postsurgical pain. As an example of the recent evolution of exotic animal soft tissue surgery, consider the changes in chelonian intracoelomic procedures, with greater attention paid to prefemoral approaches, rather than plastron osteotomy. Over the past 10 years, it has been reported that this technique is suitable for a variety of surgical procedures, including ovariectomy, salpingectomy, salpingotomy, and cystotomy among others. The patient benefits associated with the prefemoral approach are significant, and include decreased post-surgical pain and shortened duration of tissue healing. As veterinarians, it is our

Vet Clin Exot Anim 19 (2016) xiii–xiv
http://dx.doi.org/10.1016/j.cvex.2015.09.002
1094-9194/16/$ – see front matter © 2016 Published by Elsevier Inc.

vetexotic.theclinics.com

duty to continue to investigate surgical techniques that are less invasive, but equally effective, when compared with standard techniques.

We believe that our invited contributors have achieved the difficult task of providing up-to-date summaries of exotic animal surgeries and presenting novel or improved surgical techniques. We would like to thank our talented contributors for their time and commitment to our issue of the *Veterinary Clinics of North America: Exotic Animal Practice*. We are honored that we could convince contributors from 10 different institutions, with a global representation, to share their personal experiences with us and provide thorough reviews of the current literature. We believe that the articles included in this issue will be of great interest to veterinarians treating exotic animals in various settings, and we hope that we have provided a thorough update on soft tissue surgery with respect to the previously published issue in of the *Veterinary Clinics of North America: Exotic Animal Practice*.

Furthermore, we owe our gratitude to the editorial team from Elsevier, particularly, Meredith Clinton, for all of her help and patience throughout the process.

Kurt K. Sladky, MS, DVM, DACZM, DECZM (Herpetology)
Department of Surgical Sciences
School of Veterinary Medicine
University of Wisconsin–Madison
2015 Linden Drive
Madison, WI 53706, USA

Christoph Mans, Dr med vet, DACZM
Department of Surgical Sciences
School of Veterinary Medicine
University of Wisconsin–Madison
2015 Linden Drive
Madison, WI 53706, USA

E-mail addresses:
sladkyk@svm.vetmed.wisc.edu (K.K. Sladky)
cmans@vetmed.wisc.edu (C. Mans)

Updates in Perioperative Care: Ideas from the Human Field

Joerg Mayer, Dr med vet, MSc, DABVP (ECM), DECZM (Small Mammal), DACZM[a,*],
Molly Shepard, DVM, DACVAA[b,c]

KEYWORDS

• Patient preparation • Environmental adjustment • Monitoring • Evaluating

KEY POINTS

• Knowledge of the natural history is a key point in the preparation of the patient.
• Providing adequate care prior, during, and after the anesthetic event is of equal importance.
• Being able to read the patient, and signs of discomfort, is important to avoid a crisis.

INTRODUCTION

The art of medicine consists of amusing the patient while nature cures the disease
—*Voltaire (1694–1778)*

In order to provide adequate surgical service, the focus on adequate perioperative care is of utmost importance for the exotic animal patient. In order to address this topic within the context of veterinary medicine, it is important to understand the definition, the basics, and the consequences of perioperative care. It is hoped that the following text provides proper guidelines and insight on how to improve patient care during this vulnerable period of the hospital stay. Many of the newer ideas regarding perioperative care in veterinary medicine have already been implemented successfully in human medicine. Because humans can easily communicate what and how they felt prior, during, and after the anesthetic event, recommendations on how to minimize human discomfort or anxiety can be implemented faster and easier than in veterinary medicine, whereby the patient-doctor communication is less straightforward. This

The authors have nothing to disclose.
[a] Zoological Medicine, University of Georgia College of Veterinary Medicine, 2200 College Station Road, Athens, GA 30605, USA; [b] Anesthesiology, University of Georgia College of Veterinary Medicine, 2200 College Station Road, Athens, GA 30605, USA; [c] Chicago Veterinary Emergency & Speciality Center, 3123 N Clybourn Avenue, Chicago, IL 60618, USA
* Corresponding author.
E-mail address: mayerj@uga.edu

article borrows a significant number of recommendations from human medical texts and ideas, in the hope of inspiring a new way of approaching perioperative management of veterinary patients. The article tries to highlight a few of these ideas, which can easily and should be partly incorporated into the routine of a modern veterinary clinic.

DEFINITION OF PERIOPERATIVE PERIOD AND CARE

In human medicine, the term perioperative refers to the total surgical experience of a patient and includes the preoperative, intraoperative, and postoperative phases of the patient's surgical journey.[1] For the purpose of this article, the term perioperative period is defined as the minute plans begin to anesthetize a patient for a surgical, medical, or diagnostic imaging procedure through the moment of hospital discharge.

Patient Preparation

Patient hospitalization

It has been shown in human medicine that visitation of patients in the preoperative period can reduce anxiety,[2] so the same fact is most likely true for many exotic veterinary patients. Many exotic pet species are prey animals and naturally nervous in a novel area where other sounds, smells, and views dictate the daily routine. Due to the fact that many veterinary patients are heavily driven by their senses, appropriate considerations before the surgical event can have a tremendously positive impact on patient well-being. Preparing the perioperative environment in order to minimize potential sources of stress should start before the patient arrives. Turner and colleagues[3] described the perioperative environment for humans as potentially one of the most hazardous of all clinical environments.[3] It could be argued that this is equally, if not more, important for exotic pets, which are prey species. Allowing the mate of a bonded pair to be in the same cage or in close proximity might provide additional psychological comfort for the sick animal.

Housing a rodent or rabbit in a quiet, calm, and darkened area before the surgery can help to provide an adequately soothing environment (**Fig. 1**). Housing prey animals away from barking dogs will help decrease stress. Housing a rabbit in close proximity to a ferret might cause anxiety for the rabbit. Many rodents have a limited visibility of the red light spectrum and this fact can be used to optimize a calm and secure

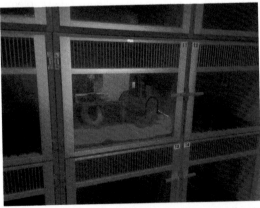

Fig. 1. A rabbit housed under a red light environment. Many small animals are not able to see red light spectrum and it appears dark to them, potentially reducing stress. (*Courtesy of* Dr J. Mayer, UGA.)

environment for those species. When rats were housed under red light versus white light, the findings of the study suggest that the basal metabolic rates of rats maintained in red-tinted cages were somewhat lower than those of rats housed in clear cages.[4] The same study also revealed that the rats housed in red compared with clear cages had significantly lower fluctuation amplitude of plasma corticosterone through the course of their circadian cycle. This finding can be interpreted as a lesser stress response and lesser effect on homeostasis for the animals in red cages. Reductions in the overall illumination during the night also correlated with a significant health benefit in this study population.[5] In the research setting, it has been shown that appropriate animal facility lighting protocols are essential for maintaining the health and well-being of laboratory animals and ensuring the credible outcome of scientific investigations.[5] This management strategy can clearly be applied to animals in the hospital setting. Undetectable levels of light-at-night[5] contamination in the animal quarters (ie, complete darkness) restored normal circadian regulation of rodent arterial blood melatonin, glucose, total fatty and linoleic acid concentrations, tumor uptake of oxygen, glucose, total fatty acid, and carbon dioxide production and tumor levels of cyclic adenosine monophosphate, triglycerides, free fatty acids, phospholipids, and cholesterol esters. Extracellular signal-regulated kinase, mitogen-activated protein kinase, serine–threonine protein kinase, glycogen synthase kinase, and proliferating cell nuclear antigen were also restored to normal levels when animals were kept in complete darkness.[5] An appropriate, strict lighting protocol in the ward area, where animals are housed before surgery, will have a significant impact on their well-being and should be

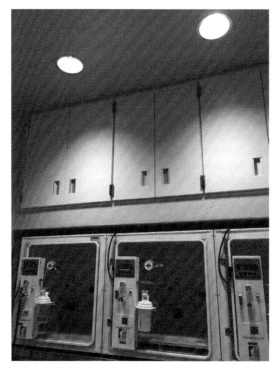

Fig. 2. Bright LED lights used to house avian patients. Many avian species require brighter conditions when compared with humans. The flicker effect of florescent lights can be distracting to the avian patient. (*Courtesy of* Dr J. Mayer, UGA.)

one of many factors adopted to reduce stress for hospitalized patients. In rabbits, it has been demonstrated that simply switching a light on during the normal period of darkness caused one rabbit to stop producing feces for 10 days in a study of caecotrophic rhythm.[6] Adequate lighting can also extremely important for avian husbandry. Recent studies have shown that birds require 5 to 20 times the light humans do in order to visualize colors in their environment.[7] The brightness of the sun in the tropics at midday is about 130,000 lux. Housing birds in an overly bright room for the human eye might be of significant benefit for many species.

A different but equally important aspect of avian vision is their ability to see strobing lights where humans do not see any strobing effect. Humans have a critical flicker fusion rate (CFF) around and less than 60 Hz, meaning that less than a frequency of 60 Hz, lighting motion appears continuous for humans, but this is seen as a continued flood of flickering images for birds. Common fluorescent lights usually flicker at 100 to 120 Hz. Studies show that some birds have a CFF around 100 Hz, but this depends on the type of bird and even differs individually.[8] A potential solution to increase illumination and flickering is to use light-emitting diode (LED) lights in areas where avian patients are housed for longer periods (**Fig. 2**). Although the topic of using LED lights versus incandescent light is still controversial, some evidence exists that the use of LED lighting has beneficial effects on poultry.[9]

These examples are only a few of how a clinician's knowledge of their patient's unique anatomy and physiology may impact the quality of their care in the hospital. The reader is advised to critically evaluate the natural history of the patient and to consider what factors of hospitalization might interfere with their well-being. Updating or adjusting a suboptimal hospital setting may require additional expenses but could increase the well-being of the patient significantly.

The Principles of Care During Anesthesia

Intra-anesthetic care is another very important part of the perioperative care period. Intra-anesthetic management requires preparation of the anesthetic equipment and more importantly applying species-specific knowledge and species-specific skills of anesthesia related to the patient's signalment, medical history, and the specific surgical procedure to ensure that the patient's individual needs are met. If the patient is a geriatric rat, for example, then additional precautions are needed to screen for subclinical disease such as renal or respiratory disease in this animal. In this respect, hospitalization on the day before a scheduled surgery can offer a significant benefit for the patient. Diagnostics, such as imaging, blood work, or fecal analysis, may be done on the day before surgery, in order to more accurately assess the patient's ASA physical status (risk analysis classification system according to the American Society of Anesthesiologists) and likely risk for complications. In addition, supportive therapies such as parenteral fluid support can be easily initiated and maintained through the moment of anesthetic induction, in the event of dehydration or renal insufficiency.

Anesthesia is a Greek word for no feeling and *analgesia* means without pain. The aim of any successful anesthetic procedure is to achieve analgesia as well as some degree of narcosis, depending on the depth required for the procedure. When making a decision about the anesthetic technique to be administered, that is, general or regional, the anesthetist should consider the species and signalment of the patient but also the patient's comorbidities and past responses to anesthesia, monitoring capabilities, and drug availability of the practice, the surgical approach, and experience level of the surgeon. Less invasive procedures, for example, or procedures involving tissues easily desensitized with local anesthetic techniques, may be performed using only sedation and regional anesthesia. More invasive procedures, however, or procedures that increase the risk of aspiration (ie, oral surgery) may require general anesthesia, that is, a deeper state of narcosis, in addition to adjunctive regional anesthetic techniques. Besides risk factors associated with the patient, facility, and surgeon, the client's preference or wishes need to be considered.

Anesthetists must assess their patients preoperatively in order to devise an optimal plan for each patient. Preoperative assessment should include a thorough physical examination (when possible, depending on the species and temperament of the patient), review of the medical record, if available, and any additional diagnostics that would improve the safety of anesthesia for that patient. The necessity of preanesthetic blood work is a controversial topic in both veterinary and human medicine. Although most adult humans can report their feelings to their physician regarding general health, veterinary patients, particularly those considered among a prey species, can be quite stoic and have adapted means of hiding subtle (or even severe!) illness from human observation. This phenomenon has been described in iguanas who did not show signs of pain when the animals realized that an observer was in the room.[10] Given this limitation, the authors of this article recommend preanesthetic complete blood count and biochemistry, if venipuncture can be achieved preoperatively with minimal stress.

The general goals of anesthesia can be divided into 3 components, a scheme that is referred to as the triad of anesthesia. These 3 elements are hypnosis (sleep), analgesia, and muscle relaxation. Although different surgical procedures require differing degrees of each factor, most surgical procedures performed on veterinary patients require all 3 factors adequately. In human medicine, care is taken during the induction of anesthesia that all personnel are calm and that noise, disruption, and disturbance are minimal, because hearing is the last sense to be depressed as the patient loses consciousness. Such ambience will aid the patient's state of mind at this time.[2] It would be difficult to produce scientific evidence that these observations apply to veterinary patients, but given the similarities in neuroanatomy and physiology that humans share with nonhuman mammals, as well as some degree of ethics-driven anthropomorphism, it is acceptable to assume that these considerations would benefit exotic veterinary patients as well. Exotic pet species are frequently less accustomed to human contact, resulting in fractious or aggressive behavior, so efforts to create a soothing environment are paramount. Although stress does not, in itself, cause pain, the state of anxiety associated with that stressful stimulus may amplify or suppress the animal's perception of nociceptive stimuli.

Surgical stimulation and pain can cause a series of physiologic changes related to the stress response, including catecholamine release and acute hemodynamic changes (eg, tachycardia, hypertension), acute behavioral responses (eg, flight, sweating, vomiting, aggression), immunologic changes adapted to maintain homeostasis, such as activation of the renin-angiotensin aldosterone system and cortisol secretion, insulin resistance and hyperglycemia, release of acute phase proteins and cytokines followed by white blood cell proliferation, accelerated catabolism of muscle, and subsequent weight loss. Analgesics often reduce the body's response to such stimulation. In rats, it has been shown that stresses imposed during anesthesia can lead to posttraumatic stress disorder (PTSD) symptoms in the distant future, and these can be prevented with sufficient concentrations of inhaled anesthetic.[11] It is therefore important to adequately assess the patient under anesthesia to make sure that the patient is not too light to avoid a potential PTSD. An unexplained and infrequent phenomenon in human medicine is awareness with recall after general anesthesia, which may result in PTSD.[12] A retrospective study found that in human medicine this happens at a rate of 1 to 2 cases per 1000 patients and that the awareness was associated with increased ASA physical status.[12] It is clearly difficult to assess if this phenomenon may also be possible in veterinary medicine. In order to objectively assess the cortical activity in human anesthesia, the bispectral index (BIS) is considered an adequate monitoring tool and its usefulness in monitoring human anesthesia is well established.[13] Unfortunately, this monitoring tool has not been validated in veterinary medicine. Although some data for different species exist to date, the BIS has been shown to produce a paradoxic increase during deep anesthesia in New Zealand white rabbits, rendering its usefulness in exotic species questionable.[14] In addition to the problem of adequately evaluating consciousness during an anesthetic event, evidence exists that general anesthesia may precipitate prolonged postanesthetic memory impairment in aged rats.[15] Although the exact mechanism of this observation is unclear, it should not be ignored that any anesthetic event has the potential to cause some postanesthetic stress on the patient.

Anesthetic monitoring

A minimum standard of monitoring during anesthesia and recovery should be established for every procedure at any given clinic. During induction of anesthesia, this can include the use of a pulse oximeter, a noninvasive blood pressure monitoring system, an electrocardiogram, and ideally, capnography to measure the CO_2 in expired air at the end of respiration (**Fig. 3**). For patients undergoing complex, invasive procedures, which require a longer anesthetic episode or are considered at high risk because of comorbidities, additional monitoring might be very beneficial. This additional monitoring can include invasive monitoring such as invasive blood pressure and central venous pressure and measurement of urine output. The monitoring of body temperature is of utmost importance because most exotic patients have a high body-surface-to-mass ratio, and a significant drop in core temperature can happen within a few minutes of anesthesia. Patients lose body heat by conductive, convective, radiative, and evaporative processes. Some of the contributory factors that allow hypothermia to develop in this environment are multifold:

- Convective heat loss:
  - Inhalant anesthetics cause vasodilation, which accelerates heat loss from the body.
  - The ambient temperature of the room causes heat loss: very often the surgical theater is kept cool, mainly to suit staff comfort.
  - The most effective intervention to prevent and treat convective heat loss is forced-air heating.[16] Small exotic patients may also be placed in incubators

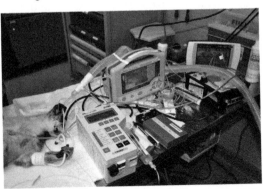

Fig. 3. Anesthetic monitoring in a ring-tailed lemur (*Lemur catta*). Note that capnography, pulse oximetry, and indirect blood pressure measurements are used to monitor this patient.

for convective heating. The advantage of the latter in the postoperative period, when the patient is no longer intubated, is that the patient may be observed without handling, and supplemental oxygen may be provided along with warmth.

- Conductive heat loss:
  - Fluids are given intravenously or under the skin without being warmed adequately. Or in case of a longer procedure, fluids are allowed to cool down while they slowly drip into the patient over a prolonged time period.
  - Patients are commonly placed on surfaces with high thermal conductivity (eg, metal gurneys or procedure tables), which draw heat away from the body.
  - Interventions for conductive heat loss include the use of heated procedure tables, placement of towels or blankets between the patient and the proce-dure table, resistive heaters,[16] and warm water blankets. Fluid warmers are not effective for this purpose in humans.[17] Although the efficacy of warming intravenous or lavage fluids has yet to be investigated in small or exotic animals; anecdotally, the use of warm lavage fluids seems very effective at conductively increasing core body temperature during open-abdominal procedures.
- Radiative heat loss
  - Failure of hospital staff to cover the patient's body with blankets, towels, or heating devices can allow the body to lose heat to the environment.
  - Prevention and treatment of radiative heat loss can be accomplished by covering the patient with blankets, when possible. Radiative heaters such as those used in human neonatal care units are also very useful, although they have the potential to cause hyperthermia in small exotic animals, if tempera-ture monitoring is not optimal.[18] Finally, reducing the time required for aseptic preparation of the patient's skin can reduce the time they are allowed to lose heat by radiation.
- Evaporative heat loss
  - Before and again after positioning in the operating theater, aseptic preparation of the surgical site is performed, which allows more heat loss as the prepara-tion solutions evaporate.
  - Fluid evaporation from open abdominal and thoracic cavities during surgery al-lows loss of heat.
  - Fluid evaporation from the respiratory tract during anesthesia (particularly when using non-rebreathing circuits and the higher fresh gas flow rates that they require) accelerates heat loss.
  - The best means of preventing evaporative heat loss seems to be limitation of anesthetic duration. When feasible in patients greater than 3 kg in body weight, a circle (rebreathing) system should be used to reduce evaporative heat loss from the respiratory tract. Heat and moisture exchangers designed to humidify gas in the breathing circuit have not been shown effective in mammals greater than 15 kg in body weight[19] and may increase resistance to breathing for smaller patients.

Within the intraoperative phase, the patient is extremely vulnerable and totally reliant on perioperative staff and other members of the team to ensure that they come to no harm. Communication and keen observation of the patient are key factors in assuring a safe recovery from anesthesia and are addressed later. The authors recommend the use of transparent drapes for small exotic patients in order to facilitate visual monitoring of the patient during the procedure. Intraoperatively, clinical risks are associated with patient positioning (eg, may affect ventilation and venous return), the risk of infection, risk of hypothermia, surgical procedure (eg, hemorrhage), and risks associated with use of anesthesia equipment. Although a procedure-specific list is not exhaustive, it identifies those potential risks to each individual patient undergoing surgery. For each risk identified beforehand, strategies should be discussed to minimize any risk to patients and staff alike.

Risk management

As in other high-risk industries (eg, aviation, oil, nuclear), the incidence of serious events has been reduced by several orders of magnitude through a focus on safety, communication, and individual behaviors (human factors). Identification and focused reform of the contributory elements of safety have reduced the incidence of disasters in these high-risk industries. A recent book in the popular media has highlighted this strategy in the context of the medical industry.[20] The author states that human surgery has 4 big killers: infection, bleeding, unsafe anesthesia, and the unexpected.[20] Although a checklist alone will not insure safe practice, communication, teamwork, and discipline are also equally crucial for a successful outcome. Within human medicine, it has been shown that the implementation of a checklist was associated with concomitant reductions in the rates of death and complications among patients who were undergoing noncardiac surgery in a diverse group of hospitals.[21] One recent study in veterinary medicine showed that the use of a short perianesthetic checklist in a veterinary teaching hospital significantly reduced the number of incidents such as medication errors, esophageal intubation, and closed adjustable pressure limiting valves.[22] This checklist should include preparation of all equipment and emergency drugs before induction in order to avoid any delay in treatment, should an emergency occur.

Immediate Postoperative Care

The same concept of adequately preparing the patient before the procedure also applies to the period after the surgical procedure. The main objectives of adequate recovery care are to continue to critically evaluate and stabilize the patient postoperatively. The immediate recovery phase is one of the most critical time points during the perioperative episode, as the patient slowly regains consciousness and becomes aware of the surroundings. Staff must anticipate and prevent potential complications in order to safeguard the patient's well-being until they are conscious and able to do so themselves. The recovering animal should be placed in a room, which is easily accessible, quiet, and monitored throughout the whole recovery process. The patient should be monitored by a skilled and knowledgeable staff, which is able to deal quickly and efficiently with any changes in the patient's condition. During the recovery process, a patient's airway must be kept patent, clear of blood or mucus. Staff must continuously monitor the patient, to ensure that adequate ventilation is achieved, and this may require support or assistance with the position of the head or neck or an airway adjunct such as a facemask, ambu bag, or air sac cannula. The patient should be repositioned in lateral recumbency or supine, depending on the situation. Oxygen therapy should be available via an oxygen mask or endotracheal tube if needed. One has to observe the movements of the chest and auscultate each hemithorax to ensure bilateral, even air movement, and feel the air flowing in and out of the mouth. Stridor or stertor are often indications of airway obstruction and indicate immediate action to relieve the obstruction. Regurgitation is often observed during the recovery phase. However, obstructed breathing is not always noisy, as complete obstruction is characterized by silence and occurs easily in smaller patients. Although the color of the mucus membranes may indicate oxygenation, subtle changes in mucous membrane color may not be noticeable, despite significant hypoxemia, and true cyanosis may not occur in anemic patients, or until hypoxemia is dangerously severe. The respiratory rate and pattern (rhythm, depth, and apparent effort on expiration or inspiration) should be serially monitored in recovery, because these changes could also be an early indication of impending respiratory or cardiac failure.

After the airway has been established and is monitored, additional parameters such as blood pressure and pulse rate should also be monitored during the recovery phase. When relying on monitors during the recovery phase, it must be remembered that electronic monitors alert staff to changes in condition, but are not a replacement for the ongoing physical, visual assessment and observation of the patient, which will allow trained staff to detect subtle changes in condition without relying on monitors. It has been shown that a human patient may be hypoxic despite a 98% reading on the pulse oximeter.[2]

The visual inspection of the patient should include checking for the return of protective reflexes and consciousness. It is not uncommon to see a state of renarcotization after the patient has been aroused at the end of anesthesia and then allowed to relax. If the patient is receiving intravenous fluids, the fluid type, drip rate, and the patency of the catheter site should be verified regularly. All postoperative assessments and observations should be recorded in the patient's documentation at the time of the observation. The recovering patient has a high potential for complications during the immediate postoperative period, and the person monitoring the recovery plays a vital role in detecting, preventing, and managing dangerous or even life-threatening conditions. The authors know from the accounts of human patients that waking up from an anesthetic episode can be a frightening experience. Animals and especially prey animals are likely to experience a similar state of confusion and fright. Unnatural external stimuli like bright lights, uncharacteristic noises, lack of familiarity with the surroundings, and pain may trigger an additional stress response in the vulnerable patient. Awareness of these potential stressors and efforts to avoid them might be of significant benefit to the patient. Various research has shown that normal, healthy exotic animals will respond to handling with a stress response.

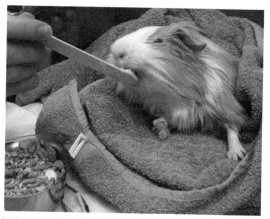

Fig. 4. A guinea pig is recovering from anesthesia. Providing nutritional support once the animal is awake is important to stimulate the gastrointestinal tract function.

Animals that are expected to exhibit this response include reptiles,[23] birds,[24] and mammals.[25] Based on these findings, it would make sense to also minimize handling during the recovery phase while exotic animal patients are vulnerable to stress.

Providing nutritional support to once the animal is awake is important to stimulate the gastrointestinal tract function, in particular in rabbits and rodents (**Fig. 4**).

Managing a Patient's Pain

Being familiar with the clinical manifestation of pain in various exotic animals is of utmost importance during the perioperative period (**Fig. 5**). Various references exist to date on how to score pain in reptiles, mammals, and birds and in recognizing pain and distress in laboratory animals.[26–29] The reader should be familiar with these specific behaviors, because signs of pain can be subtle and easily missed or misinterpreted. The objective of effective pain management is to apply a preemptive and multimodal analgesic approach. From human medicine, it is known that pain is a highly subjective experience, and an accurate assessment in veterinary medicine can be difficult to achieve. Assessment of the source and severity of pain in animals can only be made by the observation of the patient's behavior. Just providing a recommend dose might not be good enough, given the individual variability in any noxious stimulus or the individual animal's sensitivity to that stimulus. Repeated assessment is imperative for the individual care of the patient. Pain assessment in the postoperative period can be very difficult if the patient is drowsy or sedated: states of narcosis may confound the behavioral cues of pain for that animal. Even in human medicine, the recovery nurses are instructed to observe nonverbal clues, such as restlessness, grimacing, and hyperventilation.[2] Hypoxia, hypothermia, anxiety, nausea, fatigue, and pain are all symptoms of a human's stress response to surgery.[2] These findings are most likely all applicable to exotic pet patients as well. It is known that pain has many detrimental effects on the recovering body, including a delay of return to normal function as well as impaired wound healing and predisposition to infection.[2] Beyond the recognition of pain, responsiveness to analgesics can have individual variability as well as a great deal of variability between species. For example, one study comparing the pharmacokinetics of 3 different nonsteroidal anti-inflammatory drugs in various bird species showed

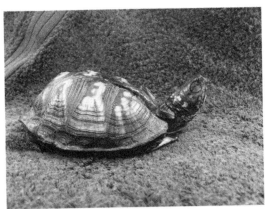

Fig. 5. The turtle is exhibiting signs of severe pain (opisthotonus); knowledge of species-specific behavior is a key element in order to provide adequate analgesia. (*Courtesy of Dr J. Mayer, UGA.*)

a significantly longer half-life of meloxicam in chickens and pigeons than in ostriches.[30] The zoo and exotic animal veterinarian must therefore realize the danger in extrapolating drug recommendations between species.

SUMMARY

In order to provide the safest perioperative experience for the exotic patient, one has to consider the species-specific anatomy and physiology of the patient. The authors described the appropriate housing, preparation, monitoring, and recovery strategies, which should be considered for the exotic patient undergoing an anesthetic procedure. The key to a successful anesthetic procedure is thorough assessment and preparation before the procedure, and optimal monitoring during and after anesthesia. Thorough preparation and appropriate monitoring are the foundation of good anesthetic technique and are imperative for the success of any anesthetic procedure.

REFERENCES

1. Phillips NF, Berry EC, Kohn ML. Berry & Kohn's operating room technique. 11th edition. St Louis (MO): Mosby; 2007. p. xvi, 1024.
2. Gilmour D. Perioperative care. In: Pudner R, editor. Nursing the surgical patient. London: Elsevier Science; 2005. p. 17–33.
3. Turner S, Wicker P, Hind M. Principles of safe practice in the perioperative environment. In: MW, Hind P, editors. Principles of safe practice. Edinburgh (Untied Kingdom): Churchill Livingstone; 2000. Available at: http://japr. oxfordjournals.org/content/17/2/211.full.
4. Dauchy RT, Wren MA, Dauchy EM, et al. Effect of spectral transmittance through red-tinted rodent cages on circadian metabolism and physiology in nude rats. J Am Assoc Lab Anim Sci 2013;52(6):745–55.
5. Dauchy RT, Dupepe LM, Ooms TG, et al. Eliminating animal facility light-at-night contamination and its effect on circadian regulation of rodent physiology, tumor growth, and metabolism: a challenge in the relocation of a cancer research laboratory. J Am Assoc Lab Anim Sci 2011;50(3):326–36.
6. Jilge B. The response of the caecotrophy rhythm of the rabbit to single light signals. Lab Anim 1980;14(1):3–5.
7. Lind O, Kelber A. The intensity threshold of colour vision in two species of parrot. J Exp Biol 2009;212(Pt 22):3693–9.
8. Lisney TJ, Rubene D, Rózsa J, et al. Behavioural assessment of flicker fusion frequency in chicken Gallus gallus domesticus. Vision Res 2011;51(12):1324–32.
9. Cao J, Liu W, Wang Z, et al. Green and blue monochromatic lights promote growth and development of broilers via stimulating testosterone secretion and myofiber growth. J Appl Poult Res 2008;17(2):211–8.
10. Fleming GJ, Robertson SA. Assessments of thermal antinociceptive effects of butorphanol and human observer effect on quantitative evaluation of analgesia in green iguanas (Iguana iguana). Am J Vet Res 2012;73(10):1507–11.
11. Rau V, Oh I, Laster M, et al. Isoflurane suppresses stress-enhanced fear learning in a rodent model of posttraumatic stress disorder. Anesthesiology 2009;110(3):487–95.
12. Sebel PS, Bowdle TA, Ghoneim MM, et al. The incidence of awareness during anesthesia: a multicenter United States study. Anesth Analg 2004;99(3):833–9. Table of contents.

13. Glass PS, Bloom M, Kearse L, et al. Bispectral analysis measures sedation and memory effects of propofol, midazolam, isoflurane, and alfentanil in healthy volunteers. Anesthesiology 1997;86(4):836–47.
14. Romanov A, Moon RS, Wang M, et al. Paradoxical increase in the bispectral index during deep anesthesia in New Zealand white rabbits. J Am Assoc Lab Anim Sci 2014;53(1):74–80.
15. Culley DJ, Baxter M, Yukhananov R, et al. The memory effects of general anesthesia persist for weeks in young and aged rats. Anesth Analg 2003;96(4): 1004–9. Table of contents.
16. Roder G, Sessler DI, Roth G, et al. Intra-operative rewarming with Hot Dog((R)) resistive heating and forced-air heating: a trial of lower-body warming. Anaesthesia 2011;66(8):667–74.
17. Campbell G, Alderson P, Smith AF, et al. Warming of intravenous and irrigation fluids for preventing inadvertent perioperative hypothermia. Cochrane Database Syst Rev 2015;4:CD009891.
18. Hofmeister EH, Hernandez-Divers SJ. Anesthesia case of the month. Tachycardia. J Am Vet Med Assoc 2005;227(5):718–20.
19. Hofmeister EH, Brainard BM, Braun C, et al. Effect of a heat and moisture exchanger on heat loss in isoflurane-anesthetized dogs undergoing single-limb orthopedic procedures. J Am Vet Med Assoc 2011;239(12):1561–5.
20. Gawande A. The checklist manifesto: how to get things right. 1st edition. New York: Metropolitan Books; 2010. p. x, 209.
21. Haynes AB, Weiser TG, Berry WR, et al. A surgical safety checklist to reduce morbidity and mortality in a global population. N Engl J Med 2009;360(5):491–9.
22. Hofmeister EH. Development and implementation of a short anesthesia checklist in a university teaching hospital. Athens (GA): University of Georgia; 2013.
23. Cabanac M, Bernieri C. Behavioral rise in body temperature and tachycardia by handling of a turtle (Clemmys insculpta). Behav Processes 2000;49(2):61–8.
24. Cabanac M, Aizawa S. Fever and tachycardia in a bird (Gallus domesticus) after simple handling. Physiol Behav 2000;69(4–5):541–5.
25. Cabanac M, Dardashti M. Emotional fever in rats persists after vagotomy. Physiol Behav 1999;67(3):347–50.
26. Hawkins P. Recognizing and assessing pain, suffering and distress in laboratory animals: a survey of current practice in the UK with recommendations. Lab Anim 2002;36(4):378–95.
27. Carstens E, Moberg GP. Recognizing pain and distress in laboratory animals. ILAR J 2000;41(2):62–71.
28. Bays TB, Lightfoot T, Mayer JR. Exotic pet behavior: birds, reptiles, and small mammals. St Louis (MO): Saunders Elsevier; 2006. p. xxii, 360.
29. Stoskopf MK. Pain and analgesia in birds, reptiles, amphibians, and fish. Invest Ophthalmol Vis Sci 1994;35(2):775–80.
30. Baert K, De Backer P. Comparative pharmacokinetics of three non-steroidal anti-inflammatory drugs in five bird species. Comp Biochem Physiol C Toxicol Pharmacol 2003;134(1):25–33.

Update on Surgical Principles and Equipment

Kevin T. Kroner, DVM, Casey Budgeon, DVM, Sara A. Colopy, DVM, PhD, DACVS*

KEYWORDS

- Surgical asepsis • Surgical instruments • Draping • Hemostasis • Suture materials

KEY POINTS

- Surgery on exotic species requires a tailored approach with challenges relating to hemostasis, thermoregulation, and small body size.
- Preparation for surgery should focus on decreasing bacterial burden while minimizing time under anesthesia and permitting adequate patient monitoring.
- Unique instruments and appropriate magnification and lighting should be considered to optimize visualization, tissue handling, and dissection.
- Advances in electrosurgery and laser technology have improved hemostasis during surgery and offers diversity to the surgeon.

INTRODUCTION

Surgery on small mammals, reptiles, and avian species poses unique challenges to the veterinary surgeon. The variety of tissue characteristics, blood volume, thermoregulatory properties, and susceptibility to anesthesia and perioperative medications requires a tailored approach to each patient. Because of their large surface area-to-volume, most exotic species are at risk of rapid hypothermia, and their relatively small blood volume can result in hypovolemia after seemingly minimal blood loss. Precise, efficient patient preparation, meticulous hemostasis, close patient monitoring, and brief operative periods are best to overcome these challenges.

PATIENT PREPARATION

Aseptic technique is paramount in all aspects of surgery and should be strictly followed in any procedure. Removal of fur and feathers decreases the bacterial burden and aids in visualization, but the process can be challenging and should be done with caution. Small mammals such as rabbits have particularly fragile skin that can be

The authors have nothing to disclose.
Department of Surgical Sciences, School of Veterinary Medicine, University of Wisconsin-Madison, 2015 Linden Drive, Madison, WI 53706, USA
* Corresponding author.
E-mail address: colopys@svm.vetmed.wisc.edu

Vet Clin Exot Anim 19 (2016) 13–32
http://dx.doi.org/10.1016/j.cvex.2015.08.011
1094-9194/16/$ – see front matter © 2016 Elsevier Inc. All rights reserved.

damaged during clipping, increasing the risk of blood loss and postoperative infection. Small and delicate clipper blades should be used, and the skin should be stretched so that a flat taut surface is achieved to minimize the risk of iatrogenic laceration.

In avian species, smaller feathers can be plucked in groups of 3 to 4. Gentle outward pressure is applied in the orientation of the follicle to avoid damage. These smaller feathers will be replaced quickly. Removal of larger flight feathers should be avoided. If there is soft tissue damage surrounding the follicle of large feathers, you may cut the feather, understanding that they will not regrow until the next molting cycle.[1]

Evaluation of the method and timing of hair removal has provided conflicting results in the literature. Currently, it is recommended to perform this process immediately preoperatively (less than 2 hours before surgery) via electronic clippers (in patients with hair or fur).[1–3] The surgical field should be free from fur and feathers; however, extensive loss can lead to a decrease in insulation and subsequent hypothermia. Therefore, it is recommended that approximately 2- to 3-cm margins be achieved in small patients.[1]

Whether to wash or bathe the patient before surgery also remains controversial. Most existing studies in human and veterinary literature suggest only a transient decrease in bacterial numbers and potential damage to surrounding skin, which may actually predispose the patient to infection. Therefore, preoperative bathing is not currently recommended in veterinary medicine.[4]

ANTISEPTICS

Following the removal of hair and fur, the skin is aseptically prepared using an antiseptic solution to reduce normal skin flora. The ideal antiseptic should be nontoxic, should not cause skin reaction, and should not interfere with the normal protective function of the skin.[3,5]

Alcohols

Alcohols have strong bactericidal properties but are less effective at eliminating viral and fungal organisms. The bactericidal activity of alcohols is attributed to denaturation of proteins, alteration of metabolism, and direct cell lysis. Alcohols are most effective at concentrations greater than 60%.[5] Undesirable effects of alcohols include skin irritation and decreased efficacy in the face of organic debris. For smaller patients, alcohols may also cause hypothermia, so judicious use is advised.

Iodophors

The antiseptic activity of iodophors (eg, povidone-iodine) is derived from the presence of molecular iodine and hypoiodic acid. Free iodine has broad-spectrum activity against bacteria, viruses, and fungi. There are few undesirable effects associated with iodophor antiseptics but may include adverse skin reactions or systemic iodine toxicity when used in open wounds.[5] Iodophors are minimally affected by organic debris when compared with other antiseptic solutions. Dilution to concentrations of 0.001% to 0.1% may still possess antiseptic properties while decreasing the risk of complications.

Chlorhexidine

Chlorhexidine is a broad-spectrum antiseptic that is most effective against bacteria, with variable efficacy against most virus and fungal organisms. Concentration of chlorhexidine greatly influences its efficacy, with higher concentrations (2%–4%) being more bactericidal.[6] At lower concentrations, the mechanism of action is attributed to disruption of the bacterial cell membrane, whereas at higher concentrations, chlorhexidine causes coagulation of cellular contents. Chlorhexidine is somewhat inhibited by the presence of organic debris; however, at least one study documented superior antiseptic properties in the face of blood when compared with povidone-iodine. Chlorhexidine binds to the tissue, leading to a long residual effect after application when compared with other antiseptic agents, making it an appealing alternative to other antiseptic agents.[3] Chlorhexidine, particularly at doses of 0.05% or less, does not cause significant cytotoxicity; however, at higher concentrations, it has been found to produce neurotoxic and ototoxic effects, making its use in areas surrounding the ear and eyes questionable.[6] In exotic species, it is commonly recommended to use a warm, dilute 0.05% chlorhexidine solution for surgical preparation to avoid the hypothermic effects of alcohol-based or cold antiseptic solutions.

Comparison of Antiseptic Agents

Aseptic techniques commonly used before surgery involve use of a chlorhexidine- or iodine-based scrub (**Fig. 1**) in alternation with alcohol. Despite these recommendations, approximately 20% of the normal flora still remain, emphasizing the importance of intraoperative aseptic technique.[3] Recent studies have found similar results when using a one-step process using a combination of isopropyl alcohol with an iodophor (DuraPrep 3M, St. Paul, MN, USA) (**Fig. 2**).[7–9] Direct comparisons between iodophor and chlorhexidine preparations have revealed similar efficacy in reducing bacterial burden, with a slightly higher rate of skin irritation when using povidone-iodine.[3,10] Combinations of different antiseptic solutions have been shown to be effective in

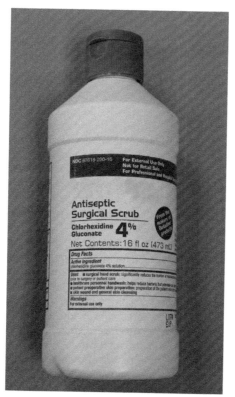

Fig. 1. Chlorhexidine (4%) surgical scrub.

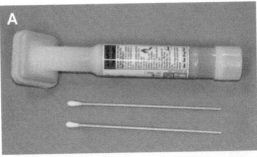

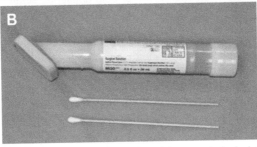

Fig. 2. Application device with 0.7% iodine and 74% isopropyl alcohol. Top (*A*) and side (*B*) view of surgical prepping solution application device containing 0.7% iodine and 74% isopropyl alcohol.

certain circumstances at decreasing bacterial load.[11] Impermeable adherent drapes impregnated with iodophors have been used following aseptic skin preparation to minimize contamination from neighboring tissue.[6]

SURGICAL DRAPES

The concept of local barrier protection has led to the development of a vast array of different techniques with the goal of preventing microbial spread from the patient into the surgical field. Ideal draping material should be impermeable to fluid, resistant to mechanical damage, and remain in place during manipulation.[5] The initial boundary should surround the planned incision site. An additional superficial layer extends to cover the body beyond the preparation site to minimize risk of contamination and allow surgical personnel to maneuver while abiding by aseptic technique. Historically, this has been achieved with the use of woven and nonwoven cloth drapes that can be either recycled or discarded after initial use.[12]

Draping poses a unique challenge in exotic species due to small body size and need for constant visual monitoring. Clear plastic drapes are commonly used in exotic surgery, allowing more precise patient monitoring and better thermoregulation (**Fig. 3**). Clear adherent drapes are also available; however, recent evidence suggests these drapes may increase the risk of surgical site infections.[13] Adhesive drapes can be challenging to maneuver due to the adhesive backing and can damage the delicate integument of smaller patients when removed. Therefore, adhesive drapes should be used with caution in exotic species. As mentioned previously, some adherent drapes are impregnated with antiseptics to further prevent bacterial contamination, although evidence that these drapes decrease the incidence of surgical site infection is lacking.[14]

The recommendation of the authors is to apply a primary layer of barrier drapes, covering the inner borders of the prepared surgical field, secured to the patient with

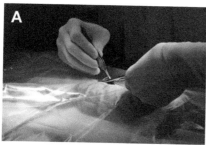
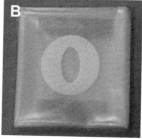

Fig. 3. Application of a clear plastic drape with fenestration for laparotomy on a green iguana (*Iguana iguana*) (*A*). Example of prefenestrated drape with adhesive border (*B*).

towel clamps. A transparent drape with a fenestration made to match the size of the proposed incision site can then be placed to cover the remainder of operative table. For smaller patients, a single fenestrated adherent plastic drape may be used to optimize patient monitoring and prevent iatrogenic trauma from towel clamps.

SURGICAL INSTRUMENTATION

Standard surgical instruments may be used for most exotic animal surgeries, especially on larger patients. In smaller patients, however, small instruments are required for better surgical precision. The surgeon may consider using ophthalmic or microsurgery instruments. Microsurgery instruments are generally preferred over ophthalmic instruments. Microsurgery instruments are longer, reaching the surgical site within the patient, while allowing the surgeon to rest the hands outside the body for stabilization. The microsurgery instruments should be comfortable in the surgeon's hand to limit fatigue and allow fine control of instrument manipulation.[1]

Microsurgery instruments have many other attributes that make them an ideal choice for exotic animal surgery. They are counterbalanced for better hand control and more precise movement. The locking mechanisms, or lack thereof, tend to allow more precise control, preventing sudden movements and forces that can bend and break smaller needles and suture. Microsurgery instruments are available with rounded handles, allowing the instrument to be rolled between the thumb and index finger while holding the instrument with the preferred pencil grip. Microsurgery instruments most often have a satin finish for reduced glare.[15] Many of the attributes that make microsurgery instruments excellent for small exotic animal surgery also require experience in using them. Therefore, the surgeon should practice using them before attempting surgery in a live animal.

Basic surgery packs have been proposed for use in small mammals and exotics, including the following instruments: Jones towel clamps (6), Adson dressing forceps (1), Adson tissue forceps (1), Bard-Parker scalpel blade number 3 (1), blunt, curved tenotomy scissors (1), curved LeGrange scissors (1), Olsen-Hegar needle holder (1), Hartmann straight mosquito forceps (2), and Hartmann curved mosquito forceps (2). Jacobson or Packer mosquito forceps may replace the Hartmann forceps given their finer tips, which are advantageous for the extremely small vessels encountered with exotic animals.[16,17]

Small scalpel blades are preferred for small, exotic species, such as a number 3 scalpel handle with a number 11 or 15 blade. Another option is a Beaver blade. These blades are smaller than number 11 and 15 blades and come in a variety of configurations (**Fig. 4**).

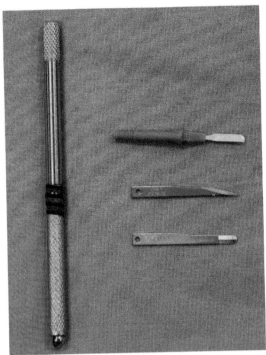

Fig. 4. Beaver blades have an advantage of being much smaller than standard number 11 or 15 blades and come in a variety of configurations. Three different blade styles are shown with a handle.

Small gauze pads may be included in the pack as well as cotton-tipped applicators. Cotton-tipped applicators may be used for gentle tissue manipulation as well as hemostasis. For tissue manipulation in very small animals, microbrushes may be adapted from dentistry use for very fine and delicate work (**Fig. 5**).

Retractors are an essential piece of equipment used during surgery. A surgical assistant may be of great value; however, an assistant's hands may impede the surgeon's visualization in very small surgical fields.[16] Tissue retraction is necessary, but

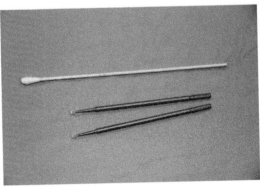

Fig. 5. Microbrushes may be adapted from dentistry for gentle tissue manipulation. Two microbrushes are shown here next to a standard cotton-tipped applicator.

tension must be controlled to avoid morbidity associated with the retractor. Ring retractors are often the recommended retractor for exotic animal surgery. The most common is the Lone Star Retractor System (Jorgenson Laboratories). This system uses a plastic ring or frame that surrounds the operative field and has notches to accommodate individual stays. A hook is applied to retract the tissue as needed, and the elastic band is then pulled to appropriate tension and inserted into one of the notches in the ring. Stays are added and adjusted as needed to achieve visualization (**Fig. 6**).[18]

Other options for retraction include small self-retaining retractors. Commonly recommended retractors are the Alm and Heiss retractors. These instruments are small adjustable retractors that tension can be adjusted to the size of the wound. The Alm retractor uses a thumbscrew adjustment, whereas the Heiss retractor uses a ratchet mechanism (**Fig. 7**). For extremely small patients or wounds, one may consider retractors such as the Agricola or the Trigger Finger Self-Retaining Retractor (buxtonbio.com). These retractors are lighter and less than 4 mm in total length and have a thumbscrew to adjust tension. Eyelid retractors have been proposed for use in exotic animal surgery; however, these are not recommended because they are maintained in an open position by a spring mechanism, and tension is not adjustable.[18]

MAGNIFICATION

Magnification is strongly recommended for proper visualization of the surgical field in small mammals and exotic species. Various forms of magnification exist, including surgical loupes or operating microscopes. Surgical loupes offer magnification ranging from 2.5 to 5× from many manufacturers, whereas operating microscopes offer magnification from 5 to 40×. For most patients, surgical loupes will be sufficient; however, an operating microscope may be worthwhile for very small patients or delicate procedures. Magnification decreases the field of vision, depth perception, and fine-motor movements, and thus, training is required to become proficient in the use of magnification during surgery.

Loupes may range from inexpensive hobby loupes to more costly high-resolution loupes with or without an attached focal light source. Newer loupes have either Galilean or prismatic (Keplerian) lenses mounted on a pair of glasses (**Fig. 8**). Surgical loupes differ in the degree of magnification and size of the telescope. Prismatic

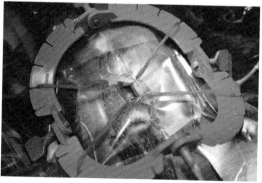

Fig. 6. Ring retractor used in a macaw undergoing ventral midline coeliotomy. The ring retractor uses hooks on adjustable stays attaching to the ring frame.

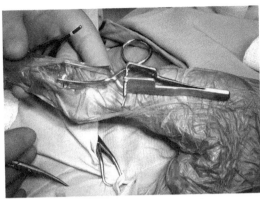

Fig. 7. The Heiss retractor is a small self-retaining retractor that uses a ratchet mechanism to maintain retraction. This can be adjusted to appropriate tension for the tissue it is retracting.

telescopes in general have higher magnification but more substantial telescope size and weight. Galilean telescopes, although lower in magnification, are sufficient for most applications, while providing decreased weight and user fatigue. The telescope may be mounted on or within the lens (through-the-lens technology) or front-mounted on the bridge of the glasses. Surgical loupes are custom-made for the user to fit inter-pupillary distance and focal working length. They should fit comfortably such that the surgeon does not have to bend over or strain to work. In general, the field width decreases with an increase in magnification. However, this does not hold true between telescope types as a prismatic loupe would have a larger field width than a Galilean telescope of the same magnification.

Surgical microscopy is an attractive option for magnification in surgery of small patients. Surgical microscopes have become more economically feasible and have been described in use outside of the teaching hospital setting.[19] Studies in human medicine including neurosurgery and dentistry have shown that operating microscopes provide better outcomes for patients because they offer better visualization and comfort for the surgeon (**Fig. 9**).[20,21]

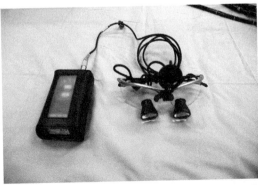

Fig. 8. Through-the-lens (×2.5) surgical loupes with an attached headlight. Surgical loops provide from ×2.5 to ×6 magnification, and the headlight provides bright focused unobstructed lighting on the surgical field.

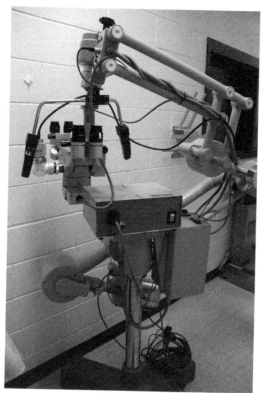

Fig. 9. Surgical microscope. Surgical microscopy provides greater magnification than surgical loops. Better patient outcome has been demonstrated with microscopy while providing better visualization and surgeon comfort.

FOCAL LIGHT SOURCE

As visualization of the surgical field is improved through tissue retraction and magnification, appropriate lighting should also be available. Often overhead lighting cannot be aimed or focused onto the patient. A focal light source allows the surgeon to direct the light into the patient and the surgical field, reducing shadows, glare, and artifact and is accomplished best when the light source is attached to the magnification used as in surgical loupes (see **Fig. 8**). With the advent of light-emitting diode technology, newer light sources offer improved brightness and decreased heat and weight over earlier light sources.

HEMOSTASIS
Electrosurgery

Electrosurgery has been refined over the past 100 years, yet the fundamental principles remain the same: heat from a developed electrical circuit causes collagen denaturation and tissue shrinkage.[5] Electrosurgical technology transfers energy from electrons in the instrument to electrolyte-rich living tissues. Electrosurgery should not be confused with electrocautery, which coagulates or cuts local tissues by using heat from an electrical current.

Electrosurgery can be applied using either a monopolar or a bipolar instrument. Monopolar electrosurgery requires the use of an inactive electrode or grounding pad that creates an electrical circuit. Radiofrequency generated within the circuit causes cells to dehydrate and vessels to coagulate. Because of the larger circuit, higher settings are required in comparison to bipolar cautery. The frequency and amplitude of the waveforms can generate different outcomes. Continuous, low-amplitude current results in a tissue cutting, whereas an interrupted, high-amplitude current results in coagulation of tissues. The field must be dry and the electrode kept free from debris to function properly. The instrument may be applied directly to the tissue, or indirectly by touching the electrode tip to an instrument holding tissue. Indirect application results in greater precision and less collateral tissue damage.[5,22]

Bipolar cautery consists of a single instrument that has dispersive and active electrodes at the tip, which allows for more isolated energy transfer (**Fig. 10**). The circuit is contained within the tips of the instrument, negating the need of a grounding pad. Additional benefits include efficacy in the face of moisture and less peripheral tissue damage due to the confines of the current application. Thermal dissipation into surrounding tissues can lead to collateral damage to neurovascular structures, warranting caution in certain areas. However, direct comparisons between skin incisions made by cold scalpel and electrosurgery have found no difference in postsurgical infection or cosmesis in human patients.[23]

There are a wide variety of tips and instrument types for use in exotic species but the most commonly used include fine-tip bipolar cautery units such as the Harrison forceps with one bent tip; this is primarily used as a method of coagulation in mammalian species but can also be used for skin incisions in birds.[1]

Laser

The term laser is an acronym standing for Light Amplification by Stimulated Emission of Radiation. All lasers work by delivering energy in the form of light. A laser beam is created from a substance called an active medium, which when stimulated by light or electricity produces photons of a specific wavelength. The light produced by a laser is both monochromatic (of one wavelength) and coherent (all waves are in phase with one another in both time and space). Medical lasers emit light anywhere from ultraviolet light, to visible light, to the infrared portions of the electromagnetic spectrum. They can deliver a large amount of energy to a focal source without actually touching the tissue. The tissue effect of lasers results from a complex interaction of the light

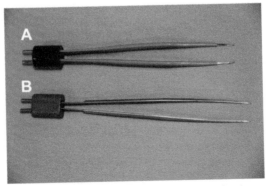

Fig. 10. Bipolar electrosurgical forceps coated with a non-conductive nylon coating (*A*) or uncoated (*B*).

emitted from the laser with the tissue, resulting in photochemical, photothermal, and photomechanical effects. Most surgical lasers have a photothermal effect on tissues, resulting in coagulation, cutting, cauterization, vaporization, or welding of tissues.

There are many types of surgical lasers, typically named by the type of lasing material used. These surgical lasers include gas lasers (CO_2, helium, or argon-ion), excimer lasers (eg, argon-fluoride or xenon-monochloride), solid-state lasers (neodymium:yttrium-aluminum garnet [Nd:YAG] or holmium:YAG [Ho:YAG]), or semiconductor lasers (diode lasers), each producing a different wavelength of light. CO_2 laser technology is the most commonly used laser in small animal surgery and has gained popularity in exotic animal surgery (**Fig. 11**). It produces its effect through instantaneous heating of intracellular water, resulting in cellular vaporization and ablation that can seal vessels measuring less than 0.6 mm in diameter.[17] Other reported benefits include simultaneous sealing of nerve endings and lymphatics, resulting in less discomfort and swelling postoperatively.[22]

More recently, the use of a diode laser has been evaluated for use in exotic species and offers unique benefits, including the ability to function in fluid environments, improved hemostasis, and capability of sealing vessels as large as 2 mm.[24] The diode lasers are in the near-infrared spectrum, typically with a wavelength of 810 nm. They can be used in direct contact with tissue (contact mode) or at a distance from tissue (noncontact). Penetration into tissue can be up to 4 mm in noncontact mode and 0.3 mm in contact mode with greater efficacy in muscle and nonkeratinized tissues.[24] Another intriguing feature of the diode laser is that it has the ability to be used in both endoscopic and open procedures. The contact mode is particularly useful to aid in hemostasis during endoscopic procedures, a technique gaining popularity in exotic animal surgery. Its use has been explored in reptiles, birds, small mammals, amphibians, and even fish due to its the efficacy in aqueous environments. Diode lasers may lead to delayed primary intention healing.

The potential for retinal damage requires all surgical personnel to wear appropriate protective eyewear when using any medical lasers in surgery.

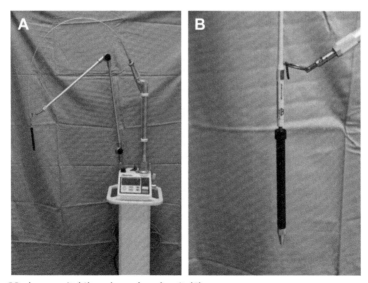

Fig. 11. CO_2 laser unit (*A*) and pen hand unit (*B*).

Electrothermal Bipolar Vessel Sealing Devices

Bipolar vessel-sealing devices provide hemostasis by denaturing collagen and elastin of the vessel wall and surrounding connective tissue, without reliance on thrombosis. These units have been used extensively in human and veterinary medicine, offering a rapid and safe alternative to suture or clip ligation of vessels. Other applications include the sealing and removal of hollow organ structures less than 9 mm in diameter in general urologic, thoracic, plastic, and reconstructive procedures.[25]

The most commonly used bipolar vessel-sealing device in veterinary surgery is the LigaSure (ValleyLab, Boulder, CO, USA; a division of Covidien), which includes a bipolar electrosurgery generator and a dedicated bipolar electrosurgery instrument (**Fig. 12**).[26] The LigaSure is able to seal vessels up to 7 mm in diameter. The more recently developed SurgRx EnSeal device (Ethicon Endo-Surgery, Inc, Cincinnati, OH, USA; a division of Johnson & Johnson, Somerville, NJ, USA) is also able to seal vessels up to 7 mm, but also limits thermal spread to 1 mm, thereby preventing damage to neighboring tissues.[4,27]

Bipolar vessel-sealing devices are often used in a minimally invasive manner during endoscopic procedures of people and animals; however, they can also be used in open abdominal or thoracic surgery. The size of instrumentation may limit its utility in many small exotic species. Use in procedures such as castration and hysterectomy in a variety of species, including lizards and chinchillas, documents the versatility and potential application in exotic species.[28]

Ultrasonic Energy: The Harmonic System

The Harmonic (Ethicon Endo-Surgery) device system delivers ultrasonic waves to tissue and can be used in both open and laparoscopic procedures. High-frequency vibrations cause an oscillating saw effect as well as vibration-induced heat and coagulation. The unit consists of a current generator, a hand piece that houses the ultrasonic transducer, an instrument with an end effector used to cut the tissue, a foot pedal, and a hand-switching adaptor. The Harmonic device is able to seal vessels up to 5 mm in diameter. The primary advantage of the Harmonic system is that it is able to cut and coagulate tissue by using lower temperatures than those used by electrosurgery, resulting in potentially less lateral thermal spread and tissue damage.[22,26]

Stapling Devices

Staplers have been used widely for 50 years and offer a rapid sealing of vessels and organ parenchyma. Their use is limited by the size of the device and finite sizes of clip

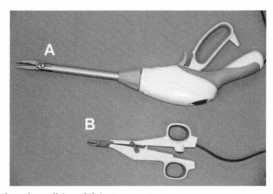

Fig. 12. Impact (*A*) and small jaw (*B*) instruments.

cartridges. Guidelines for the use of stapling equipment have been previously outlined but include[29]

1. Do not staple tissues that are inflamed or edematous or that lack a vascular supply.
2. Every staple must penetrate all tissue layers.
3. Staple size should be accurate; tissues should not be too thick to be penetrated or too thin to support the staple.
4. Tissues should be inspected thoroughly before stapler application to ensure proper alignment and no capturing of inadvertent tissues.
5. Stapling devices should be removed carefully to avoid disrupting the staples.

Tissues should be grasped gently before removal of the stapler to check for hemorrhage, leakage, or loose staples. The thoracoabdominal (TA) stapler comes in 30-mm, 45-mm, 60-mm, or 90-mm cartridge sizes that apply staggered rows of metal staples into tissues (**Fig. 13**). Several studies have documented the effectiveness of TA staplers by decreasing operative time, hemorrhage, and necrosis of tissue. There is concern for incomplete ligation of vascular tissues that may require reinforcement by oversewing the exposed pedicle to prevent leakage. The use of surgical staples has been described in a multitude of organ systems.

The GIA, or gastrointestinal and intestinal linear anastomosis, stapler can provide a linear communication between neighboring tissues by using a cutting function (**Fig. 14**). Examples of described uses include gastropexy, lobectomies, and end-to-end anastomosis.

The LDS, or ligate-divide stapler, has the ability to sever tissue while providing 2 titanium staples, one on either side of the cut ends, and is useful in procedures that require the transection of multiple vessels.

The size of all of the surgical stapling devices makes their use potentially challenging in smaller exotic species.

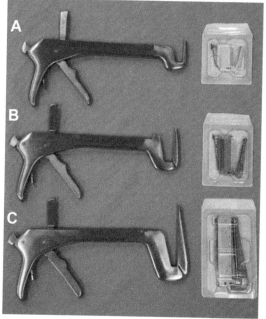

Fig. 13. TA 30 (A), TA 55 (B), and TA 90 (C) staplers with cartridges.

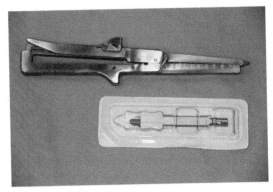

Fig. 14. Linear stapler with cartridge.

Hemostatic Clips

In an effort to expedite the ligation of smaller vessels, the use of vascular clips can be used. This advantage, however, is coupled with a reduction in strength and security when compared with traditional suture or electrosurgery techniques. They can be composed of metal in the traditional chevron design (**Fig. 15**) (Hemoclip; Weck, Triangle Park, NC, USA) or polymer composition (Absolak extra clips; Ethicon Endo-Surgery), which lock in place after deployment and can withstand a greater weight (>950 g) and intravascular pressure (>300 mm Hg) when compared with single and double Hemoclip placement.[30] Polymer designs also have the advantage of preventing interference during higher diagnostic imaging such as computed tomography or MRI and are absorbable over time.[30] To optimize security, the vessels should be carefully dissected from neighboring tissue, and the size should not be greater than two-thirds and no less than one-third than the size of the clip used.[31] Arteries and veins should be separated and clipped individually before application, allowing several millimeters between placement of the clip and the cut end of the vessel.[5] The application of vascular clips in endoscopic surgery has been well documented and offers an appealing alternative to other traditional techniques.

Hemostatic Agents

Many techniques can be used to ameliorate hemorrhage before, during, and after surgery. Decreasing blood flow to the region of interest can be achieved through the

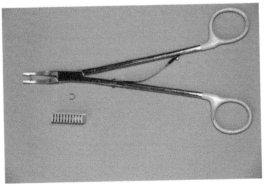

Fig. 15. Metal chevron design hemoclip with applicator.

applications of direct pressure or tamponade, decreasing perfusion via hypothermia or hypotension, or the use of tourniquets to control distant blood flow. Similarly, the use of systemic medications, such as serine protease inhibitors, lysine analogues, desmopressin, and ethamsylate, can aid in preventing blood loss by decreasing fibrinolysis, providing synthetic coagulation factors, and increasing platelet adhesiveness and aggregation. This section, however, concentrates on the use of topical hemostatic agents in the clinical setting.

The advent of hemostatic agents has gained popularity in the veterinary community in the effort to minimize blood loss in patients with small volumes. It is important to note that most agents used rely heavily on the patient's own hemostatic potential, and factors deterring this process will make them less efficacious. Products can be classified as mechanical agents, active agents, or hemostatic sealants. The appropriate selection of agent should be based on many factors, but availability and cost are often the limiting factor. None of these agents are without the potential for complication and may include local swelling, exothermic reactions, immunogenic reactions, foreign body reactions, and delayed healing.

Mechanical agents

Mechanical agents are absorbable materials that promote blood stasis and absorption at the site of hemorrhage and provide a matrix for clot formation and stabilization. They are widely available and can be combined with procoagulants to optimize hemostasis as is the case of thrombin added to porcine gelatin. Gelatin products are commonly used (Gelfoam; Pharmacia and Upjohn Co, Kalamazoo MI, USA) and are available in a foam-based medium (**Fig. 16**) in addition to a powder-based form. The main disadvantage is the occurrence of swelling, foreign body reactions, and inhibition of healing. They are not involved in active platelet aggregation and are absorbed over several weeks by granulomatous inflammation.[32]

Bovine collagen is another agent that not only acts as a mechanical activator but also enhances platelet aggregation, resulting in a superior hemostatic response.[32,33] It is available in sheets or a powder form and has similar complications and risks when compared with gelatin but the cost-prohibitive nature of the product makes it less commonly used in veterinary medicine.

Another type of topical hemostatic agent includes oxidized regenerated cellulose (Surgicel; Ethicon, Inc, Johnson and Johnson). Not only can this cause clot formation independent of the coagulation pathway but it also has antibacterial properties. The mechanism of action is not well understood, but it is generally considered to be a weaker hemostatic agent due to the inactivation of thrombin.[33]

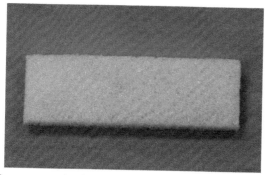

Fig. 16. Absorbable compressed gelatin sponge.

Bone wax is a variant of beeswax that can be used to decrease hemorrhage on osseous surfaces. It has been associated with a higher risk of infection and delayed bone healing according to certain reports. A newer formulation of alkylene oxide copolymer, called Ostene, is available and does not possess the same risk of infection and delayed healing and may also adhere better to moist surfaces.[34]

Active agents

Active agents can be used solely or in combination with other mechanical agents as described. Thrombin is the most active common agent, which works by converting fibrinogen to fibrin. Thrombin is available in bovine, human, and recombinant forms. Its use in humans has led to coagulopathic reactions following repeated administration, and therefore, frequent use is not recommended.

Alginate is a seaweed-derived protein that is most often used as a wound dressing, but it also has hemostatic properties, relating to the release of calcium, enhancing activation of the coagulation cascade and platelet activation.[35] It should not be used in open body cavities and must be removed before closure to prevent foreign body reactions.

Hemostatic sealants

Hemostatic sealants act as glue on tissues, creating a barrier for additional hemorrhage, and therefore, do not rely on normal hemostatic factors. Fibrin sealants provide both thrombin and fibrinogen to the site and can be derived from pooled plasma sources or can be obtained from the patient's own plasma by mixing with collagen and thrombin.[5,36] They are not widely available in veterinary medicine. Synthetic sealants such as Coseal (Baxter) and Duraseal (Covidien) consist of polyethylene polymers that form hydrogels to seal tissue. The major concern is swelling at the application site. More and more products are becoming available for use, but the lack of prospective analysis, particularly in veterinary medicine, warrants caution for the surgeon when debating their use in the clinical setting.

Suture materials

As with other species, wounds and surgical incisions of exotic species will often be closed with suture. The ideal suture material should have high tensile strength to resist fragmentation and provide sufficient time to allow tissue healing, have good knot security, resist infection, and cause minimal inflammatory reaction. Although suture material used is the same as other species, often ranging from 3-0 to 8-0, the technique

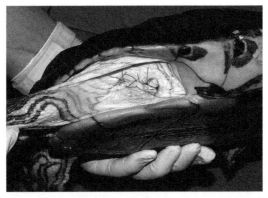

Fig. 17. Everting horizontal mattress suture pattern for closure of a prefemoral skin incision in red-eared slider turtle (*Trachemys scripta elegans*).

Table 1
Suture characteristics for commonly used materials in veterinary medicine

Suture Trade Name	Composition	Configuration	Reduction in Tensile Strength	Complete Absorption	Relative Knot Security	Tissue Reactivity
Surgical gut (chromic)	Intestinal serosa/submucosa	Twisted monofilament	33% at 7 d	60 d	—	+++
Vicryl	Polyglactin 910	Braided	25% at 14 d	56–70 d	++	+
Vicryl Rapide	Polyglactin 910	Braided	50% at 5 d	42 d	++	+
Dexon	Polyglycolic acid		35% at 14 d	60–90 d	++	+
Polysorb	Glycolide/lactide		20% at 14 d / 70% at 21 d	60 d	+++	—
Perma-Hand	Silk	Monofilament	30% at 14 d / 50% at 1 y	>2 y	—	—
Caprosyn	Polyglytone 6211	Monofilament	40%–50% at 5 d	56 d	+++	+
Monocryl	Poliglecaprone 25	Monofilament	40%–50% at 7 d	90–120 d	++	+
Biosyn	Glycomer 631	Monofilament	25% at 14 d / 60% at 21 d	90–110 d	++	+
PDS II	Polydioxanone	Monofilament	14% at 14 d / 31% at 42 d	180 d	++	+
Maxon	Polyglyconate	Monofilament	30% at 14 d / 45% at 21 d	180 d	++	+
Prolene	Polypropylene	Monofilament	—	Nonabsorbable	+++	—
Ethilon	Polyamide (Nylon)	Monofilament	30% at 2 y	Nonabsorbable	+	—

Relative knot security: (−), poor (<60%); (+), fair (60%–70%); (++), good (70%–85%); (+++), excellent (>85%).
Tissue reactivity: (−), minimal to none; (+), mild; (++), moderate; (+++), severe.
Data from Bennett RA. Preparation and equipment useful for surgery in small exotic pets. Vet Clin North Am Exot Anim Pract 2000;3:563–85; and Tobias KM, Johnston SA. Veterinary surgery: small animal. 1st edition. St Louis (MO): Elsevier Saunders; 2012.

may vary.[17] Rabbits and rodents tend to traumatize incisions and intradermal patterns with or without the additional use of tissue adhesive, or skin staples may be used.[37] In reptiles, the skin is the holding layer and it is recommended to close with an everting pattern (**Fig. 17**). An Aberdeen knot may be used instead of a square knot to minimize suture material while achieving a higher breaking.[38] A significant variety of suture materials are available, and selection should be based on tissue characteristics and expected healing times (**Table 1**).[1,5]

In closing wounds in reptiles, cyanoacrylate glue should be considered as an alternative to sutures. It should be noted that although the overall process of wound healing in reptiles is similar to that in mammals, it is slower, and certain aspects of wound healing are unique that should be taken into consideration. In particular, it is thought that the responding inflammatory cells and proteolytic enzymes involved in wound healing in reptiles may be different than that of mammals, leading to altered breakdown of suture materials. A recent study evaluated the histologic reaction to commonly used suture materials, including cyanoacrylate tissue adhesive, in the musculature and skin of ball pythons. The cyanoacrylate glue did not cause a significant inflammatory response compared with the negative control; however, all suture materials let to a significant inflammatory response. None of the sutures were absorbed by the end of the 90-day study period, and several sutures appeared to be in the process of extrusion. The authors concluded that cyanoacrylate glue should be considered to close small superficial wounds in snakes with minimal inflammatory response associated. Because of slower absorption, the authors suggest that shorter-acting suture materials may be more appropriate for use in reptiles; however, it is important to note that healing time and complications of surgery were not analyzed in this study.[39]

SUMMARY

The general principles of surgical technique, patient preparation, and instrumentation are similar between exotic species and mammals. However, due to small patient size, small mammals, reptiles, and avian species are prone to rapid hypothermia, life-threatening blood loss, and challenges in adequate tissue visualization. Furthermore, unique wound-healing processes necessitate the use of different suture materials and patterns to optimize wound healing. Recent availability of high-power magnification with focal lighting sources, novel methods of hemostasis, and small, precise surgical instruments allow for safe completion of advanced surgical procedures in exotic species. These advances have been highlighted in this article, focusing on recent literature that assesses performance in exotic animal species. Each exotic patient poses a unique challenge to the veterinary surgeon, and a tailored approach to each patient is required.

REFERENCES

1. Bennett RA. Preparation and equipment useful for surgery in small exotic pets. Vet Clin North Am Exot Anim Pract 2000;3:563–85.
2. Alexander JW, Fischer JE, Boyajian M, et al. The influence of hair-removal methods on wound infections. Arch Surg 1983;118:347–52.
3. Bhavan KP, Warren DK. Surgical preparation solutions and preoperative skin disinfection. J Hand Surg Am 2009;34:940–1.
4. Ayliffe G. The effect of antibacterial agents on the flora of the skin. J Hosp Infect 1980;1:111–24.
5. Tobias KM, Johnston SA. Veterinary surgery: small animal. 1st edition. St Louis (MO): Elsevier Saunders; 2012.

6. DeBaun B. Evaluation of the antimicrobial properties of an alcohol-free 2% chlorhexidine gluconate solution. AORN J 2008;87:925–33.
7. Gibson KL, Donald AW, Hariharan H, et al. Comparison of two pre-surgical skin preparation techniques. Can J Vet Res 1997;61:154–6.
8. Jacobson C, Osmon DR, Hanssen A, et al. Prevention of wound contamination using DuraPrep solution plus Ioban 2 drapes. Clin Orthop Relat Res 2005;439: 32–7.
9. Moen MD, Noone MB, Kirson I. Povidone-iodine spray technique versus traditional scrub-paint technique for preoperative abdominal wall preparation. Am J Obstet Gynecol 2002;187:1434–6.
10. Osuna DJ, DeYoung DJ, Walker RL. Comparison of three skin preparation techniques in the dog. Part 1: experimental trial. Vet Surg 1990;19:14–9.
11. Guzel A, Ozekinci T, Ozkan U, et al. Evaluation of the skin flora after chlorhexidine and povidone-iodine preparation in neurosurgical practice. Surg Neurol 2009;72: 207–10.
12. Garibaldi RA, Maglio S, Lerer T, et al. Comparison of nonwoven and woven gown and drape fabric to prevent intraoperative wound contamination and postoperative infection. Am J Surg 1986;152:505–9.
13. Webster J, Alghamdi A. Use of plastic adhesive drapes during surgery for preventing surgical site infection. Cochrane Database Syst Rev 2015;(4):CD006353.
14. Dewan PA, Van Rij AM, Robinson RG, et al. The use of an iodophor-impregnated plastic incise drape in abdominal surgery—a controlled clinical trial. Aust N Z J Surg 1987;57:859–63.
15. Boothe HW. Instrumentation. In: Tobias KM, Johnston SA, editors. Veterinary surgery: small animal. 1st edition. St Louis (MO): Elsevier Saunders; 2012. p. 152–63.
16. Capello V. Common surgical procedures in pet rodents. J Exot Pet Med 2011;20: 294–307.
17. Lennox AM. Equipment for exotic mammal and reptile diagnostics and surgery. J Exot Pet Med 2006;15:98–105.
18. Bennett RA, Mullen HS. Soft tissue surgery. In: Quesenberry KE, Carpenter JW, editors. Ferrets, rabbits and rodents: clinical medicine and surgery. 2nd edition. St Louis (MO): Elsevier Saunders; 2004. p. 316–28.
19. Ford S. Surgical microscopy and fluoroscopy in avian practice. J Exot Pet Med 2006;15:91–7.
20. Kumar SS, Mourkus H, Farrar G, et al. Magnifying loupes versus microscope for microdisectomy and microdecompression. J Spinal Disord Tech 2012;25: 235–9.
21. Mamoun J. Use of high-magnification loupes or surgical operating microscope when performing dental extractions. N Y State Dent J 2013;79:28–33.
22. Diamantis T, Kontos M, Arvelakis A, et al. Comparison of monopolar electrocoagulation, bipolar electrocoagulation, Ultracision, and Ligasure. Surg Today 2006; 36:908–13.
23. Aird LN, Brown CJ. Systematic review and meta-analysis of electrocautery versus scalpel for surgical skin incisions. Am J Surg 2012;204:216–21.
24. Hernandez-Divers SJ. Diode laser surgery: principles and application in exotic animals. Semin Avian Exot Pet Med 2002;11:208–20.
25. Mison MB, Steficek B, Lavagnino M, et al. Comparison of the effects of the CO_2 surgical laser and conventional surgical techniques on healing and wound tensile strength of skin flaps in the dog. Vet Surg 2003;32:153–60.
26. Barrera JS, Monnet E. Effectiveness of a bipolar vessel sealant device for sealing uterine horns and bodies from dogs. Am J Vet Res 2007;73(2):302–5.

27. Landman J, Kerbel K, Rehman J, et al. Evaluation of a vessel sealing system, bipolar electrosurgery, harmonic scalpel, titanium clips, endoscopic gastrointestinal anastomosis vascular staples and sutures for arterial and venous ligation in a porcine model. J Urol 2003;169:697–700.
28. Hruby GW, Marruffo FC, Durak E, et al. Evaluation of surgical energy devices for vessel sealing and peripheral energy spread in a porcine model. J Urol 2007;178: 2689–93.
29. Lipscomb V. Surgical staplers: toy or tool? In Practice 2012;34:472–9.
30. Hsu TC. Comparison of holding power of metal and absorbable hemostatic clips. Am J Surg 2006;191:68–71.
31. Toombs JP, Clark KM. Basic operative techniques. In: Slatter D, editor. Textbook of small animal surgery, vol. 1, 3rd edition. , Philadelphia: Elsevier Saunders; 2003. p. 199.
32. Solheim E, Anfinsen OG, Holmsen H, et al. Effect of local hemostatics on platelet aggregation. Eur Surg Res 1991;23:45–50.
33. Wagner WR, Pachence JM, Ristich J, et al. Comparative in vitro analysis of topical hemostatic agents. J Surg Res 1996;66:100–8.
34. Magyar CE, Aghaloo TL, Atti E, et al. Ostene, a new alkylene oxide copolymer bone hemostatic material, does not inhibit bone healing. Neurosurgery 2008; 63:373–8.
35. Segal HC, Hunt BJ, Gilding K. The effects of alginate and non-alginate wound dressings on blood coagulation and platelet activation. J Biomater Appl 1998;12:249–57.
36. Crow SS, Sullivan VV, Ayosola AE, et al. Postoperative coagulopathy in a pediatric patient after exposure to bovine topical thrombin. Ann Thorac Surg 2007;83: 1547–9.
37. Jenkins JR. Soft tissue surgery. In: Quesenberry KE, Carpenter JW, editors. Ferrets, rabbits and rodents: clinical medicine and surgery. 3rd edition. St Louis (MO): Elsevier Saunders; 2012. p. 269–78.
38. Schaaf O, Glyde M, Day RE. In vitro comparison of secure aberdeen and square knots with plasma- and fat-coated polydioxanone. Vet Surg 2010;39:553–60.
39. McFadden MS, Bennett RA, Kinsel MJ, et al. Evaluation of the histologic reactions to commonly used suture materials in the skin and musculature of ball pythons (Python regius). Am J Vet Res 2011;72:1397–406.

Principles of Wound Management and Wound Healing in Exotic Pets

Megan A. Mickelson, DVM, Christoph Mans, Dr med vet, DACZM, Sara A. Colopy, DVM, PhD, DACVS*

KEYWORDS

- Wound healing • Wound management • Topical wound therapy • Wound products
- Wound dressings

KEY POINTS

- General principles of wound healing are similar across species.
- Selection of appropriate topical therapies and bandaging is based on the phase of wound healing and amount of exudate produced in addition to patient factors.
- When addressing wounds in exotics, it is important to account for individual patient stress levels, behavior, and husbandry when considering wound management techniques and options.

INTRODUCTION

Open wounds often must be managed for several days, weeks, or even months until they can be closed or they heal by second intention. Most wounds heal without complications; however, the care of wounds in exotic animal species can be a challenging endeavor. Special considerations must be made in regard to the animal's temperament and behavior, unique anatomy and small size, and tendency toward secondary stress-related health problems. Basic wound care incorporates principles of aseptic technique and gentle tissue handling, and is similar across veterinary species. In addition, many wound care products are available that will potentially debride the wound without damaging healthy tissue, reduce infection, and increase the rate of wound healing. This article summarizes the phases of wound healing, factors that affect healing, and general principles of wound management. Emphasis is placed on novel modalities of treating wounds and species differences in wound management and healing.

The authors have nothing to disclose.
Department of Surgical Sciences, School of Veterinary Medicine, University of Wisconsin-Madison, 2015 Linden Drive, Madison, WI 53706, USA
* Corresponding author.
E-mail address: colopys@svm.vetmed.wisc.edu

PHASES OF WOUND HEALING

A wound is a physical injury disrupting the normal continuity of anatomic structures, and the wound-healing process consists of restoring continuity. Wound healing is typically a well-organized process divided into 3 to 5 overlapping phases, depending on the classification system: hemostasis (or coagulation) phase, inflammatory phase, debridement phase (often combined with the inflammatory phase), repair (proliferative) phase, and maturation (remodeling) phase (**Fig. 1**). Chronic or nonhealing wounds do not proceed through the normal phases of wound healing, often unable to make the transition from the inflammatory to the repair phase.[1,2] Knowledge of normal wound-healing physiology provides a framework for understanding factors that impair wound healing and for implementing effective wound-management strategies.

Hemostasis (Coagulation) Phase

Immediately following injury to the skin, hemostasis is achieved through vasoconstriction and platelet-mediated activation of the intrinsic clotting cascade, ending in formation of a fibrin clot. Release of proinflammatory cytokines from damaged tissue and the newly formed clot act as potent chemotactic signals to recruit neutrophils, endothelial cells, and fibroblasts to the wound. Formation of the fibrin clot is therefore an important step in promoting onset of the inflammatory and repair phases.[1,2]

Inflammatory and Debridement Phase

The inflammatory phase is characterized by increased capillary permeability and infiltration of neutrophils, macrophages, and lymphocytes into the wound (**Fig. 2**). Most modern wound-classification schemes include the debridement phase within the inflammatory phase because of the overlapping time and function of leukocytes within the wound.[1–3] After initial vasoconstriction during hemostasis, vasodilation and increased vascular permeability ensue. Increased blood flow and fluid extravasation combined with blockage of lymphatic drainage cause the classic signs of inflammation, including heat, redness, and swelling. This acute inflammatory response usually lasts for 1 to 2 days but may persist in a poor wound environment.[1,2]

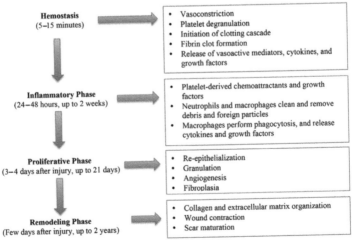

Hemostasis (5–15 minutes)
- Vasoconstriction
- Platelet degranulation
- Initiation of clotting cascade
- Fibrin clot formation
- Release of vasoactive mediators, cytokines, and growth factors

Inflammatory Phase (24–48 hours, up to 2 weeks)
- Platelet-derived chemoattractants and growth factors
- Neutrophils and macrophages clean and remove debris and foreign particles
- Macrophages perform phagocytosis, and release cytokines and growth factors

Proliferative Phase (3–4 days after injury, up to 21 days)
- Re-epithelialization
- Granulation
- Angiogenesis
- Fibroplasia

Remodeling Phase (Few days after injury, up to 2 years)
- Collagen and extracellular matrix organization
- Wound contraction
- Scar maturation

Fig. 1. Stages of wound healing. (*Adapted from* Ozturk F, Ermertcan AT. Wound healing: a new approach to the topical wound care. Cutan Ocul Toxicol 2011;30:95; with permission.)

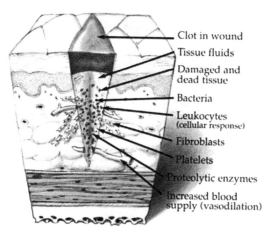

Clot in wound
Tissue fluids
Damaged and dead tissue
Bacteria
Leukocytes (cellular response)
Fibroblasts
Platelets
Proteolytic enzymes
Increased blood supply (vasodilation)

Fig. 2. Stage 1 of wound healing: inflammation (vasodilation). (*From* Sherris DA, Kern EB. Essential surgical skills. 2nd edition. Philadelphia: WB Saunders; 2004. p. 13; with permission of Mayo Foundation for Medical Education and Research. All rights reserved.)

Wound debridement begins with migration of white blood cells into the wound. Platelets within the fibrin plug release growth factors and cytokines, which recruit inflammatory cells to the wound.[2] Circulating neutrophils begin entering the wound within minutes of injury, peaking within the first 24 hours and are primarily responsible for bacterial phagocytosis.

Monocytes accumulate within 12 hours after injury and undergo differentiation to mature wound macrophages under the influence of local cytokines. Macrophages are the dominant inflammatory cell within 3 to 5 days of injury and play a pivotal role in transitioning from inflammation to repair. Macrophages are responsible for phagocytosis of apoptotic cells, tissue debris, and microbial organisms. In addition, they release proinflammatory cytokines that propagate the inflammatory response, and growth factors that stimulate conversion of mesenchymal cells to fibroblasts and also promote collagen synthesis and angiogenesis.[1,3]

Lymphocytes appear later, peaking at approximately 7 days. Although the exact role of lymphocytes in wound healing is unknown, it is thought that they produce growth factors, interferons, interleukins, and tumor necrosis factor, which recruit fibroblasts and promote wound healing.[1,3]

Proliferative (Repair) Phase

The proliferative or repair phase begins approximately 3 to 4 days after injury and is characterized by fibroplasia, angiogenesis, and epithelialization (**Fig. 3**). Under the influence of growth factors (predominantly platelet-derived growth factor [PDGF]), dermal fibroblasts proliferate, migrate, and differentiate into contractile myofibroblasts. Fibroblasts are critical for the production of extracellular matrix (ECM), which comprises collagen, glycosaminoglycans, proteoglycans, fibronectin, and elastin. Transforming growth factor β (TGF-β) is one of the most important mediators of collagen matrix formation. TGF-β stimulates fibroblasts to produce fibronectin, which is critical to the facilitation of cell binding and fibroblast movement.[2]

Angiogenesis refers to new vessel growth by the sprouting of preexisting vessels adjacent to the wound.[2] Angiogenesis occurs as dermal endothelial cells migrate into the new ECM under the influence of macrophage-derived angiogenic factor

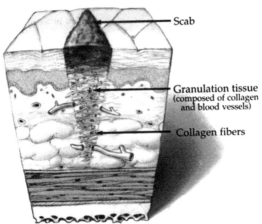

Fig. 3. Stage 2 of wound healing: proliferation. (*From* Sherris DA, Kern EB. Essential surgical skills. 2nd edition. Philadelphia: WB Saunders; 2004. p. 13; with permission of Mayo Foundation for Medical Education and Research. All rights reserved.)

and vascular endothelial growth factor.[1] The combination of fibroblasts, new capillaries, and fibrous tissue forms bright red granulation tissue.

Epithelialization involves proliferation and migration of epidermal keratinocytes from the wound edges, differentiation of epithelial progenitor cells into a stratified epidermis, and restoration of the basement membrane connecting the epidermis to the underlying dermis.[2,3] Epithelial cells move to the wound center by sliding over the fibrin deposits or basal lamina. The epithelial cells migrate under the wound clot and over granulation tissue, causing the scab to separate from the wound via secretion of proteolytic enzymes. As cells have migrated further from the wound edge, migration slows down and the initial layer formed is only 1 cell layer thick. Contraction typically occurs 5 to 9 days after initial injury. The existing tissue at the wound edges is pulled inward by contraction, and the surrounding skin stretches, decreasing the overall size of the wound. The process continues until the wound edges meet (contact inhibition), tension is high, or myofibroblasts are inadequate.[4,5]

Maturation (Remodeling) Phase

Maturation typically begins 1 week after injury following collagen deposition in the wound, and is the longest phase of wound healing, continuing for weeks to months after injury (**Fig. 4**). The main activity during this phase is strengthening and remodeling of the newly formed collagen. There is reduced proliferation and inflammation, and regression of the newly formed capillaries in the wound bed. Type III collagen is replaced by type I collagen. Collagen fibers remodel by aligning with tension lines of the body and gain strength through cross-linking. The scar eventually becomes less cellular, flattens, and softens. Normal tissue strength is never regained, with approximately 80% of the original strength acquired at best.[1,2]

FACTORS AFFECTING WOUND HEALING

Both systemic (host) and local factors serve as potential impediments to wound healing. Host factors include age, body condition, nutritional intake, and concurrent disease. Large wounds place animals in a catabolic state, and thus calorie and protein

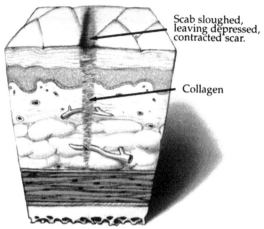

Scab sloughed,
leaving depressed,
contracted scar.

Collagen

Fig. 4. Stage 3 of wound healing: scar maturation. (*From* Sherris DA, Kern EB. Essential surgical skills. 2nd edition. Philadelphia: WB Saunders; 2004. p. 13; with permission of Mayo Foundation for Medical Education and Research. All rights reserved.)

intake should be increased to ensure that nutritional requirements are met. Hypoproteinemia (<2.0 g/dL) and diets deficient in protein delay wound healing and decrease wound strength. Underlying metabolic disease, such as diabetes mellitus, hyperadrenocorticism, and uremia, also delay wound healing.[4,6] Many medications are associated with impaired wound healing and reduced wound strength, including corticosteroids and chemotherapeutic agents.[6,7] Chemotherapeutic drugs further delay healing as they specifically target rapidly dividing cells, affecting fibroblast proliferation and wound strength.[8] Nonsteroidal anti-inflammatory drugs have been investigated with regard to their effects on wound healing; however, these medications have not been found to alter the rate of wound healing significantly.[6]

Local wound factors known to affect healing include tissue perfusion, tissue viability, infection, presence of hematoma or seroma, and mechanical factors (eg, tension, motion, wound debris). The presence of debris, dirt, hair, suture, and necrotic or devitalized tissue act as foreign material, leading to an intense inflammatory reaction that prolongs the inflammatory phase and delays the repair phase. Accumulation of fluid in the wound bed, as with a hematoma or seroma, inhibits fibroblast migration, encourages infection, and leads to wound ischemia, delaying wound healing and strength formation.[4,5] Infection of the wound also negatively affects the process of wound healing. It is generally recommended that a wound contaminated with greater than 10^5 organisms per gram of tissue not be primarily closed, as the incidence of infection is increased.[9] Other mechanical factors that impede normal healing include tight bandage placement, tension, and motion, all of which may lead to impaired blood supply, tissue ischemia and necrosis, increased risk of infection, and dehiscence.[6] Following Halsted's surgical principles (gentle tissue handling, strict aseptic technique, sharp anatomic dissection, meticulous hemostasis, obliteration of dead space, avoidance of tension, preserved vascularity, and careful approximation of tissues) will reduce negative local factors in wound healing.

WOUND CLASSIFICATION

Wounds are classified in many ways, based on whether they are open or closed, duration since injury, underlying etiology, degree of contamination, and degree of skin disruption. Class I wounds (clean) show no signs of inflammation and do not involve a hollow viscus (respiratory, gastrointestinal, or genitourinary tracts). Only skin microflora potentially contaminate the wound, and they generally have been present for only for 0 to 6 hours (**Fig. 5**). Class II wounds (clean/contaminated) are clean wounds with a higher risk of infection, such as those in which a hollow viscus has been opened under controlled circumstances without significant spillage of contents. Class III wounds (contaminated) include open accident wounds encountered relatively early after injury, and those with extensive introduction of bacteria into a normally sterile area as a result of a major break in sterile technique (**Fig. 6**). Any inflamed tissue around a surgical wound is considered contaminated. Class IV wounds (dirty/infected) include traumatic wounds for which a significant treatment delay has occurred, wounds in which a foreign object is lodged, or a wound in which necrotic tissue, pus, or fecal matter is present. Bite wounds are considered to be contaminated unless there is purulent exudate, in which case they are considered dirty. When in doubt, the worst category should be presumed for classification so as to provide optimal therapy and reduce the chance for complications. The classification of the wound, in addition to local wound factors, can help guide the type of management approach that should be taken for any given wound.[10,11]

INITIAL WOUND CARE AND MANAGEMENT

The goal of wound care is to prevent further contamination and convert contaminated or infected wounds into clean wounds for either surgical closure or second-intention healing. To fully assess an open wound, sedation or general anesthesia may be indicated. Wounds should be lavaged and debrided immediately, after which samples from the deep aspects of the wound are collected for culture and susceptibility. A biopsy should be considered for all chronic or nonhealing wounds. An aseptic technique should be used when treating wounds, including the use of sterile gloves, instruments, and bandage materials.[11] It should be noted that wound healing is faster under moist and wet conditions. Excessive wetness, however, can be problematic, so the ideal wound dressing should absorb exudate without excessively drying the wound.

Decontamination (Lavage)

The primary aim of decontamination is to remove bacteria and debris from the wound bed. Following the initial assessment, the wound should be covered with sterile water-soluble lubricant to prevent further contamination, and the surrounding wound hairs

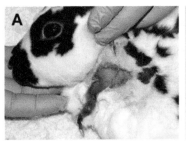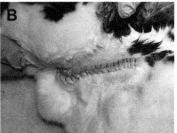

Fig. 5. Skin laceration in a rabbit. (*A*) Initial presentation of the wound, within 1 hour after infliction attributable to conspecific trauma. (*B*) The wound was lavaged the skin and edges trimmed, and skin staples were used to perform primary wound closure. The wound healed without complications.

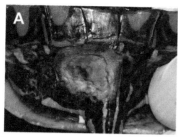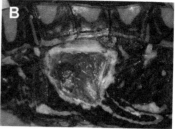

Fig. 6. Chronic wound dorsal to the tail base in a pained turtle (*Chrysemys picta*) secondary to marginal scute malformation allowing for conspecific trauma in an overcrowded enclosure. (*A*) Initial presentation. (*B*) The same wound following surgical debridement. Note the healthy granulation tissue.

should be clipped. Lavage with copious, warm, sterile isotonic fluids, such as lactated Ringer solution or phosphate-buffered saline, should be performed as soon as possible (**Fig. 7**). Use of sterile tap water or prolonged exposure to normal saline has been shown to be cytotoxic to fibroblasts in vitro.[6] Adequate irrigation pressure can be achieved with the use of a 35-mL or 60-mL syringe and an 18-gauge catheter or needle, or with the use of a syringe connected to a 3-way stopcock and bag of fluids.

Use of lavage solutions containing antiseptics has not been shown to enhance the benefits of lavage.[6] If antiseptic solutions are chosen, 0.05% chlorhexidine and 0.5% or 1% povidone-iodine would be considered appropriate. Chlorhexidine solution is not impaired by organic material, has broad-spectrum activity with minimal systemic absorption, and maintains residual activity up to 2 days following application. Povidone-iodine has broad-spectrum activity against bacteria, fungi, viruses, and yeast, but is inactivated by the presence of organic matter and has little residual activity. Caution should be observed with more concentrated formulations, as they are cytotoxic, may slow granulation tissue formation, and ultimately impair or delay wound healing.[5]

Tris-ethylenediaminetetraacetic acid increases susceptibility of bacteria, especially gram-negative bacteria, to antibiotics and antiseptics. Alcohol, hydrogen peroxide, Dakin solution, and acetic acid should be avoided, as they are cytotoxic to the normal tissues.[11,12]

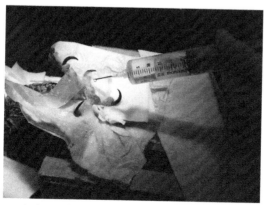

Fig. 7. Lavage of a pododermatitis wound following surgical debridement in a peregrine falcon (*Falco peregrinus*).

Debridement

Debridement entails removal of necrotic and devitalized tissue from the wound with the goal of creating a fresh, clean wound bed for primary or delayed closure. Debridement can consist of surgical, enzymatic, autolytic, or mechanical means.

Nonselective Debridement

Surgical debridement

Surgical debridement is indicated for removing large amounts of necrotic debris (see **Fig. 6**). Foreign debris is removed with thumb forceps, and necrotic tissue is removed by sharp dissection. In small exotic species, surgical debridement can be performed using sharp excision with a scalpel blade. Nonviable or necrotic tissue often appears purple or black in color, or is loose yellow to brown if sloughing. Care should be taken to avoid removal of viable tissue. Tissue with questionable viability should be left for reassessment the next day. Typically the extent of tissue necrosis will be apparent within 24 to 48 hours following tissue injury, and repeat debridement can be done at that time. The subdermal vascular plexus and supply to the skin should be preserved when possible.

Mechanical debridement

Mechanical debridement is achieved through the use of adherent dry-to-dry or wet-to-dry bandages. The dressings, usually gauze, are allowed to adhere to the wound. Debridement is nonselective because once dry, the dressings are removed while pulling off debris along with the superficial layers of the wound bed. The removal of adherent dressings can be painful, and typically need to be changed multiple times daily for the first few days.[5,11,13,14] The use of wet-to-dry bandages is controversial because of the nonselective nature of debridement and pain associated with removal. If selected, debridement with gauze sponges should only be performed during the inflammatory phase of wound healing.[6]

Selective Debridement

Enzymatic debridement

Enzymatic debridement refers to the use of enzymatic agents to selectively destroy necrotic tissue and liquefy coagulum and bacterial biofilm.[6] The most common enzymatic agents currently on the market contain either collagenase or papain-urea, and are typically available as ointments or gels. Advantages of enzymatic agents include that they are not painful and do not require anesthesia. Furthermore, they can be used as an adjunct to surgical debridement when excision could harm healthy tissues that must be preserved.

There are several disadvantages to enzymatic debridement. Enzymatic debridement is slow, which is not practical for large wounds, and the products may be cost prohibitive. Furthermore, they cause a local inflammatory and pyogenic reaction and should not be used for long-term management. Enzymes can damage or dehydrate normal tissue and, if in contact with adjacent healthy tissue surrounding the wound bed, may cause maceration. These ointments or gels are typically applied to the wound bed, covered with a nonadherent dressing, and changed every 12 to 24 hours.[12,13]

Autolytic debridement

Autolytic debridement is the natural process that occurs in a moist wound environment where the enzymes present in the wound fluid debride necrotic tissue. The process is facilitated by placement of hydrophilic, occlusive, or semiocclusive bandages to maintain wound moisture and allow wound exudate to remain in contact with the wound (**Fig. 8**). Wound exudate contains endogenous enzymes, cytokines, and growth factors that digest necrotic debris while stimulating granulation tissue formation, angiogenesis, and epithelialization. This mechanism is often preferred in wounds with questionable tissue viability, but should be avoided in infected wounds.

TOPICAL PRODUCTS

Most wounds will heal well with basic wound-management techniques and proper bandage application; however, for chronic, nonhealing wounds, topical products may be considered as an adjunct. Nonhealing wounds are arrested in one of the phases of healing, typically the inflammatory phase.[2] Thus, novel wound-care products promote transition from the inflammatory to the proliferative phase. It is important to acknowledge, however, that there is little information about the efficacy of topical wound products in veterinary medicine, and even less about exotic animal species.

Topical Antimicrobials

Topical antimicrobials include antiseptics, silver-based dressings, hyperosmotic dressings, and other dressings. These products reduce the number of microorganisms present in the wound bed and promote autolytic debridement. These agents do have cytotoxic effects and, thus, their potential benefits should outweigh the risks; they should therefore be discontinued once a granulation bed is present. Topical antimicrobials are often narrower in spectrum and may promote the creation of "super-infections" or nosocomial infections with continued usage.

Triple-antibiotic ointment

Triple-antibiotic ointment containing bacitracin zinc, neomycin sulfate, and polymyxin B sulfate has broad-spectrum antimicrobial activity and is one of the most commonly used topical antimicrobials. It is not cytotoxic and is thought to actually enhance epithelialization, although it may inhibit wound contraction.[5,11,12,15,16] Bacitracin is not recommended for use in rodents or rabbits because of the risk for dysbacteriosis of the enteric flora.

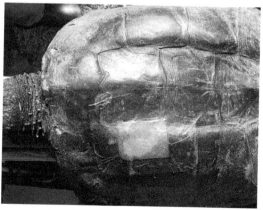

Fig. 8. Dressing of a carapacial wound in a common snapping turtle (*Chelydra serpentina*). A hydrogel sheet is applied to the wound and secured in place by a waterproof transparent film dressing. The animal was allowed full access to water because the dressing was waterproof.

Gentamicin sulfate

Gentamicin sulfate ointment is particularly active against gram-negative bacteria, including *Pseudomonas* and *Staphylococcus* species. It is also available as a solution, which promotes epithelialization and does not inhibit contraction as seen with use of the cream-based ointments.[5,11,12,15,16]

Silver

Silver is an important and widely adopted antimicrobial agent that has been shown to have effects against methicillin-resistant *Staphylococcus aureus*, fungi, and a variety of other bacteria, and does not lead to antibiotic resistance.[17] The most common topical silver formulation is silver sulfadiazine cream (SSD) (1%) (**Fig. 9**), which can penetrate necrotic tissue and enhance wound epithelialization; however, SSD cream has been shown to impede wound contraction and cause bone marrow suppression if used in larger wounds. SSD has historically been the topical wound treatment of choice in human burn patients.[5,11,12,15,16] Newer products combining a biological dressing or polymeric nanofilms with silver to immobilize silver at the wound bed show promise in reducing bacterial burden in full-thickness wounds without impeding wound contraction (see **Fig. 8**; **Fig. 10A**).[17,18]

Nitrofurazone

Nitrofurazone has broad-spectrum activity and is hydrophilic in nature, drawing fluid from the wound and decreasing edema in highly exudative wounds. However, it is known to delay epithelialization and is a known carcinogen. Furthermore, it has reduced antibacterial activity in the presence of organic matter.[5,12,15,16]

Aloe vera

Aloe vera gel has antiprostaglandin, antithromboxane, and antibacterial properties, allowing it to prevent dermal ischemia. Allantoin, a component of aloe vera, promotes epithelial growth and stimulates tissue repair. Acemannan, available as a hydrogel or freeze-dried form (eg, Carravet [Veterinary Products Labs, Phoenix, AZ, USA]; Carrasorb [Carrington Labs, Irving, TX, USA]), is another component of aloe vera that stimulates macrophages to increase cytokine production, increasing fibroblast proliferation, epidermal growth, and collagen deposition. This agent is best applied in the early inflammatory phase of wound healing. It can cause excess granulation tissue formation, especially in the freeze-dried form, which inhibits wound contraction.[5,12,15,16] Aloe vera was shown to stimulate fibroblast replication in an experimental study with guinea pig burn wounds.[19] The gel enhanced wound healing

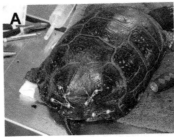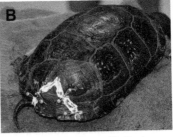

Fig. 9. (*A*) Carapacial fracture repair followed by application silver sulfadiazine cream (*B*) to the fracture site following reduction, to prevent contamination in a Blanding turtle (*Emys blandingii*).

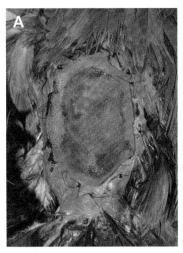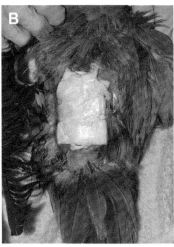

Fig. 10. Large full-thickness wound over the dorsum in a blue and gold macaw (*Ara ararauna*). (*A*) A hydrogel sheet is placed on the wound as the primary dressing. Note the loose suture loops placed in the periphery of the wound to facilitate the tie-over bandage. (*B*) Gauze has been used as the secondary bandage layer. Umbilical tape is used to create a tie-over bandage. For additional support a waterproof transparent film dressing was applied.

at 7 days compared with triple-antibiotic and control groups in dogs with pad wounds.[20]

Tripeptide-copper complex

Tripeptide-copper complex (TCC) gel (eg, Iamin-Vet Skin Care Gel, Covington, GA, USA) serves as a chemoattractant for macrophages and mast cells, which stimulates debridement, angiogenesis, collagen deposition, and wound contraction. Copper is used for collagen cross-linking, and is thus best used in the late inflammatory and early repair phases of wound healing.[5,15,16] TCC was shown to significantly decrease overall wound-healing time in ischemic wounds of rats when compared with controls.[21]

Maltodextrin NF

Maltodextrin NF, a ᴅ-glucose polysaccharide with 1% ascorbic acid (eg, Intracell; Techni-Vet, Albuquerque, NM, USA), is a hydrophilic powder or gel that provides glucose for cell metabolism, draws fluids from the wound, acts as a chemoattractant, and has antibacterial and bacteriostatic properties. It can be used in the early inflammatory phase to reduce exudate, swelling, and infection in the wound bed.[5,15,16,20]

Honey

Honey has historically been used in wound management, with the benefits of decreasing inflammatory edema, enhancing wound debridement via stimulation of macrophage migration, and acceleration of tissue slough, providing a protective layer of protein to the wound bed along with improvement in wound nutrition, and promoting granulation tissue formation. In addition to these benefits, it is reported to have antibacterial properties resulting from its high osmolarity, low pH, and enzymatic production of hydrogen peroxide from glucose. Although honey is readily available, the use of medical-grade honey is recommended.[5,11,15,16,22] Honey is widely used in wound management of exotic animals, particularly chelonians and birds (**Figs. 11** and **12**).

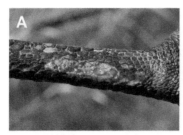
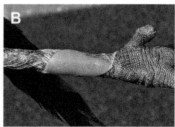

Fig. 11. (*A*) Full-thickness wound of the distal tarsometatarsus of a wattled crane (*Bugeranus carunculatus*). (*B*) Application of a commercial honey dressing sheet to the same wound. A waterproof transparent film dressing is applied as the secondary layer to secure the honey dressing in place. An elastic bandage was applied as the tertiary layer (not shown).

Sugar

Sugar has a high osmolality, which reduces wound edema, attracts macrophages, accelerates sloughing of devitalized tissue, provides an energy source for cells, promotes formation of a protective protein layer over the wound, and enhances formation of granulation tissue. Granulated sugar should be applied at least 1 cm thick over the wound and covered with an absorbent bandage.[5,15,16,23] When using sugar and honey, caution should be taken to ensure the patient maintains normal hydration, electrolytes, and protein levels given the hydrophilic nature of the 2 topical therapies. Both honey and sugar can be applied throughout the inflammatory phase of wound healing, but should be discontinued once granulation tissue is present.

Hypertonic saline

Hypertonic saline–soaked dressings composed of 20% sodium chloride can be used for their osmotic effect, which draws fluid from the wound into the dressing, desiccating necrotic tissue and bacteria in the process.[11] These dressings are only recommended for infected, heavily exudative, and necrotic wounds that require aggressive debridement, as debridement is nonselective. Such dressings are only appropriate in the initial few days of the inflammatory phase, and should be changed at least every 3 days. Following initial treatment with hypertonic saline, the wound bed can be further treated with an alginate, hydrogel, or foam dressing.[5,24]

Growth factors

Growth factors regulate many of the key cellular activities involved in the normal wound-healing process, including cell division and migration, angiogenesis, and

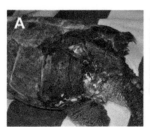
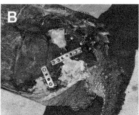
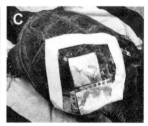

Fig. 12. Multiple carapacial fractures and bone loss in a common snapping turtle (*C. serpentina*). (*A*) Initial presentation. (*B*) Following surgical debridement and stabilization of the fractures, sterile gauze strips soaked in raw honey were applied to the soft-tissue wounds. (*C*) A waterproof transparent film dressing is applied as the outer layer, and the edges are secured with medical tape.

synthesis of the extracellular matrix. Applying a single growth factor is likely not efficacious without knowing which specific growth factors are deficient at the time. Recombinant human-derived PDGF (Regranex Gel; Ortho-McNeil Pharmaceutical, South Raritan, NJ, USA) is available, and is thought to promote chemotactic recruitment and proliferation of cells for wound repair, accelerate wound healing via promotion of granulation tissue formation, wound contraction, and remodeling, and stimulate angiogenesis and recruitment of macrophages, neutrophils, and fibroblasts.[5,12,15] It has been shown to accelerate wound healing in humans with diabetic and neurotropic ulcers.[25]

Platelet-derived products are available as a source of growth factors. Platelets can be harvested and concentrated to produce platelet-rich plasma (PRP), which can be used to enhance fibroblast proliferation and epithelialization. Gel derived from PRP has been shown to speed the healing of chronic decubital ulcers in dogs when compared with controls with paraffin-impregnated gauze.[26]

Chitosan

Chitosan is a polysaccharide derived from chitin, a component of the exoskeleton in shellfish, which contains the active ingredient glucosamine. It accelerates wound healing by enhancing the function of inflammatory cells, growth factors, and fibroblasts. A reported side effect in dogs is fatal hemorrhagic pneumonia at doses greater than 50 mg/kg subcutaneously.[11,12,15,16,27]

WOUND-CLOSURE TECHNIQUE

Factors considered when deciding how to close a wound include the degree of contamination present, the time from injury, the presence of devitalized tissue, the amount of tissue tension and extent of dead space, the amount of soft-tissue loss and adjacent tissue available for closure, the blood supply and status of the wound vasculature, hemostasis, location and ability to close, and overall patient stability for general anesthesia.

Primary Wound Closure

Primary wound closure (first-intention healing) is considered appositional healing whereby closure is achieved by fixing the edges of the wound in contact with one another. Class I wounds and those that can be completely excised and converted to a surgical wound are managed by primary closure. Primary closure is often recommended in cases where the wound is clean, has minimal trauma and contamination, and is less than 6 to 8 hours old following lavage and debridement.[5,11]

Secondary Wound Closure

Secondary wound closure (second-intention healing) is used for large skin defects in which the wound edges cannot be approximated, or wounds with extensive tissue devitalization. Secondary closure requires formation of a granulation tissue matrix, wound contracture, and epithelialization. Disadvantages of this technique include an increased length of time to healing or incomplete healing, significant time and energy in wound management, formation of a fragile epithelial scar, and creation of scar tissue.[5,11]

Delayed Primary Wound Closure

Delayed primary closure (tertiary-intention healing) is a combination of primary and secondary closure. This type of closure is preferred when a wound is heavily contaminated, to reduce the risk of the wound becoming infected. The wound is cleansed and watched for several days to ensure no infection is apparent. When the wound appears to be clean and on its way to healing, it is closed surgically. Closure may be elected before or after the presence of granulation tissue. The granulation bed offers the benefit of microbial resistance and increased vascularity once closure is elected.[5,11] Certain injuries almost always become infected (eg, bite wounds); these types of injuries are frequently left open and closed only if the infection is controlled.

BANDAGING

The purpose of bandage application is multifactorial, including protection of the wound from contamination and mechanical forces exerted by the external environment or the patient, management of wound exudate, elimination of dead space, immobilization of injured tissue, support and comfort, prevention of wound contamination, minimization of scar tissue, and promotion of healthy wound environment that ultimately promotes healing.[5,12,24,28] Bandages are an important adjunct when considering open wound management. A bandage typically consists of 3 main layers, the contact, intermediate, and outer layers, with each layer serving a specific purpose. As mentioned previously, keeping the wound bed moist has been shown to accelerate both the inflammatory and proliferative phases of wound healing.

Primary Contact Bandage Layer (Wound Dressings)

Potential functions of the primary contact layer of a bandage include debridement of necrotic debris, delivery of medications, absorption of wound exudate, or formation of an occlusive seal that maintains a moist wound environment. The choice of dressing depends on the condition of the wound (cause, size, location, degree of exudate, and level of contamination), stage of healing, and the activity level or special needs of the patient (**Fig. 13**).[2] Considerations in choosing the contact layer include whether it is adherent or nonadherent, and the permeability and absorptive capacity of the material. Adherent dressings are those that adhere to the wound surface, leading to nonselective debridement of necrotic tissue, bacteria, and some normal tissue from the wound. Nonadherent dressings serve to maintain a moist wound environment and encourage epithelialization once a granulation bed is present. Nonadherent dressings are typically semiocclusive (allowing permeability of fluid and air) or occlusive (impermeable to fluid and air, keeping the wound humidified during the repair phase) and include films, foams, hydrogels, hydrocolloids, and alginates (see **Fig. 10**A). Contrary to previous belief, occlusive dressings are associated with faster wound healing and better cosmetic outcomes.[2,6]

Semiocclusive dressings

Semiocclusive dressings allow penetration of air and exudate from the wound surface because of their porous nature. These dressings are the most common primary layers in use, and are typically used on less exudative wounds to maintain moisture in the early repair phase.[5,11] Traditional choices include cotton nonadherent bandages, such as polyethylene (eg, Telfa Adhesive Pads; Kendall, Mansfield, MA, USA), moisture- and vapor-permeable dressings (eg, Tegaderm; 3M Animal Care Products, St Paul, MN, USA) (see **Figs. 8** and **12**C), and petroleum-impregnated gauze (eg, Adaptic; Ethicon, Arlington, TX, USA).[5,16,28] Petroleum can slow wound contraction and epithelialization.[28]

Films

Films are thin membranes that are also semiocclusive, permitting the exchange of oxygen and water vapor between the wound and the environment while remaining

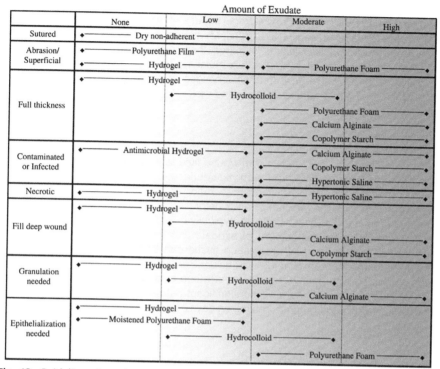

Fig. 13. Guidelines for selection of primary wound dressings based on wound type and amount of wound exudate. (*From* Campbell BG. Dressings, bandages, and splints for wound management in dogs and cats. Vet Clin Small Anim 2006;36:764; with permission.)

impermeable to liquid and bacteria. These dressings are nonabsorbent, in that they manage moisture by vapor transmission only. Films are not ideal for wounds with heavy exudate.[2]

Foams

Polyurethane foams are composed of synthetic polymers (eg, Hydrasorb; KenVet Animal Care Group, Ashland, OH, USA). These highly absorptive, hydrophilic, and non-adherent dressings promote autolytic debridement, stimulate the formation of granulation tissue, and promote epithelialization.[5,28,29] Polyurethane foam is recommended for wounds with moderate to heavy levels of exudate and can be used cases of infected wounds. Dressings should be replaced every 1 to 5 days while avoiding that they dry out, as they can become incorporated into the wound bed and become difficult, painful, and traumatic to remove.

Hydrogels

Hydrogels consist of a fibrous network of polymers and humectants combined with 90% to 95% water, which forms a sheet or gel. Hydrogels are able to absorb small amounts of fluid but are capable of donating significant amounts of moisture to the wound bed, rehydrating the wound, facilitating autolytic debridement, and removing a dried eschar. These gels are useful in the later phases of wound healing that have healthy granulation tissue and initiation of epithelialization. Hydrogels are flexible and can fill dead space, but present problems similar to those with hydrocolloids, whereby maceration of surrounding tissue is possible if they are not cut to the size of the open wound bed.[5,12,24,28,30] A hydrogel sheet and gel form with sustained release of silver ions (SilvaSorb; Medline Industries, Mundelein, IL, USA) has been used extensively in exotic and wildlife patients (see **Figs. 8** and **10A**). These products provide up to 7 days of antimicrobial control and a moist wound environment. The sustained release of silver allows for less frequent changes of dressing, which results in less handling and restraint-related stress, and risk of injury, for exotic and wildlife patients.[31]

Hydrocolloids

Hydrocolloids are composed of hydrophilic polymers, such as carboxymethylcellulose with gelatin or pectin, that interact with wound fluid to form a gel, maintaining a moist wound environment that facilitates autolytic debridement. The dressings are cut to the size and shape of the wound to avoid maceration of the wound edges. The dressing can be prewarmed in the clinician's hands before application to soften it for improved wound contouring.[24] The dressings are typically designed to be changed every 3 to 7 days, depending on the amount of exudate and the manufacturer guidelines. If used for too long, exuberant granulation tissue can form.[5,12,24,28,29] Hydrocolloids are not recommended for wounds with heavy exudate or when infection is present. When compared with hydrogels and polyethylene oxide dressings for open wounds in dogs, they were shown to have no significant difference early on (days 4 and 7), but demonstrated less complete healing on days 21 and 28 compared with the hydrogel group.[30]

Alginates

Alginates consist of fibers derived from seaweed arranged in sheets or ropes. Sodium ions in the wound fluid exchange with calcium ions in the dressing, converting the material into a gel that is capable of absorbing up to 20 times its own weight.[32,33] The calcium ions released activate prothrombin in the clotting cascade, promoting hemostasis.[34] Alginates impregnated with silver are available for its antimicrobial properties. Alginates are best suited for heavily exudative wounds in which they promote autolytic debridement and formation of granulation tissue. Sheets are cut to fit the size of the wound bed, and ropes can be placed within deep wounds. The dressings are changed when strike-through of exudate occurs, which can take up to 7 days.[5,23,24,28,32] With use of an occlusive dressing that converts to a gel a mild odor or yellow, purulent appearance is often seen at bandage changes, which should not to be confused with infection.[29,32,33]

Other products

Other products available include bioactive dressings that originate from living tissue, such as those derived from fibroblasts, keratinocytes, amnion, and submucosa of porcine small intestine or urinary bladder. These agents are thought to accelerate wound repair by provision of an ECM for cellular migration, and can thus be used as a scaffold for tissue ingrowth.

Hydrolyzed bovine collagen (eg, Collamand; BioVet, Topeka, KS, USA) serves as a template of collagen fibers for fibroblasts, epithelial cells, and endothelial cells to enter and migrate across.[5,15,24] Bovine collagen has been shown to enhance early epithelialization in comparison with controls in dog wounds, which could be due to its hydrophilic nature.[35]

Porcine small intestinal submucosa (PSIS) (eg, VetBioSIST; Cook, West Lafayette, IN, USA) consists of collagen, fibronectin, hyaluronic acid, chondroitin sulfate A, heparin, and various growth factors.[5,15,16,24] In a study of open wounds with bone exposure in dogs, there was no difference in wound healing, epithelialization, contraction, inflammation, or angiogenesis between PSIS-applied wounds and control wounds.[36] These scaffolds are cut slightly larger than the area of the wound with the edges tucked underneath the wound edges, sutured, and left in place to be incorporated within the host tissues. Over 2 weeks following placement the neutrophils break down the scaffold, releasing cytokines and growth factors that promote healing and neovascularization.[37]

Equine amnion has been used as an occlusive dressing that was shown to increase wound contraction and epithelialization when compared with hydrogel and polyethylene nonadherent dressings in a canine study.[38] Because of cost concerns, these dressings are reserved for chronic, nonhealing wounds in which granulation tissue is needed.

Secondary (Intermediate) Bandage Layer

The secondary or intermediate layer is often minimized or avoided in exotic species to limit the bulkiness of the bandage. This layer holds the contact layer in place, and functions in exudate absorption, pressure, support, and reduction of mobility. This layer should be thick enough to collect the amount of exudate anticipated and serve as a pad to prevent movement (see **Fig. 10**B). Materials commonly used include cast padding, combine rolls, or absorbent bulk roll cotton. The inner, absorbent layer is typically followed by an outer, stabilizing layer. When indicated, a splint or stabilizing rod can be placed between these layers to provide immobilization. The outer stabilizing portion is typically achieved using roll gauze.

Tertiary (Outer) Bandage Layer

The tertiary or outer layer primarily functions to hold the other layers of the bandage in place and to protect the wound and underlying bandage from external contamination. Materials most commonly used for this layer include elastic adhesive tapes, stockinette, surgical adhesive tape, or spandex garments.[5,24,28] Care should be taken that the bandage is not placed too tight when using bandage material with elastic properties. In exotic patients, adhesive films (eg, Tegaderm) can be effective outer layers and are frequently used, especially in birds and reptiles (see **Figs. 8**, **10**B, and **12**).

Tie-Over Bandages

In cases where a circumferential bandage is not possible, a tie-over bandage can be used. Several sutures are loosely placed in the skin surrounding the periphery of the primary wound (see **Fig. 10**A). The primary wound is covered with an appropriate dressing over which an absorbent layer of gauze or laparotomy pads is placed. The bandage is secured using umbilical tape or suture threaded through the suture loops in the skin and knotted (see **Fig. 10**B). When bandages are changed the suture loops remain in place, limiting additional stress placed on the patient. To prevent additional contamination an adhesive film can be placed over the entire bandage, limiting environmental exposure.[5]

Bandage Changes

The level of exudate present should determine the timing of bandage changes. The ideal timing of a bandage change may be daily initially; however, in exotic species it is imperative to consider the risks of stress and frequent sedation or anesthesia indicated. Therefore, bandage choices, such as hydrogels, which can potentially be changed less frequently because of their ability to maintain wound moisture, may be better options in these species. Efforts should be made to protect the bandage.

Elizabethan collars (E-collars) are the most common method to protect the bandage from patient-induced damage, such as licking or chewing. It is imperative that the bandage be kept dry, away from fecal and urinary contamination. This action may merit separation of group-housed animals temporarily. Proper selection of bandage materials and topical wound dressings should be catered according to the individual patient, and consideration should be given to the behavior of the species along with the nature of the wound.

NEGATIVE PRESSURE WOUND THERAPY

Negative pressure wound therapy (NPWT) is an adjunctive wound management technique that locally applies subatmospheric pressure across a wound in a closed environment. Open-pore polyurethane foam sponges are placed within the wound bed following debridement, and a semiocclusive adhesive dressing is placed over the foam extending a few centimeters beyond the edge of the wound margin to create a complete seal. A hole is created in the dressing over the center of the foam, and the suction port with tubing is attached to the suction-pump canister. The unit is set to either continuous or intermittent suction. If no leaks in the system are present, the foam should visibly collapse beneath the adhesive.[11,39]

NPWT is proposed to increase wound healing by promoting wound contraction, stimulating granulation tissue formation, increasing tissue perfusion, reducing edema, removing exudate, and decreasing bacterial colonization.[40] Large, comprehensive reviews have revealed that insufficient or contradictory evidence currently exists regarding the mechanisms of action of NPWT.[40] However, reports of clinical success have been published for exotic species including birds and chelonians, and experimentally in rabbits and rats. NPWT should not be used when there is potential for the wound to contain neoplastic cells or when there are exposed organs, nerves, or large vessels, whereby negative pressure could result in hemorrhage or erosion.[40,41] Initially the dressings may need to be changed daily, but can later be changed every 2 to 3 days.

CONSIDERATIONS FOR WOUND MANAGEMENT IN EXOTIC ANIMAL SPECIES

Although the underlying concepts of wound healing detailed herein are similar across the board, variations among species do exist with regard to healing.

Birds

Avian integument is thinner and more delicate than mammalian skin, while also being dry and inelastic. It comprises 2 layers, the dermis and epidermis. The dermis is the site of feather development from dermal papilla, and contains striated muscle that functions to control skin tension. Dense dermal capillary beds contribute to the red coloration of wattles, combs, and appendages in some species. The epidermis contains living and dead cells, with the outer keratinized stratum corneum consisting of horny dead cells. One must bear in mind that wounds of the distal extremities have reduced vascular supply and thus heal more slowly. In avian species, bruising may develop 2 to 3 days after injury, characterized by a green discoloration of the skin caused by biliverdin pigment accumulation following breakdown of hemoglobin.

Caution should be observed with the use of topical therapy because of the thin dermis, which is predisposed to increased absorption of topical medications with the potential for systemic effects. Oil-based products should be avoided in birds because they can be preened into feathers, affecting thermoregulation. Causes of open wounds are most often traumatic, bite wounds from other animals, or self-inflicted wounds, but constriction injuries, infections, and cutaneous neoplasms are also seen. Chronic, nonhealing wounds of the medial wings and patagium are difficult to manage primarily because of the dynamic movement of muscles, tendons, and skin of the wings during flight. It is often necessary to immobilize the limb to allow healing, but care should be taken to limit the risks of permanent inability for wing extension and prevention of flight.

Pododermatitis, or bumblefoot, is an especially large problem in captive raptors and waterfowl species. Management is best achieved with aggressive surgical debridement with primary closure followed by postoperative protective foot casting, in addition to local and systemic antimicrobial therapy.[42] Often both feet need to be bandaged, owing to the risk of weight shifting onto the other limb during healing. The casts should be removed every 7 days to re-evaluate the foot.

Reptiles

Reptiles have dry skin, devoid of glands, with scales of epidermal origin arranged in regular geometric patterns. As reptiles are ectotherms, the wound-healing process depends highly on the environmental temperature. Lower temperatures will delay cell migration and, thus, wound healing.[43] In addition, as in other species, stress has a negative effect on wound healing.[44] In snakes, antibiotic ointments have been shown to delay wound healing of experimentally induced skin wounds, whereas occlusive polyurethane film (Op-Site Spray Bandage; Smith and Nephew, Lachine, QC, Canada) resulted in more advanced wound healing.[45] Consideration should be made for semiaquatic or aquatic reptiles (eg, turtles), as these open wounds should be closed primarily despite common wound-healing principles. Causes of open wounds are often abscesses or abrasions secondary to poor husbandry, conspecific trauma (see **Fig. 6**), thermal burns from heated rocks or incandescent light bulbs, abnormal shedding (dysecdysis) that allows tearing of the epidermis, or trauma, especially from prey species.

SUMMARY

Wound healing is a complicated process that includes overlapping phases: hemostasis, inflammation, debridement, repair (proliferation), and remodeling. Each phase is affected by various endogenous and exogenous factors. An understanding of normal wound healing, in addition to the pathogenesis of impaired or delayed healing, is critical in choosing an appropriate and successful wound-management strategy. Finally, consideration of the patient species must be made when determining appropriate wound care to achieve the best possible outcome.

REFERENCES

1. Portou MJ, Baker D, Abraham D, et al. The innate immune system, toll-like receptors and dermal wound healing: a review. Vascul Pharmacol 2015;71:31–6.
2. Ozturk F, Ermertcan AT. Wound healing: a new approach to the topical wound care. Cutan Ocul Toxicol 2011;30:92–9.
3. Pazyar N, Yaghoobi R, Rafiee E, et al. Skin wound healing and phytomedicine: a review. Skin Pharmacol Physiol 2014;27:303–10.
4. Cornell K. Wound healing. In: Tobias KM, Johnston SA, editors. Veterinary surgery: small animal, vol. 1, 1st edition. St Louis (MO): Saunders; 2012. p. 125–34.
5. Hedlund CS. Surgery of the integumentary system. In: Fossum TW, editor. Small animal surgery. 3rd edition. St Louis (MO): Mosby, Inc; 2007. p. 159–228.

6. Balsa IM, Culp WT. Wound care. Vet Clin North Am Small Anim Pract 2015;45: 1049–65.

7. Franz MG, Robson MC, Steed DL, et al. Guidelines to aid in healing of acute wounds by decreasing impediments of healing. Wound Repair Regen 2008;16: 723–48.

8. Amsellem P. Complications of reconstructive surgery in companion animals. Vet Clin Small Anim 2011;41:995–1006.

9. Tobin GR. Closure of contaminated wounds. Biologic and technical considerations. Surg Clin North Am 1984;64:639–52.

10. Brown DC. Wound infections and antimicrobial use. In: Tobias KM, Johnston SA, editors. Veterinary surgery: small animal, vol. 1, 1st edition. St Louis (MO): Saunders; 2012. p. 135–9.

11. Hosgood G. Open wounds. In: Tobias KM, Johnston SA, editors. Veterinary surgery: small animal, vol. 1, 1st edition. St Louis (MO): Saunders; 2012. p. 1210–20.

12. Davidson JR. Current concepts in wound management and wound healing products. Vet Clin Small Anim 2015;45(3):1–28.

13. Ayello EA, Cuddigan JE. Debridement: controlling the necrotic/cellular burden. Adv Skin Wound Care 2004;17:66–75.

14. Kirshen C, Woo K, Ayello EA, et al. Debridement. A vital component of wound bed preparation. Adv Skin Wound Care 2006;19:506–17.

15. Krahwinkel DJ, Boothe HW. Topical and systemic medications for wounds. Vet Clin Small Anim 2006;36:739–57.

16. Fahie MA. Evidence-based wound management: a systematic review of therapeutic agents to enhance granulation and epithelialization. Vet Clin Small Anim 2007;37:559–77.

17. Guthrie KM, Agarwal A, Tackes DS, et al. Antibacterial efficacy of silver-impregnated polyelectrolyte multilayers immobilized on a biological dressing in a murine wound infection model. Ann Surg 2012;256:371–7.

18. Herron M, Agarwal A, Kierski P, et al. Reduction in wound bioburden using a silver-loaded dissolvable microfilm construct. Adv Healthc Mater 2014;3: 916–28.

19. Rodriguez-Bigas M, Cruz NI, Suarez A. Comparative evaluation of aloe vera in the management of burn wounds in guinea pigs. Plast Reconstr Surg 1988;81:386–9.

20. Swaim SF, Riddell KP, McGuire JA. Effects of topical medications on the healing of open pad wounds in dogs. J Am Anim Hosp Assoc 1992;28:499–502.

21. Canapp SO, Farese JP, Schultz GS, et al. The effect of topical tripeptide-copper complex on healing of ischemic open wounds. Vet Surg 2003;32:515–23.

22. Matthews KA, Binnington AG. Wound management using honey. Compend Contin Educ Pract Vet 2002;24:53–60.

23. Matthews KA, Binnington AG. Wound management using sugar. Compend Contin Educ Pract Vet 2002;24:41–52.

24. Campbell BG. Dressings, bandages, and splints for wound management in dogs and cats. Vet Clin Small Anim 2006;36:759–91.

25. Knighton DR, Ciresi K, Fiegel VD, et al. Stimulation of repair in chronic, nonhealing, cutaneous ulcers using platelet-derived wound healing formula. Surg Gynecol Obstet 1990;170:56–60.

26. Tambella AM, Attili AR, Dini F, et al. Autologous platelet gel to treat chronic decubital ulcers: a randomized, blind controlled clinical trial in dogs. Vet Surg 2014;43: 726–33.

27. Uneo H, Mori T, Fujinaga T. Topical formulations and wound healing applications of chitosan. Adv Drug Deliv Rev 2001;52:105–15.

28. Campbell BG. Bandages and drains. In: Tobias KM, Johnston SA, editors. Veterinary surgery: small animal, vol. 1, 1st edition. St Louis (MO): Saunders; 2012. p. 221–30.
29. Kannon GA, Garrett AB. Moist wound healing with occlusive dressings. A clinical Review. Dermatol Surg 1995;21:583–90.
30. Morgan PW, Binnington AG, Miller CW, et al. The effect of occlusive and semi-occlusive dressings on the healing of acute full-thickness skin wounds on the forelimbs of dogs. Vet Surg 1994;23:494–502.
31. Mans C, Guincho M, Smith D, et al. Application of a sustained-release silver hydrogel dressing sheet in avian wound management. Exot DVM 2007;9:21–4.
32. Dissemond J, Augustin M, Eming SA, et al. Modern wound care-practical aspects of non-interventional topical treatment of patients with chronic wounds. J Dtsch Dermatol Ges 2014;12:541–54.
33. Eaglstein WH. Moist wound healing with occlusive dressings: a clinical focus. Dermatol Surg 2001;27:175–81.
34. Segal HC, Hunt BJ, Gilding K. The effects of alginate and non-alginate wound dressings on blood coagulation and platelet activation. J Biomater Appl 1998;12:249–57.
35. Swaim SF, Gillette RL, Sartin EA, et al. Effects of a hydrolyzed collagen dressing on the healing of open wounds in dogs. Am J Vet Res 2000;61:1574–8.
36. Winkler JT, Swaim SF, Sartin EA, et al. The effect of porcine-derived small intestinal submucosa product on wounds with exposed bone in dogs. Vet Surg 2002;31:541–51.
37. Badylak SF. Xenogeneic extracellular matrix as a scaffold for tissue reconstruction. Transpl Immunol 2004;12:367–77.
38. Ramsey DT, Pope ER, Wagner-Mann C, et al. Effects of three occlusive dressing materials on healing of full-thickness skin wounds in dogs. Am J Vet Res 1995;56:941–9.
39. Howe LM. Current concepts in negative pressure wound therapy. Vet Clin Small Anim 2015;45(3):565–84.
40. Moues CM, Heule F, Hovius SE. A review of topical negative pressure therapy in wound healing: sufficient evidence. Am J Surg 2011;201:544–56.
41. Marin ML, Norton TM, Mettee NS. Vacuum-assisted wound closure in chelonians. In: Mader DR, Divers SJ, editors. Current therapy in reptile medicine and surgery. St Louis (MO): Elsevier Saunders; 2014. p. 197–204.
42. Remple JD. A multifaceted approach to the treatment of bumblefoot in raptors. J Exot Pet Med 2006;15:49–55.
43. Smith DA, Barker IK, Allen OB. The effect of ambient temperature and type of wound on healing of cutaneous wounds in the common garter snake (Thamnophis sirtalis). Can J Vet Res 1988;52:120–8.
44. French SS, Matt KS, Moore MC. The effects of stress on wound healing in male tree lizards (Urosaurus ornatus). Gen Comp Endocrinol 2006;145(2):128–32.
45. Smith DA, Barker IK, Allen OB. The effect of certain topical medications on healing of cutaneous wounds in the common garter snake (Thamnophis sirtalis). Can J Vet Res 1988;52(1):129–33.

Fish Surgery
Presurgical Preparation and Common Surgical Procedures

Kurt K. Sladky, MS, DVM, DACZM, DECZM (Herpetology)[a,*],
Elsburgh O. Clarke III, DVM[b]

KEYWORDS

- Fish • Teleost • Elasmobranch • Surgery • Surgical • Coelom • Bath anesthetic

KEY POINTS

- Fish are among the most diverse of all phyla, and a knowledge of anatomy, behavior, and natural history of the individual species greatly facilitates the ability to perform successful surgery.
- Basic surgical procedures used across fish species maintain surgical principles and instruments similar to those used in mammalian species, with some important adaptations.
- Fish surgery requires knowledge of bath and recirculating anesthetic applications and an understanding of basic analgesic principles. Fish must be kept moist during all surgical procedures.
- Common surgical procedures in fish include integumentary mass excision, intracoelomic mass removals, reproductive system procedures, gastrointestinal foreign body removal, ocular procedures, and radiotransmitter implantation.

INTRODUCTION

Many fish species are commonly maintained as pets, in zoos and aquaria, and in research facilities. With the burgeoning interest in fish medicine in recent years, the importance of developing, refining, and performing fish surgical procedures has increased dramatically. A considerable number of displayed fish species are valuable, from aesthetic, emotional, public interest, endangerment, and economic perspectives. Therefore, the application of surgical techniques to fish species has become critical to aquarium, zoo, wildlife, and exotic pet veterinarians.

The authors have nothing to disclose.
[a] Department of Surgical Sciences, School of Veterinary Medicine, University of Wisconsin, 2015 Linden Drive, Madison, WI 53706, USA; [b] Audubon Nature Institute, 1 Canal Street, New Orleans, LA 70130, USA
* Corresponding author.
E-mail address: sladkyk@svm.vetmed.wisc.edu

Vet Clin Exot Anim 19 (2016) 55–76
http://dx.doi.org/10.1016/j.cvex.2015.08.008
vetexotic.theclinics.com

Surgical techniques performed on terrestrial animals can be similarly applied, and/or extrapolated, to fish across all sizes and species, from a 1-g zebrafish to a 500-kg tiger shark. If an elective surgical procedure is performed, the general guidelines of asepsis, hemostasis, good technique, and care, as with terrestrial animal surgery, should be followed. Of significance, is developing an understanding the natural history, behavior, and anatomy of the species considered for surgical procedures. During presurgical patient evaluation, if possible, the clinician should visually assess the animal in its home aquarium or primary enclosure to understand the individual or species behavior, movement, attitude, and general health condition. This assessment is vital to gauging a patient's postsurgical recovery and determining when it is safe for an animal to be placed back into its enclosure. Clinical observations of a healthy patient include normal species-specific swimming behavior patterns, strong rhythmic opercular movement suggesting adequate oxygenation, and no excessive mucus shedding or visible skin or ocular manifestations of disease. Presurgical health assessment should include a physical examination, bloodwork (complete blood cell count and serum biochemical profile), and imaging (eg, radiographs, CT scan, or ultrasound) as necessary. Presurgical and postsurgical supportive care should be considered in fish and may include fluid therapy and appropriate antimicrobial, analgesic, and anti-inflammatory medications. Perioperative antibiotics are commonly used in fish surgical procedures because of the general microbial contamination associated with the aquatic environment. The most common choices of antibiotics include oxytetracycline (10 mg/kg, intramuscularly [IM], every 24 hours); enrofloxacin (5–10 mg/kg, IM, every 24 hours); ceftazidime (30 mg/kg, IM, every 48–72 hours); and florfenicol (40 mg/kg, IM, every 24–48 hours). Antibiotics can be continued postoperatively if deemed necessary and may be administered parenterally, with immersive baths, or orally, in medicated feed or medicated gel food.[1,2] There are times when immediate surgical intervention is necessary regardless of a patient's health status. In these circumstances, it is important that the patient be given the best possible outcomes for survival, which include properly oxygenated water, excellent water-quality parameters that minimize or exclude infectious agents present within the system, and medically appropriate supportive care.

PRESURGICAL CONSIDERATIONS
Anesthesia and Analgesia

Regardless of species, a safe and effective anesthetic protocol is a key component of a successful surgical outcome. There is a vast difference between fish and terrestrial animal anesthesia, with most fish anesthetic procedures involving bath anesthetic drugs. Because a majority of fish surgeries occur out of the water, the animal must be placed on a recirculating water apparatus (commonly referred to as fish anesthetic delivery system [FADS]),[3] typically containing a bath anesthetic, such as tricaine methanesulfonate (MS-222) (**Fig. 1**). This apparatus allows simultaneous anesthesia in conjunction with the ability to keep the skin moist during prolonged procedures (**Fig. 2**). Select procedures can be performed, however, while the fish patient is partially submerged in water. Most of these partial submersion procedures are reserved for 1 of the following: (1) minimally invasive procedures, (2) large animals that make it logistically challenging for removal from the water column, and/or (3) inadequate space for out-of-water procedures. The primary disadvantages of partial submersion procedures are that there is increased chance of surgical site contamination and lack of adequate space for surgical equipment to be aseptically maintained.

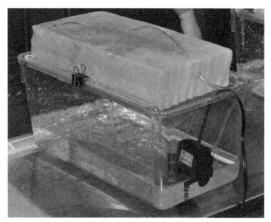

Fig. 1. Fish Anesthesia Delivery System (FADS). This system is used for small to medium-sized fish and is designed from a plastic laboratory rat cage on the bottom as an anesthetic water receptacle and a plastic platform fastened to the rodent cage using binder clips. An aquarium pump is placed in the water with constant flow from 2 aquarium tubes (1 tube is placed in the oral cavity of the fish to bathe the gills in anesthetic solution and the other tube is used for keeping the skin moist during long procedures). A wet foam pad is placed on top of the Plexiglas platform on which the fish is placed.

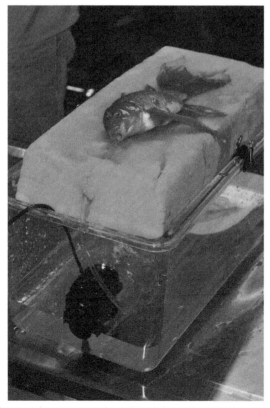

Fig. 2. Fish Anesthesia Delivery System (FADS) with koi in lateral recumbency. The aquarium tubing is visible in the oral cavity of the koi.

The arsenal of drugs that can be used as anesthetic agents for fish patients has significantly increased over the past decade. Anesthetics drugs, such as tricaine methanesulfonate (MS-222), eugenol (the active ingredient in clove oil), and isoeugenol (AQUI-S), are most commonly used as bath anesthetic agents for induction and maintenance.[2] The authors, however, caution any clinician using eugenol and isoeugenol products that there is some evidence that these anesthetic drugs may not provide analgesia during surgical procedures.[4] More recently, propofol and alfaxalone were demonstrated as effective bath anesthetics in some species, and multiple injectable anesthetic agents, such as α_2-agonists (eg, dexmedetomidine and medetomidine) and ketamine, are available for parenteral administration.[2] There are excellent reviews of fish anesthesia techniques in the published literature.[1,2] The water-quality parameters used during anesthesia should be similar to those in the aquarium from which the fish is housed. The constant flow of water over the gills during bath anesthesia plays an important role in maintaining appropriate oxygenation during the surgical procedure as well. Delivering water to the patient is often achieved by inserting a flexible plastic tube (eg, aquarium tubing) of appropriate size to fit in the patient's mouth, which is attached to an adequate-sized aquarium pump. The specific pump size should be selected to provide constant water flow over the gills and exiting through the operculum. This is to ensure that all gill arches are adequately oxygenated and the bath anesthetic appropriately delivered. The flow rate should not be high enough, however, to cause anesthetic water to enter the incision site or cause excess water to enter the gastrointestinal tract through the oral cavity. This is frequently observed when the oropharyngeal tube is placed caudal to the operculum as well. When building larger FADS, the use of ball valves or similar types of plumbing equipment can be used to adjust flow rate to appropriate levels for the individual species.

Preemptive analgesia is an important consideration, and any analgesic drugs should be administered prior to making the first incision. Although some investigators argue that fish do not experience pain, and few data are available with respect to analgesic efficacy and safety across fish species, it is the authors' opinion that fish experience pain and analgesic use is imperative. Although the published literature regarding fish pain and analgesia is scant, μ-opioids in concert with nonsteroidal anti-inflammatory drugs should be considered the current standard of practice.[2,5–8] Dosage regimens, duration of effect, and analgesic safety are unknown for most species and vary across species. Therefore, the administration of opioids and nonsteroidal anti-inflammatory drugs is still considered empirical.[5]

Surgical Preparation

Once sedated or anesthetized, unlike their terrestrial counterparts, fish patients do not require an extensive surgical preparation. Like mammalian surgery, aseptic practices should always be exercised and patients must be provided a clean surgical area. Securing patients in a proper surgical position is critical. Foam fabric upholstery blocks of various sizes are commonly used for this purpose (**Fig. 3**). Foam pads can be readily acquired from mattress and furniture manufacturers/distributors and the foam material cut into an appropriate size and shape, and a V-shaped wedge can be cut into 1 side of the foam to secure the fish patient in dorsal recumbency. Foam is minimally abrasive to fish skin and has the advantage of absorbing water, which contributes to keeping the fish skin moist.[9]

Once the fish has been securely positioned on the foam, surgical preparation of the incision site can be completed. All fish species have a coat of mucus covering the body. The mucus layer is protective, containing immunoglobulins and aids in osmoregulation. This must be considered when applying any type of surgical scrub

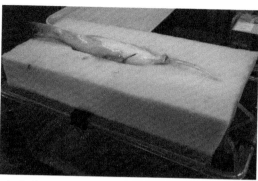

Fig. 3. Fish Anesthesia Delivery System (FADS) with an elliptical divot cut into 1 side of the foam and a koi placed in dorsal recumbency in preparation for a ventral midline incision.

(eg, povidone-iodine, chlorhexidine, or alcohol) to prepare the incisional site.[9] The chemicals can disrupt the mucus layer on the nonsurgical portions of the fish's body and potentially irritate the skin. Frequently, sterile, physiologic saline (0.9%) can be used to gently wipe the incision site, which is most commonly the ventral midline. Some veterinarians choose to use dilute povidone-iodine on cotton-tipped applicators to minimally wipe the skin. In addition, in some of the large-scaled fish species, individual scales may need to be removed along the planned incision site to facilitate ease of cutting through the skin. This can be accomplished by using aseptic hemostats and/or forceps to grab and secure the distal tip of the scale and exert force caudally, away from the base of the scale insertion point. Small-scaled or scaleless fish and elasmobranchs do not require removal of such scales and the incision can be made directly into the integument.

Choice of surgical instruments depends on size and species of patient; standard small mammal surgical packs are selected for medium to large species, and minisurgical or microsurgical and ophthalmic packs may be most appropriate for smaller patients. Surgical loupes are beneficial for magnification under most circumstances, regardless of size and species of fish patient.

General Surgical Approach in Fish

Once the surgical site is prepared, a plastic drape (stick or nonstick) can be cut to an appropriately sized shape for access to making the incision and placed over the fish (**Fig. 4**). Some sticky drapes can be placed over the fish and the incision made directly

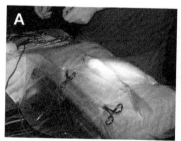
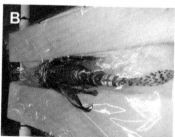

Fig. 4. (*A*) A plastic, sticky drape placed over a koi during presurgical preparation. (*B*) A lionfish presurgically prepared with a commercial plastic wrap that has been sterilized.

through the drape and into the skin. Plastic drapes have the advantages of providing constant visualization of the patient and promoting moisture retention during prolonged procedures. Alternatively, conventional cloth drapes can be used but frequently become water-laden and are abrasive, removing more mucus from the fish skin. Towel clamps can be placed as with terrestrial animals, but caution should be used in small species or those species without scaled skin. In most fish species, a #15 or #10 blade can be used to make the ventral midline incision through the skin and coelomic membrane. To adequately access a fish's coelomic cavity, it is generally recommended to make an incision large enough to provide good visualization of most coelomic organ systems (**Fig. 5**). In some species, such as cyprinids (koi, carp, and goldfish), the cartilaginous pectoral girdle, associated with the pectoral fins, is best incised using a pair of scissors.[5] Retractors are frequently necessary in most fish species, because the skin and underlying muscles tend to invert, contract, and obstruct the surgical view (**Fig. 6**). Conventional surgical retractors (eg, Weitlaner, Gelpi, Heaney, Alm, eyelid, and Lone Star [Cooper Surgical, Inc., Trumbull, CT, USA]) can be used, depending on the size and species of fish. Once in the coelomic cavity, hemostasis can be facilitated by use of cautery devices (unipolar or bipolar), hemostats, and Hemoclips (Teleflex Medical, Morrisville, NC, USA) of varying sizes (**Fig. 7**). When using cautery devices, be mindful of potential tissue damage to adjacent tissues, particularly in small patients.

Closure of the incision may require 1 or 2 layers depending on size and species of fish. Synthetic, monofilament absorbable suture material can be used and is preferred, primarily because the tissue reaction is minimized and integrity of the suture holding power maximized.[10] Unlike mammalian skin, the fish immune system does not readily degrade absorbable suture and it tends to stay intact for weeks or months. A continuous or interrupted suture pattern can be used, and the pattern is typically firmly apposing or slightly everting, because incised fish skin tends to naturally invert. In koi, the authors use a Ford interlocking, horizontal mattress, or cruciate pattern, and it is critical to get complete apposition of the cartilaginous pectoral plate (**Fig. 8**).[5] With a 2-layer closure, a simple continuous pattern using monofilament, absorbable suture material can be used to close the coelomic membrane, and the skin and muscle can be closed, as described previously. It is best to allow the sutures to remain in place for several weeks (typically 4–8 weeks). Once a fish is recovered, the authors typically lower or raise the salinity,

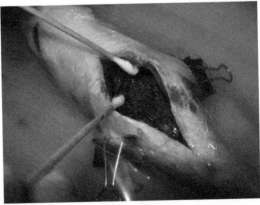

Fig. 5. Ventral midline incision in a koi. Koi have a cartilaginous pectoral plate, which is firm, and may require Metzenbaum scissors for extending the incision cranially for excellent intracoelomic exposure.

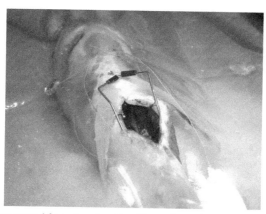

Fig. 6. Eyelid retractor used for retracting the skin and muscle layers of a small koi. Fish skin has a tendency to invert once incised, so retractors are useful in any fish surgical procedure.

depending on the animal's environmental preference. This is considered a part of the initial healing process. In freshwater fish, the salinity is slightly raised, whereas in marine dwelling fish, salinity is slightly decreased. The thought is that this approach to regulating salinity helps decrease microorganisms within the environment, stimulate skin mucus production, and decrease osmotic stressors on the animal due to the compromised integument layer, postoperatively.

COMMON SURGICAL PROCEDURES IN TELEOST AND ELASMOBRANCH FISH

The majority of published literature on fish surgery describes a variety of procedures across a variety of teleost species.[5,9,11–15] The few elasmobranch surgical procedures described in the primary literature focus on foreign body removal in shark species or reproductive surgery in ray species.[13,14,16,17] Details of surgical procedures in elasmobranchs are limited, however, and, therefore, there is a need for descriptive clinical reports and systematic surgical research in captive and free-ranging elasmobranch species.

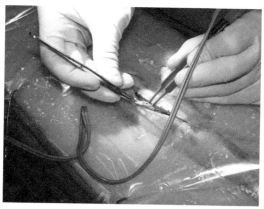

Fig. 7. Bipolar cautery used during a koi surgery for hemostasis. Unipolar or bipolar cautery is useful during fish surgical procedures for rapid hemostasis and cutting through vessels after ligatures or Hemoclips are placed.

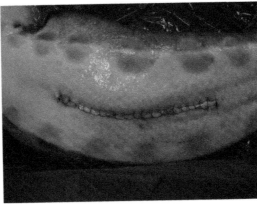

Fig. 8. A continuous Ford interlocking suture pattern in a sturgeon. Ford interlocking and horizontal mattress suture patterns work well in most fish species to close muscle and skin.

For elasmobranchs, the logistics associated with providing proper anesthesia, a clean surgical environment, and postoperative care can be challenging, especially with larger species. Creative and improvised approaches may be necessary to accommodate these procedures and are planned with the particular layout of the facility housing the animal (**Fig. 9**). Due to the ability of some elasmobranch species to cause bodily harm, when possible, detailed staff planning should be performed.[9,18,19] Small elasmobranch species can be easily transported to appropriate hospital facilities, whereas larger elasmobranchs are frequently managed in close proximity to their exhibit. Despite being able to recover quickly from minor surgical procedures,[20] when possible, elasmobranchs should be placed in an isolated area postoperatively until fully recovered.[19] Once adequate recovery is determined, the animal can be released back into the main exhibit area. This reduces conspecific aggression if a patient is normally housed with other elasmobranch or teleost species and potentially reduces risk trauma to the incision site from enclosure décor.[19]

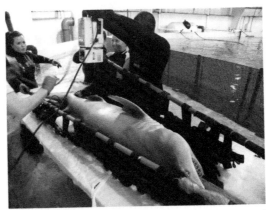

Fig. 9. Large tigershark undergoing portable radiographs. This image illustrates the logistical and facility manipulations necessary for performing procedures on large fish species.

Integumentary Mass Removal

In clinical practice, the most common fish surgical procedures encountered are those involving the integumentary system, in particular, cutaneous masses (**Figs. 10** and **11**). Complete excision of cutaneous masses can be challenging due to the nonelastic nature of fish integument. Although it is easy to excise masses at the level of the dermis, it is frequently difficult to completely excise masses in total owing to the depth of excision required. Although many integumentary masses are benign in fish, simply snipping the cutaneous mass almost certainly results in recurrence. In addition, many skin masses in fish have an underlying viral cause.[9,21] Deep tissue excisions require healing by second intention and antimicrobial coverage because of the likelihood of opportunistic microorganisms invading the open surgical wound. Electrocautery can be used for both hemostasis and destruction of the abnormal tissue. In a unique case requiring surgery for impaired vision in an oranda goldfish, it was necessary to surgically excise greater than 50% of the wen, which was completely covering the eyes of the fish, causing complete anorexia and wasting (**Figs. 12** and **13**). Electrocautery was used to cut the wen tissue and expose the eyes (**Fig. 14**). The fish recovered uneventfully and started to eat immediately after discharge. Cryotherapy is another option for integumentary mass and abnormal tissue destruction (**Fig. 15**).[22]

Intracoelomic Mass and Foreign Body Removal

Intracoelomic masses are commonly diagnosed in fish species and can be associated with any organ system.[23] Intracoelomic masses are most commonly associated, however, with reproductive organs, liver, or swim bladder.[23] A variety of presurgical imaging modalities (CT, ultrasound, and fluoroscopy) may help characterize the organ system with which the mass or masses are associated, but frequently an exploratory laparotomy is necessary for confirming and treating/excising the mass. In teleost fish, a ventral midline approach is performed, as described previously. Retractors are essential in visualizing the mass(es) and associated organ system(s) as well as the degree to which the mass is or is not invasive or metastatic. Electrocautery, Hemoclips (Teleflex Medical, Morrisville, NC, USA), and ligatures can be used for hemostasis prior to and during surgical removal of intracoelomic masses. Blunt dissection of surrounding soft tissues using hemostats is frequently necessary. In some cases, for example, swim bladder masses or metastases to the swim bladder, the swim bladder must be partially resected and closed using a 2-layer inverting suture pattern (eg, Cushing-Connell). In those species with a bilobed swim bladder (eg, cyprinids), care

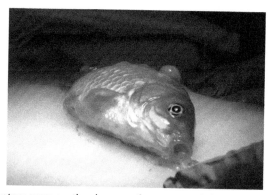

Fig. 10. Integumentary mass on the dorsum of a comet goldfish.

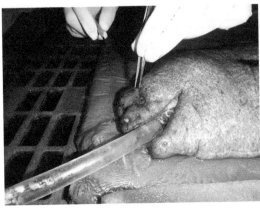

Fig. 11. Integumentary mass dorsal to the left eye of a green moray eel.

must be taken to attempt to preserve the bilobed integrity; otherwise, abnormal buoyancy issues may ensue.[9,24] The skin/muscle layer incision can be closed, as described previously, in either 1 or 2 layers using a monofilament, absorbable suture material. All masses should examined and dissected after removal, with part preserved in formalin, and the remainder frozen for future diagnostics, if necessary.

Ingestion of foreign bodies is common in elasmobranchs and some teleosts.[9,13,14,16,25] Elasmobranchs tend to ingest metallic foreign bodes, such as fishhooks, which can cause fistulas within the coelomic cavity and lead to secondary peritonitis, pericarditis, and septicemia.[13,16,19,20,25,26] The hooks tend to corrode within the coelom, and surgical excision is necessary for curative treatment.[13] Teleosts tend to ingest aquarium furniture, including substrate, tank material, plastic plant materials, rubber suction cups, and so forth. The surgical approach to gastrointestinal foreign bodies is similar in both teleost and elasmobranch fish species. Presurgical imaging is imperative for localizing the foreign body. In addition, presurgical antimicrobials and analgesics should be administered, because coelomic contamination with gastrointestinal contents is possible. Once a surgical plane of anesthesia is achieved, typically, a ventral midline incision is made, which may or may not incorporate the

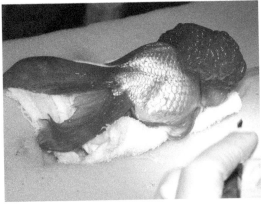

Fig. 12. Oranda goldfish, presurgery, with its wen completely occluding vision.

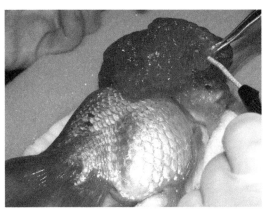

Fig. 13. Unipolar cautery device used to cut away the wen of an oranda goldfish.

cartilaginous pectoral girdle, depending on the organ location of the foreign body. Consider making a large incision through the skin, muscle, and coelomic membrane for best visualization within the coelomic cavity. Once the appropriate gastrointestinal organ is localized (eg, stomach or small intestine), stay sutures are placed on each side of the proposed incision site, and the organ is gently elevated out of the coelomic cavity (**Fig. 16**).[13] The incision is made in the location of the foreign body and the foreign body removed. If vascular integrity of the stomach or intestine has been compromised, resulting in tissue devitalization, a resection and anastomosis procedure, as in mammals, should be performed.[9,27] As with mammalian gastrointestinal surgical procedures, the stomach or intestine is closed in 2 layers using monofilament, absorbable suture material in an inverting pattern (eg, a Cushing-Connell pattern). The second layer should close over the top of the first. The integrity of the suture line can be tested by infusing sterile saline into the gastrointestinal organ and observing the suture line for leakage. Once satisfied that the 2-layer closure is intact, the coelomic cavity can be flushed multiple times with sterile saline and the remaining saline can be suctioned from the coelomic cavity. Depending on the species and size of the animal, the coelomic membrane, muscles, and skin can be closed in 1 or 2 layers using

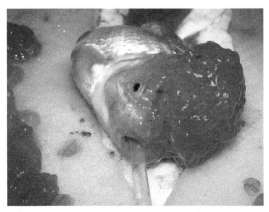

Fig. 14. Oranda goldfish, postsurgery, with its wen excised using a unipolar cautery device to expose both eyes and restore vision.

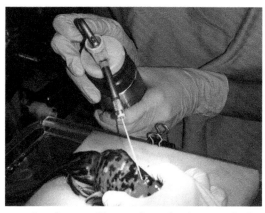

Fig. 15. Cryosurgery used to freeze a fibroma from the dorsum of a butterfly koi.

absorbable, monofilament suture material in appositional patterns, such as horizontal mattress, Ford interlocking, cruciate, and simple continuous or interrupted patterns. The authors generally use simple continuous for an inner muscle/membrane closure and a continuous Ford interlocking or cruciate pattern for closing skin. Silver sulfadiazine cream or gel or an iodine-based ointment can be applied over the suture line for further protection.

Ophthalmic Surgery

Ocular disease is common in pet and displayed fish and can be due to trauma, microorganism infection, or neoplastic diseases (**Fig. 17**).[28–30] Severe ocular diseases are unsightly in displayed or pet fish, and, therefore, enucleation is a common procedure and is easy, with generally less hemorrhage than a similar procedure in a reptile or mammal.[28,31] There is a single research report describing the surgical process association with prosthetic eye placement in hybrid striped bass after enucleation.[31] This report provides an excellent description of the enucleation procedure, which can be readily applied across fish species, as well as ocular prosthetic placement, which can be considered in display fish for aesthetic reasons. Briefly, for enucleation, the

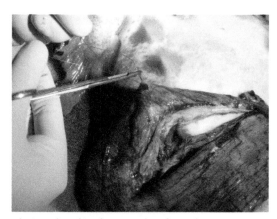

Fig. 16. Stay sutures being placed in the serosal surface of a sturgeon stomach prior to making a gastrotomy incision.

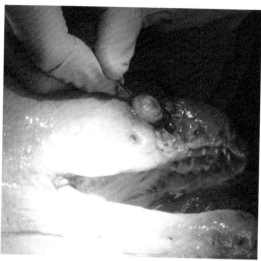

Fig. 17. Ocular trauma in a green moray eel. Ocular trauma is common in captive fish and frequently requires enucleation.

fish should be placed in lateral recumbency with the surgical eye exposed to the surgeon. The surgical eye can be prepped by irrigating the eye and swabbing the periocular tissues using dilute povidone-iodine (1:10 dilution with water). Using a dorsal approach, a small pair of scissors can be used to incise around the circumorbital sulcus and the globe bluntly dissected from the orbit. Ocular muscles are transected and blunt dissection is continued. Hemostasis can be maintained by applying direct pressure using sterile swabs and Gelfoam (Pharmacia and Upjohn Co. Kalamazoo, MI, USA). A small amount of phenylephrine hydrochloride (2.5%) can be used to vasoconstrict orbital vessels if there is excessive hemorrhage.[31] Bipolar electrocautery may be useful during this phase as well, but extreme care must be taken so as not to damage adjacent tissues. Once the optic nerve and adjacent connective tissue are visible, these tissues and remaining connective tissue can be transected and the globe removed as well as remaining conjunctivae, fat, and extraocular muscle tissues. The orbital and facial bones are fragile, so a gentle surgical technique is imperative. If a prosthetic implant is considered, it is useful to leave the periorbital skin intact, which facilitates holding the prosthesis in place.[31] Stainless steel sutures and polyvinyl siloxane can be used to hold the prosthetic eye in place.[31] If a prosthesis is not used, the orbital sulcus can be left open to heal by second intention; antimicrobial therapy should be considered. Parenteral, immersive baths or oral antibiotics can be administered to prevent secondary infection of the sulcus, and/or water quality can be altered by increasing salinity in freshwater fish species or by decreasing salinity in saltwater fish species.

Reproductive Surgery

Elective gonadectomies are rarely performed in clinical practice, but ovariectomies may be necessary in cases of egg-bound female fish or for population control in larger aquaria or pond situations. Gonadectomies may also be performed in research settings, especially in the disciplines of endocrinology, reproductive physiology, behavioral endocrinology, and clinical analgesia.[5,9,27] In most teleost species, once anesthetized, the fish is placed in dorsal recumbency and a ventral midline incision performed. Due to the large size/length of fish gonads, in particular the ovaries, the incision is started at the level of the pectoral fins, cranially, and extended caudally to just cranial to the anus. This allows visualization of the blood vessels supplying the gonads and allows manipulation and exteriorization of the gonads (**Figs. 18** and **19**). In some species, the normal ovarian mass is friable and begins to fall apart because it is manually exteriorized from the coelom. Be careful not to leave ovarian material in the coelomic cavity, because it may be a persistent inflammatory nidus much like yolk coelomitis in birds and reptiles. Flush the coelomic cavity well with sterile saline if ovarian material fractures and falls back into the coelom. Suction is useful in helping to remove the saline and ovarian material. Blood vessels supplying the gonads are located toward the cranial aspect of each gonad, and either Hemoclips or monofilament absorbable suture ligatures can be used to ligate these vessels. Once the gonads are excised, the coelomic membrane, muscle, and skin can be closed in either 1 or 2 layers depending on the species and size of fish. When using a 2-layer closure, an absorbable monofilament suture material can be used in a simple continuous pattern. The skin can be closed using an absorbable monofilament suture material with a continuous Ford interlocking, cruciate, or horizontal mattress suture pattern. Once closed, silver sulfadiazine cream or an iodine-based ointment (eg, Betadine ointment [Mundipharma GmbH, Limburg/Lahn, Germany]) can be applied to cover the suture line (**Fig. 20**). This may reduce the likelihood of postsurgical infections by aquatic microorganisms.

Reproductive success of elasmobranchs in captivity has greatly increased over the years, which has led to new methods for contraception but also contributed to reproductive associated lesions that require surgical intervention. Aquariums and zoos commonly use populations of same-sex ratios as a form of contraception, with the female gender typically chosen for display. This is especially true for batoid species, such as the southern stingray (*Dasyatis americana*), a popular species exhibited throughout aquarium facilities. In the wild, these animals are continuously gravid. When maintained in same-sex captive populations, however, the lack of pregnancy and natural inhibitory processes associated with reproduction can cause excessive follicular production, which can progress into endometritis, placentitis, coelomitis, secondary bacterial infections, neoplastic diseases, and, ultimately, high mortality. Prevention of these deleterious consequences of captive population manipulation is a priority of facilities maintaining this species. Surgical ovarioectomies have been pioneered at several aquariums as possible options for this problem. Initially, surgical

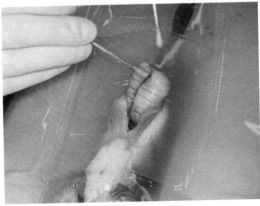

Fig. 18. Female koi with ovaries exposed during an ovariectomy procedure.

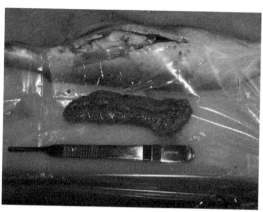

Fig. 19. Female koi postovariectomy showing the normal, excised left ovarian mass.

candidates must be chosen wisely to provide the best outcome. Animals with a disc diameter range of 50 to 60 cm seem to have the best surgical outcomes, because the internal organs are large enough to identify, but the animal is not too large, which can make surgery too cumbersome. Once fully anesthetized, the ray is placed in ventral recumbency. A drape or rolled up towel can be placed between the cranial and caudal half of the animal to prevent excess water from entering the surgical site. The left paralumbar region is surgically prepped, and a clear adhesive surgical drape is applied over the planned incision site. The initial incision is made parallel to the spinal column, approximately 2 cm lateral to the dorsal lumbar muscles (**Fig. 21**). The elasmobranch's skin is thick and durable. Purposeful forceful motions are needed to penetrate the skin along with an appropriately sized, durable scalpel blade. Once the skin is incised, the coleomic membrane is then elevated and incised for viewing of the coelomic organs (**Fig. 22**). The ovary and cranial portion of the oviduct is visualized and bluntly dissected from the surrounding tissues (**Fig. 23**). The ovarian vessels are identified, clamped using forceps, and ligated with Hemoclips or an encircling suture ligature of appropriate size. The parallel running suspensory ligament is identified and

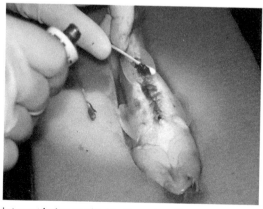

Fig. 20. Betadine ointment being applied to the suture line postovariectomy to attempt secondary microorganism infection into the suture line.

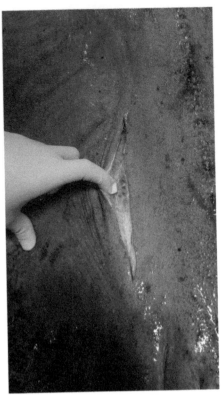

Fig. 21. Female southern stingray in ventral recumbency showing a dorsal approach to an ovariectomy with the incision made parallel to the vertebral column, approximately 2 cm lateral to the dorsal lumbar muscles.

transected. Hemostasis of the ligament is achieved by clamping the tissue with a pair of hemostats. The caudal pole of the ovary is connected to the epigonal gland. With blunt dissection, the ovary can be separated from the epigonal gland and fully excised. Typically, there is minimal hemorrhage. The coelomic cavity should then be thoroughly evaluated for any excess hemorrhage. The peritoneum can be closed with 3.0 poly-dioxanone or polyglyconate using a simple interrupted suture pattern. The muscle and integument layers are closed, using methods previously described. Recovery is typically rapid in this species, with animals interested in food within a few hours after the procedure.

Cesarean Section in Elasmobranchs

Other elasmobranch reproductive diseases in which surgical intervention may be required include dystocias and extended parturition and/or uterine inertia. These reproductive issues are documented in the cownose ray (*Rhinoptera bonasus*).[19,32] A full diagnostic work-up of the animal should precede any surgical procedures, which typically includes hematology and serum biochemical profile, ultrasononic evaluation, and estimation of gestation length from time of copulation, if known. Cownose sting-rays are viviparous, delivering young in a breach position with the tail first, curled over the head, presumably so as not to injure the dam on parturition.[33] In circumstances in which the fetal head is facing the opposite direction on parturition, or if uterine inertia

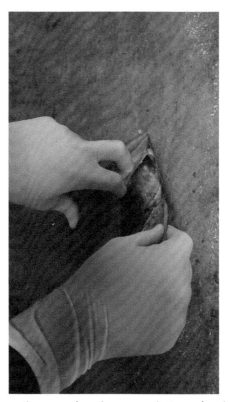

Fig. 22. Female southern stingray undergoing an ovariectomy showing the coelomic membrane and coelom through the incision.

has been diagnosed, a cesarean section may be warranted. As with any species, it is important to know normal anatomy and reproductive activity. In the case of the cownose stingrays, the left ovary is active, but this can vary by species.[33] A cesarean section approach can be performed in a fashion similar to ovarioectomy in southern stingrays, described previously.[17] The animal is placed in ventral recumbency. A longitudinal incision is made parallel to the spinal column approximately 2 cm lateral to the dorsal lumbar muscles (**Fig. 24**). The coelomic membrane is incised and the uterus visualized. On incising the uterus, the embryonic nutritional histotroph should not be allowed to spill into the coelomic cavity, which may lead to secondary coelomitis. The viability of the fetus can be determined prior to surgery using ultrasound. The fetuses can be removed from the uterus using gentle traction. When closing the uterus, similar techniques to those used in terrestrial animals can be applied: continuous inverting suture patterns (eg, Cushing-Connell) in 2 layers using a monofilament absorbable suture material. The muscular layer and integument can be closed as in teleost species, using a monofilament absorbable or nonabsorbable suture material in a continuous or interrupted Ford interlocking, horizontal mattress, or simple pattern.

Organ Prolapse Repair

Anal/cloacal prolapse, intestinal prolapse through the anus, and ovarian prolapse through the genital pore and anus have been described.[9,34] There are cases of gastric prolapse through gill slits in sand tiger sharks (**Fig. 25**).[34] In all cases, an attempt to

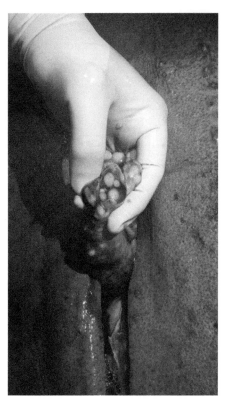

Fig. 23. Female southern stingray undergoing an ovariectomy with ovary exposed in the surgical site.

replace the organs was attempted with varying results. With anal/cloacal prolapse, a suture technique in which 2 to 3 simple interrupted sutures are placed longitudinally across the anus/cloaca can be useful. Nonabsorbable suture material and stainless steel sutures are the best choices. Stainless steel sutures can remain in place for weeks to months if necessary. Cases of gastric prolapse through the gill slits in elasmobranchs should be considered a medical emergency and an urgent response is required, because the gastrointestinal tissue rapidly becomes entrapped within the gill slits and vascular supply is quickly compromised. Swelling and ischemic necrosis of both

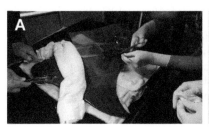
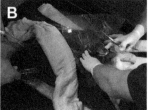

Fig. 24. Female cownose ray undergoing cesarean section. (*A*) The dorsal incision is made, just lateral to the vertebral column. (*B*) Once the uterus is incised, the baby stingrays can be manually extracted. (*Courtesy of* RH George, DVM, Ripley's Aquariums Incorporated, Orlando, FL, USA.)

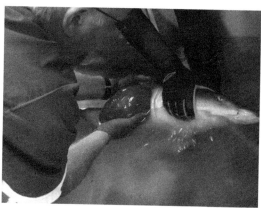

Fig. 25. Gastric prolapse through the gill slits in a sand tiger shark.

the gills and surrounding gastrointestinal tissue are common sequelae, ultimately leading to the death of the animal.[34] Manual manipulation and application of force to reduce the gastrointestinal tissue back through the gill slits, from both the oral cavity and operculum of the animal, may be successful in correcting the prolapse, if performed early in the disease process. Anecdotally, the application of topical dextrose, table sugar, or other osmotic substances to the prolapsed tissues may facilitate reducing tissue swelling for easier manipulation. In extreme cases, in which the actions discussed previously are unsuccessful, the prolapsed stomach can be incised to make 2 halves, which allows for the manipulation of the 2 stomach halves to be placed back into the oropharyngeal cavity. Simultaneously, a midline ventral laparotomy is performed, and the previously prolapsed gastrointestinal tissue is visualized within the coelomic cavity and inverted back to its normal position, and incised tissues are sutured using an inverted Cushing-Connell suture pattern. The muscular and integumentary layers are closed, as described previously (Clarke, personal observation, 2009).

Radiotransmitter Implantation

Surgical radiotransmitter placement is common in fish and is typically used in research on threatened or endangered species or, more recently, for assessing movement, migration, body temperature, and other physiologic or behavior parameters.[11] A simple rule of thumb is that transmitters should weigh less than 2% of the fish's body weight. To place a transmitter intracoelomically in fish, a ventral midline incision is made with the diameter of the transmitter in mind. The skin and coelomic membrane should be incised until there is a clear view within the coelomic cavity. A circumferential suture loop is made around the midpoint of the sterilized transmitter body and tied in place while maintaining the remaining suture material and needle intact. The transmitter is inserted through the incision and into the coelomic cavity. It is the authors' preference to place stay sutures into the inside of the body wall to prevent the transmitter from migrating. This is especially important for future retrieval operations. The antenna can be placed subcutaneously by first passing a small-diameter, plastic pipette from the incision site, cranially. The antenna can be threaded through the pipette in a cranial direction. A scalpel blade can be used to cut over the cranial end of the plastic pipette so that the pipette can be removed from the subcutaneous space, leaving the antenna to reside completely within the subcutaneous space. If the pipette diameter is small enough, either a single, simple interrupted suture can be used to close the small pipette exit wound or the wound can be left open to heal by second intention. There are no systematically derived data characterizing long-term negative sequlae associated with transmitter placement in fish.

Endoscopic Procedures

Although endoscopy has become more commonplace as a fish diagnostic tool, particularly for collecting tissue samples or determining gender of fish, endoscopic surgery is not discussed in the published literature.[35] There are a few published descriptions of endoscopic liver biopsies in sturgeon,[36] endoscopic gender determination in sturgeon,[37] endoscopic gastric biopsy techniques in a green moray eel,[38] and endoscopic procedures in sharks.[18] As endoscopic surgery becomes more routine in mammals, birds, and reptiles, fish endoscopic surgical procedures are likely to become more prominent in the clinical and scientific literature.

SUMMARY

Fish surgical procedures are becoming more commonplace in clinical veterinary medicine and research, especially with the advent of more reliable fish anesthetic protocols and a greater demand for performing surgical procedures on valuable individuals in aquaria and zoos, in pet fish, and in the show circuit. Current understanding of pain and analgesia in fish supersedes most other nonmammalian phyla, yet surgical techniques in fish are not well described. Perhaps the traditional rush to euthanize fish with medical problems is waning, as veterinarians increasingly pursue antemortem diagnostic and treatment techniques. The authors are encouraged by this trend and hope that the surgical techniques outlined in this article persuade more veterinary clinicians to take the plunge into aquatic medicine and make fish surgery a routine part of clinical practice.

REFERENCES

1. Harms CA. Anesthesia in fish. In: Fowler ME, Miller RE, editors. Zoo and wild animal medicine; current therapy 4. Philadelphia: WB Saunders; 1999. p. 158–63.
2. Neiffer DL, Stamper MA. Fish sedation, analgesia, anesthesia, and euthanasia: considerations, methods, and types of drugs. ILAR J 2009;50:343–60.
3. Lewbart GA, Harms CA. Building a fish anesthesia delivery system. Exotic DVM 1999;1:25–8.
4. Sladky KK, Swanson CR, Stoskopf MK, et al. Comparative efficacy of MS-222 (tricaine methanesulfonate) and clove oil (eugenol) in red pacu (*Piaractus brachypomus*). Am J Vet Res 2001;62(3):337–42.
5. Baker T, Baker B, Johnson SM, et al. Comparative analgesic efficacy of morphine and butorphanol in koi (*Cyprinus carpio*) undergoing gonadectomy. J Am Vet Med Assoc 2013;243:882–90.
6. Harms CA, Lewbart GA, Swanson CR, et al. Behavioral and clinical pathology changes in koi carp (Cyprinus carpio) subjected to anesthesia and surgery with and without intra-operative analgesics. Comp Med 2005;55:221–6.
7. Harms CA, Lewbart GA, McAlarney R, et al. Surgical excision of mycotic (*Cladosporium* sp.) granulomas from the mantle of a cuttlefish (*Sepia officinalis*). J Zoo Wildl Med 2006;37:524–30.
8. Nordgreen J, Kolsrud HH, Ranheim B, et al. Pharmacokinetics of morphine after intramuscular injection in common goldfish *Carassius auratus* and Atlantic salmon *Salmo salar*. Dis Aquat Organ 2009;88:55–63.

9. Harms CA, Lewbart GA. Surgery in fish. Vet Clin North Am Exot Anim Pract 2000; 3:759–74.

10. Hurty CA, Brazik DC, Law JM, et al. Evaluation of the tissue reactions in the skin and body wall of koi (*Cyprinus carpio*) to five suture materials. Vet Rec 2002;151: 324–8.

11. Brown RS, Cooke SJ, Wagner GN, et al. Methods for surgical implantation of the acoustic transmitters in juvenile salmonids. Oak Ridge (TN): United States Department of Energy; 2010.

12. Harms CA, Bakal RS, Khoo LH, et al. Microsurgical exicision of an abdominal mass in a gourami. J Am Vet Med Assoc 1995;207:1215–7.

13. Lecu A, Herbert R, Coulier L, et al. Removal of an intracoelomic hook via laparotomy in a Sandbar Shark (*Carcharhinus plumbeus*). J Zoo Wildl Med 2011;42: 256–62.

14. Lloyd R, Lloyd C. Surgical removal of a gastric foreign body in a sand tiger shark, *Carcharias taurus* Rafinesque. J Fish Dis 2011;34:951–3.

15. Lloyd R, Sham N. Surgical repair of mandibular symphyseal fractures in three Silver Arowana (*Osteoglossum bicirrhosum*) using interfragmentary wire. J Zoo Wildl Med 2014;45:926–30.

16. Borucinska J, Martin J, Skomal G. Peritonitis and pericarditis associated with gastric perforation by a retained fishing hook in a Blue Shark. J Aquat Anim Health 2001;13:347–54.

17. George RH, Steeil J, Baine K. Ovariectomy of sub-adult Southern stingrays (Dasyatis americana) to prevent future reproductive problems. In: proceedings of the International Association of Aquatic Animal Medicine. Sausalito, CA, April 21 - 26, 2013. p. 270–1.

18. Murray MJ. Endoscopy in sharks. Vet Clin North Am Exot Anim Pract 2010;13: 301–13.

19. Smith M, Warmoults D, Thoney D, et al. Elasmobranch husbandry manual: captive care of sharks, rays and their relatives. Columbus (OH): Ohio Biological Survey; 2004.

20. Gurshin CW, Szedlmayer ST. Short-term survival and movements of Atlantic sharpnose sharks captured by hook-and-line in the north-east Gulf of Mexico. J Fish Biol 2004;65:973–86.

21. Harms CA. Fish. In: Fowler ME, Miller RE, editors. Zoo and wild animal medicine. 5th edition. Philadelphia: Saunders; 2003. p. 2–20.

22. Boylan SM, Camus A, Waltzek T, et al. Liquid nitrogen cryotherapy for fibromas in tarpon, *Megalops atlanticus*, Valenciennes 1847, and neoplasia in lined sea horse, *Hippocampus erectus*, Perry 1810. J Fish Dis 2015;38:681–5.

23. Groff JM. Neoplasia in fishes. Vet Clin North Am Exot Anim Pract 2004;7:705–56.

24. Lewbart GA, Stone EA, Love NE. Pneumocystectomy in a Midas cichlid. J Am Vet Med Assoc 1995;207:319–21.

25. Chansue N, Monanunsap S. The man-made cause of death in whale shark due to foreign body in the stomach. In: Proceedings of AZWMP, Chulalong-korn UniFac. of Vet. Sci. p. 55.

26. Wilde GR, Sawynok W. Effect of hook removal on recapture rates of 27 species of angler-caught fish in Australia. Trans Am Fish Soc 2009;138:692–7.

27. Murray MJ. Fish surgery. Seminars in Avian and Exotic Pet Medicine 2002;4: 246–57.

28. Bakal RS, Hickson BH, Gilger BC, et al. Surgical removal of cataracts due to *Diplostomum* species in Gulf Sturgeon (*Acipenser oxyrinchus desotoi*). J Zoo Wildl Med 2005;36:504–8.

29. Clode AB, Harms C, Fatzinger MH, et al. Identification and management of ocular lipid deposition in association with hyperlipidaemia in captive moray eels, *Gymnothorax funebris* Ranzani, *Gymnothorax moringa* (Cuvier) and *Muraena retifera* Goode and Bean. J Fish Dis 2012;35:683–93.

30. Deters KA, Brown RS, Boyd JW, et al. Optimal suturing technique and number of sutures for surgical implantation of acoustic transmitters in juvenile salmonids. Trans Am Fish Soc 2012;141:1–10.

31. Nadelstein B, Bakal R, Lewbart GA. Orbital exenteration and placement of a prosthesis in fish. J Am Vet Med Assoc 1997;211:603–6.

32. Hamlett WC, Hysell M. Uterine Specializations in elasmobranchs. J Exp Zool 1998;282:438–59.

33. Neer JA, Thompson BA. Life history of the cownose ray, Rhinoptera bonasus, in the northern Gulf of Mexico, with comments on geographic variability in life history traits. Environ Biol Fishes 2005;73:321–31.

34. Tuttle AD, Burrus O, Burkart MA, et al. Three cases of gastric prolapse through the gill slit in sand tiger sharks, *Carcharhinus taurus* (Rafinesque). J Fish Dis 2008;4:311–5.

35. Divers SJ, Boone SS, Hoover JJ, et al. Field endoscopy for identifying gender, reproductive stage and gonadal anomalies in free-ranging sturgeon (*Scaphirhynchus*) from the lower Mississippi River. J Appl Ichthyol 2009;25(Suppl 2):68–74.

36. Divers SJ, Boone SS, Berliner A, et al. Nonlethal acquisition of large liver samples from free-ranging river sturgeon (*Scaphirhynchus*) using single-entry endoscopic biopsy forceps. J Wildl Dis 2013;49:321–31.

37. Hernandez-Divers SJ, Bakal RS, Hickson BR, et al. Endoscopic sex determination and gonadal manipulation in the Gulf of Mexico Sturgeon (*Acipenser oxyrinchus desotoi*). J Zoo Wildl Med 2004;35:459–70.

38. Meegan J, Sidor IF, Field C, et al. Endoscopic evaluation and biopsy collection of the gastrointestinal tract in the green moray eel (*Gymnothorax funebris*): application in a case of chronic regurgitation with gastric mucus gland hyperplasia. J Zoo Wildl Med 2012;43:615–20.

Surgery in Amphibians

Norin Chai, DVM, MSc, PhD, DECZM (ZHM)

KEYWORDS

- Amphibians • Surgery • Anesthesia • Analgesia • Skin surgery • Celiotomy
- Gastrotomy • Cystotomy

KEY POINTS

- Most surgical procedures described in reptiles (especially lizards) can be undertaken in most amphibians.
- A major concern of the surgery in an amphibian is to provide adequate anesthesia and analgesia.
- For any surgical procedures, it is necessary to be familiar with the anatomic and behavioral differences between amphibian species commonly kept in captivity.
- In all cases, the skin of patients must always be kept moist with dechlorinated water.
- Surgical celiotomy provides access to most of the major internal organs, and therefore is useful for a range of surgical procedures including exploration and biopsy.

INTRODUCTION

Although concentrated in the neotropical countries, amphibians are globally distributed except in the polar regions of Antarctica. They display a diversity of life history and reproductive strategies to suit almost all habitats, from rain forests to deserts. New species continue to be discovered. There are 3 orders of amphibians: Anura, Caudata, and Gymnophiona. The AmphibiaWeb database currently contains 7416 amphibian species (May 22, 2015).[1] Only amphibian species commonly maintained in captivity are discussed here; therefore, caecilians have been excluded. Clinicians should not hesitate to advocate a surgical manipulation of amphibian patients. They heal well, tolerate blood loss, and tend to have fewer postsurgical complications than do higher vertebrates. Early amphibian surgical reference goes back almost 70 years, mostly developed in research.[2] Since then, surgery in amphibian research has progressed to amazing procedures like facial transplantation in *Xenopus laevis* embryos or to participate in conservation like, for instance, implantation of radiotransmitter.[3,4] Over the past 2 decades, veterinarians have gained experience thanks in large part to the pioneering work of G.J. Crawshaw, F.L. Frye, B.R. Whitaker, D.L. Williams, and

The author has nothing to disclose.
Ménagerie du Jardin des Plantes, Muséum national d'Histoire Naturelle, 57 Rue Cuvier, Paris 75005, France
E-mail address: chai@mnhn.fr

Vet Clin Exot Anim 19 (2016) 77–95
http://dx.doi.org/10.1016/j.cvex.2015.08.004
1094-9194/16/$ – see front matter © 2016 Elsevier Inc. All rights reserved.

K.M. Wright.[5–8] Most clinicians who wrote much of the earliest veterinary work published with emphasis on clinical cases.[9–15] This overview provides the practitioner with some pragmatic advice on how to conduct routine and advanced surgery in amphibians.

INDICATIONS AND CONTRAINDICATIONS

Commonly performed surgical procedures include wound debridement and repair, skin biopsy, abscess/neoplasm/parasite removal, and prolapse replacement/repair. Celiotomy is indicated for laparotomy exploration, laparoscopy, gastrotomy, cystotomy, and reproductive surgery. Orthopedic surgery mainly includes digit and legs amputation. Ophthalmologic surgeries include eye enucleation and lens surgery.

Contraindications are mainly related to the anesthetic risks. Practical recommendations for amphibian surgery should follow the edict primum non nocere (first do no harm).

EQUIPMENT

Clear plastic drapes are generally advocated for amphibian surgery. They tend to isolate the surgical site for aseptic procedures and help to keep the surrounding skin moist by reducing evaporation. One may use a combination of cold steel, radiosurgery, or diode laser. Skin incisions in amphibian patients are best made with a number 15 or 11 scalpel blade.[16] The diode laser has been used infrequently in amphibians to remove cutaneous lesions and neoplasms. But subjective assessments indicated that postoperative skin infections were reduced compared with either radiosurgery or sharp excision.[17] Hemostasis during procedures with limited expected hemorrhage may be achieved by electrocautery or diode laser. To allow the surgeon to apply localized pressure to a small vessel and keep track of blood loss, cotton-tipped spears or applicators are less traumatic and more manageable in small confined spaces than standard gauze squares. Most amphibian patients are less than 1 kg. Microsurgical instruments, like ophthalmologic instruments, with fine, small tips, are preferred. Plastic, self-retaining retractors (eg, Lone Star retractor [CooperSurgical, Inc., CT, USA]) can be adjusted to fit different sizes of incisions. Eyelid retractors can be useful for retracting coelomic incisions. Some form of magnification may be necessary, particularly with smaller patients. Between mammals and amphibians, the absorbability and reactivity of many suture materials is not the same. X laevis has been used as a model to investigate the gross and histologic tissue reactions to 5 commonly used suture materials: 3 to 0 silk, monofilament nylon, polydioxanone, polyglactin 910, and chromic gut. Monofilament nylon elicited the least histologic reaction and, therefore, seems to be the most appropriate choice for use in amphibian skin.[18] Alternatively, it is possible to use cyanoacrylate tissue adhesives for skin closure or over sutured incisions to ensure a waterproof barrier and to prevent bacterial colonization. Absorbable sutures, such as polyglactin (Vicryl, Ethicon, Somerville, NJ) and polydioxanone (PDS, Ethicon), are appropriate for internal use including muscle.[16] Taper needles are preferable to cutting needles, and it is usually possible to remove skin sutures after 14 days.[19] Insufflation is needed in laparoscopy to improve the visibility of all organs. A simple syringe for air is practical for a simple endoscopic examination. But a carbon dioxide (CO_2) insufflator with silicone tubing is needed for endoscopic surgery. In the author's experience, the endoscopic procedure should not last more than 10 minutes. Despite the variation in size and the nature of the procedures that may be performed, the basic endoscope system consist of a 2.7-mm diameter, 18-cm length, 30° oblique rigid telescope with a 4.8-mm operating sheath, an endoscopic video camera with a monitor, a xenon light source and light cable, a 1-mm or 1.7-mm endoscopic biopsy forceps, and grasping forceps. Throughout the surgical procedure, the skin of the patients must be kept moist with dechlorinated water. A variety of devices, including syringes and intravenous bags may be used.

PATIENT PREPARATION

Amphibian patients should be handled with care, and wrapping with a wet paper towel is a good technique to restrain an animal for a quick examination or for medication administration. Wearing moistened, powder-free gloves prevents the transfer of microorganisms or chemicals from the handler as well as protection against secreted toxins. Presurgical preparations include hydration of the animal in a shallow dechlorinated water bath. Adequate presurgical hydration is essential for a successful surgical outcome; therefore, soaking amphibian patients in water for 1 hour before surgery is recommended.[7,8] Amphibians do not require fasting before anesthesia. Their larynx remains tightly closed even under general anesthesia, and the chance of aspiration is very low.[7] However, fasting large frogs and toads for 24 to 48 hours before anesthesia will assist visualization during coelomic surgery and ensures there is no gastrointestinal disruption (ileus) associated with anesthesia and decreased metabolic processes.

ANALGESIA, ANESTHESIA, PRESURGICAL PREPARATION

Frogs likely have both rapid and well-localized pain perception as well as perception of diffuse and chronic pain.[20] The author suggest that analgesia is required with any surgical procedure in amphibians, which would be deemed painful in other animals. Failure to administer adequate analgesia during surgery has been associated with delayed return of normal functions.[21] Moreover, analgesia potentates the effects of anesthetic drugs.[21] Although amphibians have kappa, mu, and delta opioid receptors, amphibian receptors are less selective than mammalian opioid receptors. In addition, amphibians require higher doses of opioids than do mammals, and opioids are longer acting in amphibians.[22] For the author, the drug of choice for sedation or anesthesia is tricaine methanesulfonate (MS-222; **Fig. 1**A–C). However, one should keep in mind that MS-222 has not been proven to be analgesic in amphibians. **Table 1** presents protocols that have been used and evaluated by the author and additional options recently published. Other doses may be found elsewhere.[23] Small amphibians are intubated with red rubber catheters (**Fig. 1**D) or uncuffed tubes (**Fig. 1**E). A classic cuffed endotracheal tube can also be used but without inflating the cuff (**Fig. 1**F). A low flow of oxygen (the author uses 0.5–0.75 L/min) may then be provided (with or without 0.5%–1.0% isoflurane; see **Fig. 1**F).

Once the amphibian has been adequately anesthetized, it may be placed in a suitable support structure for the procedure. Any material that contacts the animal's skin must be moistened before. It may be helpful to cover the amphibian's eyes as an aid to the anesthetic effects. Although there should be some form of presurgical preparation of the entry site, it should minimally disrupt the protective functions of the skin and mucus layer. The surgical field is aseptically prepared by gently wiping the surgical site with sterile cotton-tipped applicators soaked in povidone-iodine solution diluted (1:10) in sterile saline.[24] An alternative is to place a moist sterile gauze with the diluted povidone-iodine solution, for 10 to 15 seconds (**Fig. 2**A). It is also possible to apply sterile gauze soaked in 0.75% chlorhexidine solution to the surgical site for at least 10 minutes before surgery (**Fig. 2**B).[16]

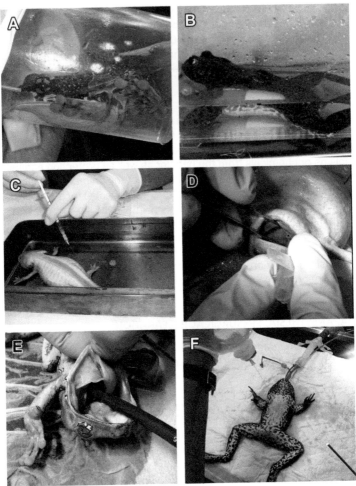

Fig. 1. Amphibian anesthesia and intubation. Anesthesia by bath with MS-222 of (*A*) a milk frog (*Trachycephalus resinifictrix*), (*B*) a bullfrog (*Lithobates catesbeianus*), and (*C*) an axolotl (*Ambystoma mexicanum*). The concentration of the anesthetic gradually increased. (*D*) Intubation of an African clawed frog (*Xenopus laevis*) with a red rubber catheter. (*E*) Intubation of a 2-colored leaf frog (*Phyllomedusa bicolor*) with an uncuffed 4-mm diameter tube. (*F*) Intubation of a bullfrog with a classic cuffed endotracheal tube without inflating the cuff. (*Courtesy of* Norin Chai, DVM, MSc, PhD, DECZM, Paris, France.)

CONTROL OF THE ANESTHETIC DEPTH AND MONITORING

Table 2 presents several reflexes that can be used to assess the anesthetic depth: escape response, righting reflex, superficial and deep pain responses, and the palpebral reflex. Surgical anesthesia is defined as the state when all recorded reflexes absent. Observing the animal trying to walk or jump away can assess escape behavior. Placing the animal in dorsal recumbency and recording the time required to correct its position can measure the righting reflex. Pinching the skin of an amphibian can assess superficial pain. Grasping a digit can assess deep pain. One should not grasp too forceful as amphibian skin is fragile (**Fig. 3**). Touching the upper or lower eyelids with a cotton-tipped applicator assesses the palpebral reflex.

Table 1		
Protocols for anesthesia and analgesia in anurans		
Drug	**Dosage and Route**	**Comments, Reference**
Alfaxalone	5 mg/L (bath)	In a Mexican axolotl (*Ambystoma mexicanum*), there was only one case.[12]
Tricaine methanesulfonate (MS-222)	Tadpoles and aquatic frogs 0.25–0.5 g/L (bath) Adult frogs and toads 1 g/L (bath)	Buffer MS-222 solutions before use. Induction times are variable. After induction, place the frog into a shallow amount of nonanesthetic water or on a wet towel. Recovery is generally achieved 30–90 min after removal from the anesthetic.
Isoflurane	5% in oxygen (inhalation or bubbling in bath) (see **Fig. 1**) 2–3 mL/L (bath) 0.01–0.06 mL/g (topical)	Gentle stimulation encourages continued respiration. Use effective but slow induction. Isoflurane is sprayed directly into the water. Dilute it in gel form or it apply directly.
M/K/Mel/But	M 0.5 mg/kg +K 50 mg/kg +Mel 0.2 mg/kg +But 1 mg/kg (IM)	It is an effective protocol in *Xenopus laevis* for heart surgery. It is reversed with atipamezol hydrochloride at equal volume to medetomidine IM.
Dexmedetomidine	0.6 mg/kg, (IM, intracoelomic)	78% of animals showed an effect of analgesia at that dose.[23]
Butorphanol	0.5 mg/L (bath)	It is from an experimental study in an eastern red-spotted newt (*Notophthalmus viridescens*).[20]
Meloxicam	0.1–0.2 mg/kg (IM)	—

Abbreviations: But, butorphanol; IM, intramuscular; K, ketamine; M, medetomidine; Mel, meloxicam.

Recording opercular movements is probably the most important method to measure the respiratory rate. Gular, branchial, and pulmonary respiratory movements are classically described as often being absent at surgical planes of anesthesia using traditional agents.[12] Amphibians have developed a highly vascular integument that can assist with respiration. There are several different methods available for measuring an amphibian's heart rate. A 3-lead system electrocardiogram (ECG) can be used as in higher vertebrates. One should never use alligator clips directly on the skin but instead connected to hypodermic needles (25 or 26 gauge) placed through the skin (**Fig. 4**A). Doppler ultrasound probes placed on the ventral pectoral girdle or axillary region of caudates or anurans is also a good way of assessment of the heart rate (**Fig. 4**B). The use of portable ECG (AliveCor Veterinary Heart Monitor devices, Vetoquinol France, Paris, France) is less traumatic and preferred over standard ECG (**Fig. 4**C, D).

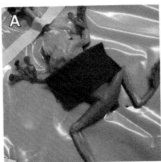 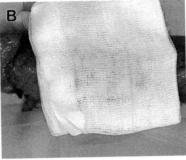

Fig. 2. Aseptically preparation of (*A*) a milk frog (*Trachycephalus resinifictrix*) with diluted povidone-iodine solution and (*B*) an axolotl (*Ambystoma mexicanum*) by the use of a sterile gauze soaked in 0.75% chlorhexidine solution. (*Courtesy of* Norin Chai, DVM, MSc, PhD, DECZM, Paris, France.)

Table 2
Reflexes that can be used to assess the anesthetic depth in amphibians

Stage	Parameter/Reflexes	Observed Effect
I: Sedation Suitable for advanced clinical examination, blood sampling	Escape behavior	Delayed
	Muscle tone	Slight decrease
	Gular movements	Slight decrease
	Cardiac rate	Normal
	Righting reflex	Delayed response
	Superficial and deep pain responses	Normal or reduced
	Palpebral reflex	Normal
II: Light anesthesia Suitable for minor invasive sampling, biopsy, noninvasive endoscopy	Escape behavior	Loss, weak response to postural changes
	Muscle tone	Decreased
	Gular movements	Normal/decreased
	Cardiac rate	Normal/decreased
	Righting reflex	Delayed, slow response/absent
	Superficial and deep pain responses	Reaction to strong stimuli present
	Palpebral reflex	Normal
III: Surgical anesthesia	Escape behavior	Absent
	Muscle tone	Very slow/absent
	Gular movements	Slow
	Cardiac rate	Absent
	Righting reflex	Total loss of reactivity
	Superficial and deep pain responses	Slow
	Palpebral reflex	
IV: Suitable for euthanasia only	Escape behavior	Absent
	Muscle tone	Absent
	Gular movements	Absent
	Cardiac rate	Cardiac arrest
	Superficial and deep pain responses	Absent
	Palpebral reflex	Absent

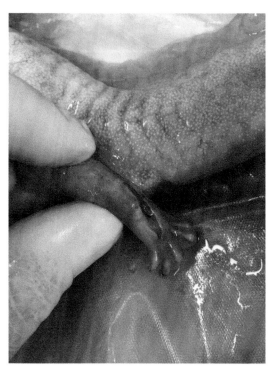

Fig. 3. Iatrogenic trauma in an axolotl (*Ambystoma mexicanum*) by pinching the hind limb for evaluating the deep pain. (*Courtesy of* Norin Chai, DVM, MSc, PhD, DECZM, Paris, France.)

A pulse oximeter with an appropriate probe (placed over a peripheral vessel) can also be used to measure the heart rate in larger amphibians. Although measuring the heart rate of an amphibian can be invaluable during an anesthetic procedure, it is important to recognize that the heart of an amphibian can beat after it is clinically dead. Because of this, it is important to recognize that heart rate should not be the only monitoring method for anesthesia in amphibians.[12]

SURGERY OF THE INTEGUMENT

In the author's experience, most of the skin amphibian surgeries involve tissue sampling and/or debulking (**Fig. 5**A, B), treatment of skin trauma (**Fig. 5**C, D), or removal of parasites (**Fig. 5**E, F) or cutaneous masses (**Fig. 5**G, H). One may use a combination of cryosurgery, radiosurgery, diode laser surgery, and scalpel blades in an attempt to perform these cutaneous surgeries.

Firm abscesses and cutaneous neoplasia should be excised with a wide margin (**Fig. 6**A–C).[8,25] Closure of these large skin defects is often impossible and can be left to close by second intention. Topical antimicrobials, such as silver sulfadiazine cream or benzalkonium chloride (Dermaflon), may be used postoperatively (**Fig. 6**D).[26] Antibiotics are warranted for large, nonhealing or infected wounds.[8]

CELIOTOMY

Surgical celiotomy provides access to most of the major internal organs and, therefore, is useful for a range of surgical procedures, including exploration and biopsy.

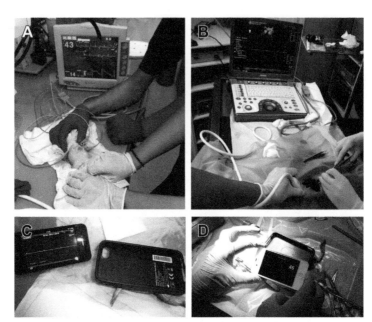

Fig. 4. Monitoring anesthesia in an African clawed frogs (*Xenopus laevis*) with (*A*) a 3-lead system ECG and (*B*) a Doppler ultrasound. (*C, D*) Monitoring of 2 amphibians with a portable ECG (AliveCor Veterinary Heart Monitor devices, Vetoquinol France, 75,009 Paris, France). (*Courtesy of* Norin Chai, DVM, MSc, PhD, DECZM, Paris, France.)

With the animal positioned in dorsal recumbency, the surgical field is aseptically prepared. Bupivacaine (2 mg/kg, use diluted 3:1 with sodium bicarbonate solution, duration 3 hours) or lidocaine (2 mg/kg, use diluted 3:1 with sodium bicarbonate solution, duration 30–60 minutes) may be swabbed onto the skin or may be infiltrated at the incision site and allowed time to absorb before surgery. For both, do not exceed 5 mg/kg total dose either topical or intraincisional.[16]

For skin incision, it is better to make one bold stroke leaving a clean incision (**Fig. 7**A). Celiotomy incisions by radiosurgery (**Fig. 7**B) or with diode laser (contact mode; see **Fig. 7**C) are essentially bloodless, but some carbonization of the wound edges may be evident.

Following the skin incision, the abdominal membrane is elevated, incised, and carefully dissected. Care must be taken to avoid puncturing the lungs (**Fig. 8**A), the gastrointestinal tract, or a distended bladder and not to damage the macroscopic glands, lymph hearts, and blood vessels, especially the midventral vein (**Fig. 8**B). Depending on the season, the presence of large fat bodies (**Fig. 8**C) and ovaries can make visualization of other organs difficult. Eyelid retractors can be useful for retracting coelomic incisions (**Fig. 8**D). The visceral organs of most reptiles are more delicate and friable than their mammalian counterparts. In all cases, one will take care to prevent dehydration of all exteriorized organs and the skin during the procedures. Celiotomy incisions are closed in 2 layers, with a simple continuous pattern for the coelomic membrane with muscle and with an interrupted, everting suture pattern for the skin.

GASTROTOMY, ENTEROTOMY, AND CYSTOTOMY

In all cases, noninvasive methods should be attempted first (**Fig. 9**). The stomach and the bladder should be stabilized with encircling ligatures before incision.

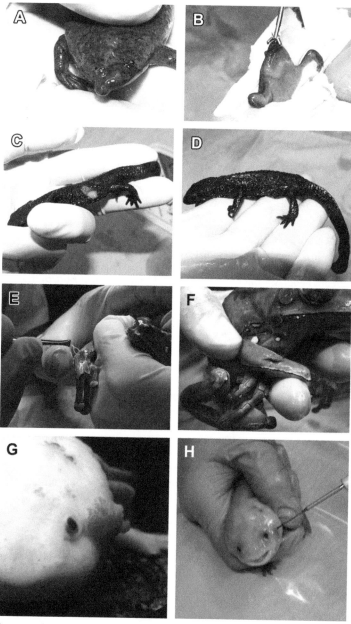

Fig. 5. Skin surgeries in amphibians. (*A*, *B*) Use of 1.7-mm endoscopic biopsy forceps for debulking surgery in an African clawed frog (*Xenopus laevis*). (*C*, *D*) Skin trauma in a ribbed newt (*Pleurodeles waltl*) treated with a single everting suture. (*E*, *F*) Removal a subcutaneous parasite in a 2-colored leaf frog (*Phyllomedusa bicolor*). An incision is made near each worm. The parasites are removed gently with ophthalmic hemostats. The skin is closed with a single everting suture. (*G*, *H*) Removal of a pedunculated lobular capillary hemangioma by radiosurgery in an axolotl (*Ambystoma mexicanum*). (*Courtesy of* Norin Chai, DVM, MSc, PhD, DECZM, Paris, France.)

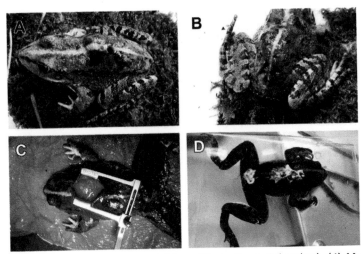

Fig. 6. Fibroma in a Riobamba marsupial frog (*Gastrotheca riobambae*). (*A*) Macroscopic appearance of the lesion. (*B*) The frog also had skin ulcers, indicating a secondary infection. (*C*) The cutaneous neoplasm was excised with a wide margin. (*D*) Closure of the crested large skin defects was impossible and, therefore, left open to allow for second-intension healing. Topical antimicrobials were used postoperatively. (*Courtesy of* Norin Chai, DVM, MSc, PhD, DECZM, Paris, France.)

When performing a gastrotomy and enterotomy, the coelom should be packed with moist gauze to avoid or minimize contamination the coelomic cavity with spilled digestive and bladder contents. As suggested in small animal medicine, 2-layer closures would be ideal for the gastrointestinal tract and urinary bladder. But except in larger amphibians specimens, in most cases, single-layer closure may be adequate. In captive waxy monkey frogs (*Phyllomedusa sauvagii*), the bladder wall was closed using 5 to 0 PDS in a simple continuous pattern.[15] Surgical cystotomy represents a viable, short-term treatment strategy for cystic urolithiasis.[15] After gastrotomy, it is recommended to withhold feeding for 1 week and to offer only small meals for the next month.

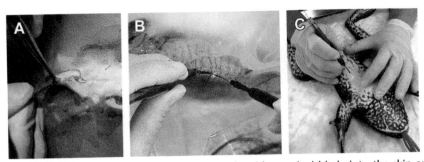

Fig. 7. Celiotomy in amphibians. (*A*) Incision made with a scalpel blade into the skin and body wall in an African clawed frog (*Xenopus laevis*). (*B*) Radiosurgery used for incision in an axolotl (*Ambystoma mexicanum*). (*C*) Diode laser used for incision in a bullfrog (*Lithobates catesbeianus*). (*Courtesy of* Norin Chai, DVM, MSc, PhD, DECZM, Paris, France.)

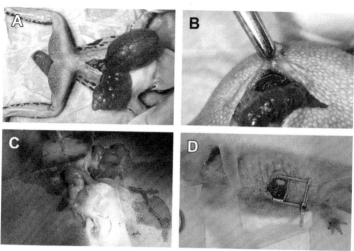

Fig. 8. Celiotomy in amphibians. Care must be taken to avoid puncturing the voluminous and fragile lungs (*A*) and the midventral vein (*B*) of this milk frog (*Trachycephalus resinifictrix*). (*C*) Large fat bodies make sometime visualization of other organs difficult (African clawed frog [*Xenopus laevis*]). (*D*) Eyelid retractors can be useful for retracting coelomic incisions, here (axolotl [*Ambystoma mexicanum*]). (*Courtesy of* Norin Chai, DVM, MSc, PhD, DECZM, Paris, France.)

REPRODUCTIVE SURGERY

Ovariectomy is a common method used in various frog species for obtaining oocytes for embryologic studies. Testicular biopsy is also a commonly used method in embryologic and reproductive studies.[8] In the author's experience, gonadectomy may also be indicated for population control and medical issue (eg, egg retention).

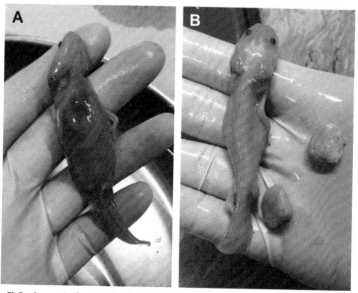

Fig. 9. (*A*, *B*) Endoscopic foreign bodies in an axolotl (*Ambystoma mexicanum*). (*Courtesy of* Norin Chai, DVM, MSc, PhD, DECZM, Paris, France.)

In some research protocols, only a portion of egg mass is needed. It is possible to excise this portion from a donor animal without ligating any blood vessels (**Fig. 10**A, B). Complete ovariectomy (**Fig. 10**C, D) and gonadectomy (**Fig. 10**E, F) require the control of hemostasis of the surrounding blood vessels. Ligation or small surgical clips work well for this purpose.[8] The author prefers the use of electrocautery (see **Fig.10** E) or diode laser (see **Fig. 10**F).

CLOACAL PROLAPSE

Cloacal prolapse (**Fig. 11**A, B) can involve various tissues and often occurs secondary to an underlying disease.[25] It is often not possible to replace such a prolapse without

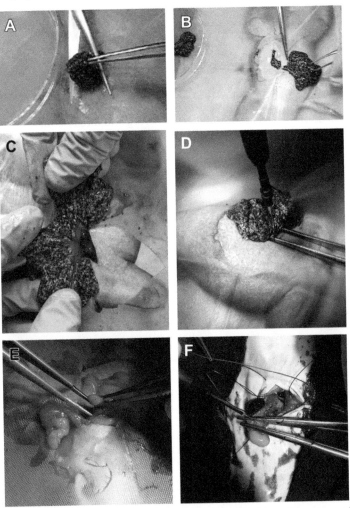

Fig. 10. Ovariectomy and orchiectomy in amphibians. (*A, B*) Excision of a portion of egg mass (for some research purposes) without ligating any blood vessels from an African clawed frog (*Xenopus laevis*). (*C, D*) Complete ovariectomy using electrosurgery in an African clawed frog. (*E*) Orchiectomy using bipolar cauterization in an African clawed frog. (*F*) Orchiectomy using a diode laser in a bullfrog (*Lithobates catesbeianus*). (*Courtesy of* Norin Chai, DVM, MSc, PhD, DECZM, Paris, France.)

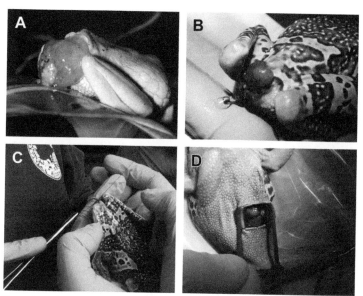

Fig. 11. Cloacal prolapse in (*A*) a Suriname golden-eyed treefrog (*Phrynohyas coriacea*), involving the cloacal membrane and, in (*B*) a milk frog (*Trachycephalus resinifictrix*), involving the reproductive and digestive tracts. (*C*) Pericloacal purse-string suture in a milk frog. (*D*) Colonopexy on a milk frog. The colon is sutured to the peritoneum. (*Courtesy of* Norin Chai, DVM, MSc, PhD, DECZM, Paris, France.)

first shrinking the hyperemic tissue with either a hyperosmotic saline or sugar solution. It is then necessary to coat the prolapsed tissue with a water-soluble lubricant before replacing it back through the cloacal opening using a cotton-tipped applicator. In all cases, the identification and management of underlying conditions must follow the reduction of exposed tissue. It may also be necessary to use a peri-cloacal purse-string suture to prevent the prolapse from recurring (**Fig. 11**C).[16] If cloacal prolapse reoccur following replacement, then, in addition to addressing the primary underlying cause, cloacopexy is recommended (**Fig. 11**D).

MINIMAL INVASIVE SURGERY

A review on endoscopy in amphibians has been recently published.[26] Endoscopic orchiectomy in a bullfrog (*Lithobates catesbeianus*) is used here as an example of minimal invasive surgery. Celioscopy is performed in intubated amphibians placed in dorsal recumbency. A 3-mm paramedian skin incision is made in the midcoelom (between the shoulders and the cloaca). After celiotomy, the telescope-sheath system is inserted into the coelom cavity, which is insufflated. Typically, CO_2 insufflation pressures of 0.5 to 2.0 mm Hg with a flow rate not exceeding 0.5 L/min are used. The coelomic cavity is evaluated and the gonads identified (**Fig. 12**A). A second entry is achieved under direct endoscopic visualization and guided by transillumination of the body wall, thereby avoiding large blood vessels (**Fig. 12**B). A simple incision with a size 11 scalpel blade is sufficient to allow the insertion of an atraumatic 5-mm rigid grasping forceps. The gonad is held with the forceps (**Fig. 12**C, D) while the surrounding blood vessels and the epididymis are cauterized with the diode laser (**Fig. 12**E–G). After cauterization, the testicle is removed from the coelom (**Fig. 12**H). Once the endoscope has been removed, the animal deflates immediately. The

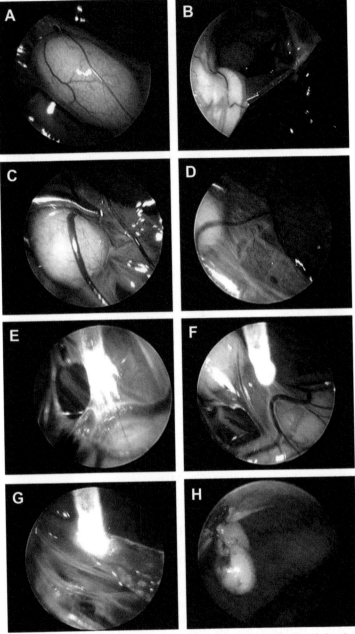

Fig. 12. Orchiectomy by minimal invasive surgery in a bullfrog. (*A*) The abdominal cavity is evaluated and the testicles identified. (*B*) A second entry is achieved with a 11 scalpel blade under direct endoscopic visualization. (*C*, *D*) The gonad is held with atraumatic 5 mm rigid grasping forceps. The surrounding blood vessels (*E*, *F*) and the epididymis (*G*) are cauterized with a diode laser. (*H*) After cauterization, the testicle is removed from the coelom. (*Courtesy of* Norin Chai, DVM, MSc, PhD, DECZM, Paris, France.)

coelomic membrane and the skin are closed in one layer with 1 or 2 interrupted sutures. Then the animal is transferred to a warm, anesthetic-free bath and rinsed copiously with fresh, well-oxygenated water.

OPHTHALMOLOGIC SURGERY

Reports of ocular surgery in amphibians are fairly uncommon in the literature. The author experienced several cases of uncompleted cataracts that do not justify a surgery. Corneal biopsy can be performed in cases of advanced corneal lipidosis (**Fig. 13**A–C). If enucleation is required in an amphibian patient, it is important to avoid damaging the membrane that separates the eye from the oral cavity. Second-intention

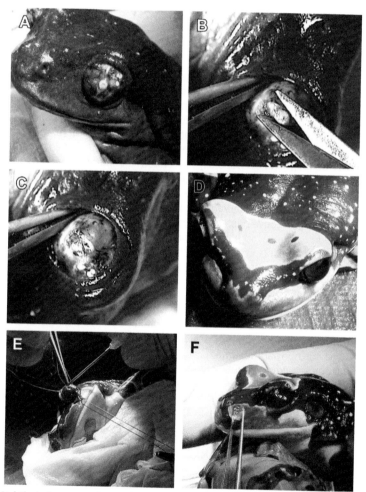

Fig. 13. Ophthalmic surgery in amphibians. (*A*) Advanced corneal lipidosis in a White's tree frog (*Litoria caerulea*). (*B*, *C*) Corneal biopsy of the same frog. (*D*) Complete lens luxation into the anterior chamber in a milk frog (*Trachycephalus resinifictrix*). (*E*) Eye position is obtained and maintained for the entire length of the surgery with encircling ligatures. (*F*) The lens was removed, and the corneal incision was closed using a 9 to 0 nylon suture in a simple interrupted pattern. (*Courtesy of* Norin Chai, DVM, MSc, PhD, DECZM, Paris, France.)

healing is often preferred following enucleation.[7] Complete lens luxation into the anterior chamber in a milk frog (Trachycephalus resinifictrix) required lens removal (**Fig. 13**D). For lens surgery, because the eyeballs can bulge out far and may sink deep, adequate eye position has to be obtained and maintained for the entire length of the surgery (**Fig. 13**E). The eyes were surgically prepared with 1% povidone-iodine solution. A clear-corneal incision was made circumferentially for approximately 180° at the limbus with a microsurgery knife. After decompression of the globe, intracameral injection of a viscoelastic substance (Provisc) helps to protect the endothelium of the cornea and maintain the anterior chamber of the eye. The lens was retrieved from the vitreal compartment using a Snellen loop. The globe was irrigated with saline solution. The corneal incision was closed using a 9 to 0 nylon suture (Ethilon, Ethicon) in a simple interrupted pattern (**Fig. 13**F). Topical antibiotics were administered for 10 days, and a single topical application of steroids was performed once after surgery. No other postsurgical treatment was given.

ORTHOPEDICS

Orthopedics in amphibians is mostly dominated by amputation. Adult urodele amphibians possess extensive regenerative abilities, including lens, jaws, limbs, and tails.[27] Amputation, when needed, is simple to perform (**Fig. 14**A, B). In anurans, strong consideration for a species' natural behavior must be taken into account before performing amputation. Some animals need both forelimbs for posture, ambulation, and manipulation of food. It is important to preserve a stump because male anurans without forelimbs may be unable to successfully reproduce.[7] Amputation of the hind limb can be performed successfully (**Fig. 14**C–F) and usually results in the return to all functions, except reproduction.[7] For amputation of the femur, the cutaneous femoral arteries, and veins, the major vessels of the anuran hind limb should be ligated.[9] Small wounds can be protected with a protective paste composed of gelatin, pectin, and sodium carboxymethylcellulose in a plasticized hydrocarbon gel (Orabase).[9]

Fracture repair is possible in larger specimens and should follow standard orthopedic practices. In smaller animals, amputation may be more appropriate.[7,8,10] A fracture of the left femur in an adult male American bullfrog (Rana catesbeiana) was successfully repaired by use of an internal fixation technique that included Kirschner wires, a positive-profile pin secured along the femur with encircling sutures, and polymethyl methacrylate molded around the entire apparatus.[10] In the bullfrog of this report, the applied internal fixation method provided effective long-term stabilization of the femur, allowed for normal movement, and enabled the bullfrog to be housed in an aquatic environment immediately after surgery.[10] Surgical spinal decompression with a dorsal laminectomy in an amphiuma (Amphiuma means) was attempted and clinically successful in the short-term.[13]

It is necessary to consider euthanasia in cases of mandibular fractures, which carry a grave prognosis.[7]

RECOVERY AND POSTOPERATIVE MANAGEMENT

Recovery from water-bath–based anesthesia (MS-222) can be accomplished by thoroughly rinsing the animal with anesthetic-free dechlorinated water. The author finds that a bath well oxygenated decreases the recovery time for aquatic species (**Fig. 15**A). Aquatic animals should have their head out of water during recovery (**Fig. 15**B). As the animal begins its recovery, the withdrawal reflex and gular respirations are the first to return followed by the righting reflex. The amphibian should be considered recovered when all of the reflexes have returned and the heart and

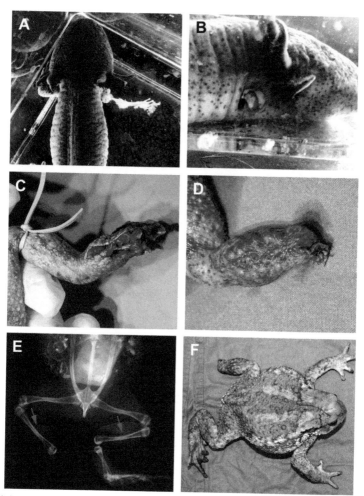

Fig. 14. (*A*) Severe wound of a foreleg due to intraspecific aggression in an axolotl (*Ambystoma mexicanum*). (*B*) Amputation was performed, and the animal regrew a completely normal new foreleg after 3 months. (*C*) Trauma of the hind limb in a common toad (*Bufo spinosus*). (*D*) The tibiotarsal junction was transected, and the skin was closed with a simple interrupted everting suture. (*E*) The bone was evaluated radiographically for secondary infection. Two asymptomatic tibial fractures (*red arrows*) were found and left untreated. (*F*) Twenty-five days later, the appearance of the wound was improved and the toad could ambulate with the help of the stump. (*Courtesy of* Norin Chai, DVM, MSc, PhD, DECZM, Paris, France.)

respiration rates have returned to preanesthetic values. The primary factors to consider postoperatively are analgesia and continued vigilance concerning hydration, nutrition, and hygiene. The continuation of preemptive analgesia using opioids and/or nonsteroidal antiinflammatory agents should be a routine part of postoperative care.

An important adjunct to maintain hydration and restore the health of ill amphibians is to soak the animals in balanced electrolyte solutions. A simple formulated solutions for use in amphibian patients consists of one part of saline (0.9% sodium chloride [NaCl]) mixed with 2 parts of 5% dextrose. Alternatively, a solution can be formulated with 7 parts of saline mixed with one part of sterile water. An appropriate dose of either

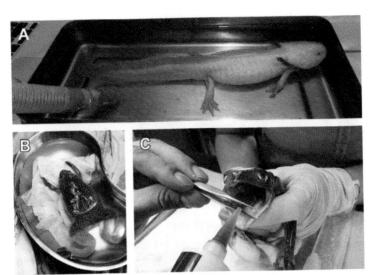

Fig. 15. (*A*) Recovery of an axolotl (*Ambystoma mexicanum*) in a well-oxygenated bath following ovariectomy. (*B*) Aquatic animals should have their head out of water during recovery (African clawed frog [*Xenopus laevis*]). (*C*) A 2-colored leaf frog (*Phyllomedusa bicolor*) is fed a highly palatable energy supplement. (*Courtesy of* Norin Chai, DVM, MSc, PhD, DECZM, Paris, France.)

solution is 25 mL/kg of body weight.[28] Two other classic formulations are amphibian Ringer solution (6.6 g NaCl, 0.15 g calcium chloride [$CaCl_2$], 0.15 g potassium chloride [KCl], and 0.2 g sodium bicarbonate [$NaHCO_3$] per liter of dechlorinated water), and Holtfreter solution (3.46 g NaCl, 0.1 g $CaCl_2$, 0.05 g KCl, and 0.2 g $NaHCO_3$ per liter of dechlorinated water). It may be necessary to assist amphibian patients with feeding for a brief period after any surgical procedure. A/D Prescription Diet (Hill's Pet Nutrition) or a highly palatable energy supplement for cats and dogs like Nutrigel are suitable choices for nutritional support in amphibians that are not self-feeding (**Fig. 15**C).

Antibiotic therapy is routinely recommended after any surgical procedure. The recommended duration of therapy is 2 weeks after an amputation, 3 weeks after fracture repair, and up to 6 weeks for open fractures.[7]

REFERENCES

1. AmphibiaWeb. Information on amphibian biology and conservation. Berkeley (CA). Available at: http://amphibiaweb.org. Accessed May 22, 2015.
2. Foote FM. Studies on hypophysectomized second year *Rana clamitans* larvae. J Exp Zool 1948;109(2):331–7.
3. Jacox LA, Dickinson AJ, Sive H. Facial transplants in *Xenopus laevis* embryos. J Vis Exp 2014;(85):50697.
4. Johnson JR. Success of intracoelomic radiotransmitter implantation in the tree frog (*Hyla versicolor*). Lab Anim (NY) 2006;35(2):29–33.
5. Crawshaw GJ. Amphibian medicine. In: Fowler M, Miller R, editors. Zoo and wild animal medicine, current therapy. 3rd edition. Philadelphia: WB Saunders; 1993. p. 131–9.
6. Frye FL, Williams DL. Self-assessment color review of reptiles and amphibians. Ames (IA): Iowa State University Press; 1995. p. 145–6.

7. Wright KM. Surgical techniques. In: Wright KM, Whitaker BR, editors. Amphibian medicine and captive husbandry. Malabar (FL): Krieger; 2001. p. 274–83.
8. Wright KM. Surgery of amphibians. Vet Clin North Am Exot Anim Pract 2000;3(3): 753–8.
9. Pizzi R, Miller J. Amputation of a Mycobacterium marinum-infected hind limb in an African bullfrog (*Pyxicephalus adspersus*). Vet Rec 2005;156(23):747–8.
10. Royal LW, Grafinger MS, Lascelles BD, et al. Internal fixation of a femur fracture in an American bullfrog. J Am Vet Med Assoc 2007;230(8):1201–4.
11. Menger B, Vogt PM, Jacobsen ID, et al. Resection of a large intra-abdominal tumor in the Mexican axolotl: a case report. Vet Surg 2010;39(2):232–3.
12. McMillan MW, Leece EA. Immersion and branchial/transcutaneous irrigation anaesthesia with alfaxalone in a Mexican axolotl. Vet Anaesth Analg 2011;38(6): 619–23.
13. Waffa BJ, Montgerard AC, Grafinger MS, et al. Dorsal laminectomy in a two-toed amphiuma (*Amphiuma means*). J Zoo Wildl Med 2012;43(4):927–30.
14. Fischer D, Lorenz N, Heuser W, et al. Abscesses associated with a Brucella inopinata–like bacterium in a big-eyed tree frog (*Leptopelis vermiculatus*). J Zoo Wildl Med 2012;43(3):625–8.
15. Archibald KE, Minter LJ, Dombrowski DS, et al. Cystic urolithiasis in captive waxy monkey frogs (*Phyllomedusa sauvagii*). J Zoo Wildl Med 2015;46(1):105–12.
16. Gentz EJ. Medicine and surgery of amphibians. ILAR J 2007;48(3):255–9.
17. Hernandez-Divers SJ. Diode laser surgery: principles and application in exotic animals. Journal of Exotic Pet Medicine 2002;11(4):208–20.
18. Tuttle AD, Law JM, Harms CA, et al. Evaluation of the gross and histologic reactions to five commonly used suture materials in the skin of the African clawed frog (*Xenopus laevis*). J Am Assoc Lab Anim Sci 2006;45(6):22–6.
19. Brown CS. Rear leg amputation and subsequent adaptive behavior during reintroduction of a green tree frog, *Hyla cinerea*. Bull Assoc Reptil Amphib Vet 1995;5:6–7.
20. Koeller CA. Comparison of buprenorphine and butorphanol analgesia in the eastern red-spotted newt (*Notophthalmus viridescens*). J Am Assoc Lab Anim Sci 2009;48(2):171–5.
21. Stevens CW. Analgesia in amphibians: preclinical studies and clinical applications. Vet Clin North Am Exot Anim Pract 2011;14(1):33–44.
22. Stevens CW. Relative analgesic potency of mu, delta and kappa opioids after spinal administration in amphibians. J Pharmacol Exp Ther 1996;276(2):440–8.
23. Wright KM, DeVoe RS. Amphibians. In: Carpenter JW, Marion CJ, editors. Exotic animal formulary. St Louis (MO): Elsevier; 2013. p. 53–82.
24. Chai N. Anurans. In: Fowler M, Miller R, editors. Zoo and wild animal medicine. 8th edition. St Louis (MO): WB Saunders; 2014. p. 1–13.
25. Poll CP. Wound management in amphibians: etiology and treatment of cutaneous lesions. J Exot Pet Med 2009;18(1):20–35.
26. Chai N. Endoscopy in amphibians. Vet Clin North Am Exot Anim Pract 2015. http://dx.doi.org/10.1016/j.cvex.2015.04.006. VAP533.
27. Dawley EM, O Samson S, Woodard KT, et al. Spinal cord regeneration in a tail autotomizing urodele. J Morphol 2012;273(2):211–25.
28. Wright KM. Overview of amphibian medicine. In: Mader DR, editor. Reptile medicine and surgery. 2nd edition. St Louis (MO): Saunders Elsevier; 2006. p. 941–71.

Reptile Soft Tissue Surgery

Nicola Di Girolamo, DVM, MSc(EBHC)[a],*,
Christoph Mans, Dr med vet, DACZM[b]

KEYWORDS

- Coeliotomy • Chelonians • Lizards • Snakes • Prefemoral fossa

KEY POINTS

- The field of surgery on reptiles is in continuous evolution, with novel, less invasive surgical techniques being progressively developed.
- Prefemoral fossa coeliotomy should be the approach of choice in chelonians, especially for reproductive surgeries.
- The paramedian approach is generally indicated in lizards that are dorsally compressed; in chameleons and other laterally compressed lizards, the coelom may be easily approached through the flank.
- A common mistake is to remove the oviduct without the respective ovary, which may lead to yolk coelomitis, and ovarian neoplasia.

INTRODUCTION

The field of reptile surgery is continuously evolving and novel surgical techniques have been reported in recent years. These innovative procedures often reduce the invasiveness of conventional interventions[1–5] or provide insightful solutions to common disorders.[6,7] Most of these novel surgical techniques are described in case reports, case series, or other observational studies, as in other medical fields.[8] However, these reports are often biased toward an overly positive representation of the effectiveness of reported techniques and ideally should be followed up by randomized controlled trials. Contrary to other fields in medicine, such research designs are underused in veterinary medicine.[9] In addition, reptile medicine is an extremely heterogeneous field, including species that have unique physiologic, anatomic, and pathologic differences. Therefore, strong supporting evidence for a specific surgical technique in the reptile species of interest is usually unavailable.

The authors have nothing to disclose.
[a] Clinica per Animali Esotici, Centro Veterinario Specialistico, Via Sandro Giovannini 53, Roma 00137, Italy; [b] Department of Surgical Sciences, School of Veterinary Medicine, University of Wisconsin-Madison, 2015 Linden Drive, Madison, WI 53706, USA
* Corresponding author.
E-mail address: nicoladiggi@gmail.com

The purpose of this review was to describe common soft tissue surgical techniques used in reptiles. Clinicians should consider the lack of high-quality evidence for the actual effectiveness of most of these interventions, and use the information provided as a guideline.

SURGERY OF THE SKIN

Surgery of the skin in reptiles is indicated for wound management, cutaneous and subcutaneous abscesses, and removal of neoplasms. General anesthesia or sedation in combination with local tissue infiltration or peripheral nerve block using lidocaine or bupivacaine can be used to desensitize skin and allows for cutaneous surgeries.[10]

Skin Sutures

Reptile skin has the tendency to invert after incision, especially in squamates.[11,12] Therefore, a slightly everting suture pattern (eg, horizontal mattress) is recommended to ensure first intention wound healing.[11] Healing of the skin can be accelerated if reptiles are maintained at the upper end of their preferred temperature range.[13] Often, definitive skin healing with disappearing of the scab occurs after the first or the second ecdysis.[12]

Suture Materials

Most suture materials used for surgery in the higher vertebrates are suitable for use in reptiles.[11] In an early study on wound healing in garter snakes (*Thamnophis sirtalis*) in which sutured and unsutured wounds were compared, unsutured linear incisions tended to have more rapid epithelial maturation and a less intense inflammatory response.[13] On this basis, the investigators suggested that suturing small incisional wounds may not be advantageous.[13] In another study, the tissue reaction to 4 suture materials (chromic gut, polyglyconate, polyglactin 910, poliglecaprone 25) was evaluated grossly and histologically in 258 loggerhead sea turtles. Among the 4 suture types, polyglyconate (eg, Maxon; Covidien Ltd, Dublin, Ireland) and poliglecaprone 25 (Monocryl; Ethicon, Inc, Sommerville, NJ) caused the least tissue reaction. However, patient outcome (eg, eversion size and amount of body weight change) did not vary significantly among suture types.[14]

Tissue adhesive and skin staples can also be used as alternatives to suture materials for closure of skin incisions in reptiles.[15] In a study, the reactions to several suture materials (polydioxanone, polydioxanone with triclosan, poliglecaprone 25, poliglecaprone 25 with triclosan, polyglactin 910, monofilament nylon, chromic gut) and to cyanoacrylate tissue adhesive were compared in the skin of 30 ball pythons.[15] The subjective histologic inflammation scores were significantly higher for suture materials compared with the values for negative control and cyanoacrylate tissue adhesive at several time points. Furthermore, sutures often underwent extrusion from tissues before complete absorption. However, the skin in reptiles needs to support most of the tensile strength of coelomic incisions.[12] Therefore, current recommendation for closure of coelomic breaches is to use absorbable synthetic monofilament suture material (eg, poliglecaprone 25, polyglyconate).

Surgical Technique for Wounds with Avulsion of the Skin from Bone in Chelonians

Traumatic wounds are common in reptiles and may result in the avulsion of the skin from the plastron or the carapace in chelonians. After proper debridement, if the loss of tissue is not exaggerated and tension-free surgical attachment is feasible, the skin can be sutured to the bony tissue (**Fig. 1**).[11] Small holes on the bony tissue are made with Backhaus towel clamps in young or nonmineralized chelonians or with a rotary tool equipped with a thin drill bit in chelonians with mineralized shells. Nonabsorbable suture material is then passed through the holes and the skin. The sutures are left in place for at least 6 weeks.[11] Final esthetic result is usually satisfactory (see **Fig. 1C**).

Subcutaneous Abscess Removal

Subcutaneous abscesses are a frequent finding in captive reptiles. Typically, subcutaneous abscesses present as single or multiple, firm, swellings of the skin (**Fig. 2**). Proper diagnostics always should be used before surgical removal. In particular, the epidemiology of certain cutaneous tumors (eg, squamous cell carcinoma in bearded dragons[16]) should be considered as differentials.

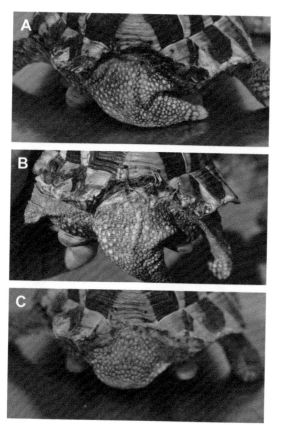

Fig. 1. Long-term outcome after suturing the skin to the edge of the carapace in an injured Hermann tortoise (*Testudo hermanni*). Multiple small holes were drilled in the bone. Sutures are then placed to attach the skin to the bone. (*A*) Appearance of the wound site at day 7. (*B*) Appearance of the wound site at day 50. (*C*) Appearance of the wound site at day 150. (*Courtesy of* Nicola Di Girolamo, Rome, Italy.)

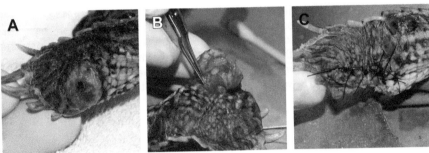

Fig. 2. (*A*) Abscess of the distal forelimb in a red-eared slider (*Trachemys scripta elegans*). (*B*) Surgical removal of the abscess in toto. (*C*) Closure of the surgical wound is performed using horizontal mattress sutures. Note the eversion of the wound edges. In semiaquatic and aquatic turtles, managing open wounds is challenging, in particular on the limbs and neck; therefore primary closure is recommended after irrigation of the wound to promote first intension wound healing. (*Courtesy of* Christoph Mans, Madison, WI.)

HEAD AND NECK SURGERY
Aural Abscesses

Aural abscesses are a common clinical presentation in aquatic turtles, characterized by unilateral or bilateral swelling of the tympanic membranes (**Fig. 3**A). The association among aural abscesses and hypovitaminosis A has been proposed but could not be proven,[17] and etiology of aural abscesses is more likely to be multifactorial.[18]

Surgical treatment consists of incision of the tympanic membrane and surgical debridement of the tympanic cavity under general anesthesia. A single vertical, 2

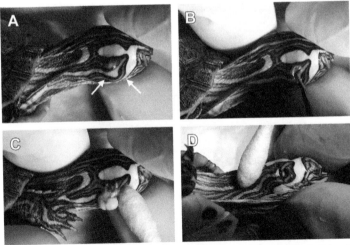

Fig. 3. Surgical management of an auricular abscess in a yellow-bellied slider (*Trachemys scripta scripta*). The animal is sedated and the neck is extended. (*A*) Typical swelling of the auricular area (*arrows*). (*B*) A vertical incision is performed with a No. 11 triangular scalpel blade on the tympanic membrane. Alternatively, a cross incision or a 360° incision around the tympanic membrane can be made. (*C*) Purulent material is gently removed from the tympanic cavity. (*D*) The tympanic cavity is left open to heal by second intention. (*Courtesy of* Nicola Di Girolamo, Rome, Italy.)

cross incisions, or a circular incision (180–360°) are made on the tympanum (see **Fig. 3**B). By use of a cotton tip, debris and caseous material in the tympanum is gently removed (see **Fig. 3**C). Culture and sensitivity testing may be performed from the debris or the tympanum. The tympanic cavity is lavaged, packed with an antimicrobial ointment, and managed as an open wound to allow healing by second intention (see **Fig. 3**D). Appropriate changes in management and diet are crucial to avoid recurrences.

Trachea

Surgery of the trachea has been performed in reptiles suffering from tracheal avulsion[19] and tracheal neoplasia.[20,21] In case of benign masses in the tracheal lumen, endoscopic removal may be preferred over more invasive surgeries (ie, tracheal resection and anastomosis). In 2 ball pythons (*Python regius*) with intraluminal chondromas, endoscopic removal with biopsy forceps resulted in amelioration of clinical signs and no recurrence of the masses was observed at a 12-month and 4-month follow-up.[20]

Temporary tracheal bypass

To temporarily relieve tracheal obstructions, saccular lung cannulation may be performed.[7] With the animal in right lateral recumbency, a skin incision is made at the level of the caudal aspect of the palpable lung field. The intercostal muscles are retracted and a small stab incision is made into the saccular lung. An appropriate-size cuffed tube is inserted into the lung and sutured in place with a purse-string pattern and a roman sandal suture.[7]

Endoscopic removal of tracheal masses

The reptile is positioned in ventral or dorsal recumbency with the neck extended, as for standard tracheoscopy. Depending on the size of the reptile and the distance of the lesion from the glottis, an endoscope of the appropriate size and type (rigid or flexible) should be used. Once the mass is located, the biopsy forceps are used to debride all the tissue that protrudes into the tracheal lumen.[20]

Tracheal resection in snakes

The snake is placed in dorsal recumbency with the neck extended. An incision on the skin at the level of the stricture is performed, and muscular layers are bluntly separated. The section of the trachea of interest is removed after placement of stay sutures orally and aborally. Anastomosis of the orad and aborad segments of the trachea is then performed encompassing 1 or 2 tracheal rings with monofilament absorbable sutures in a simple interrupted pattern.[21]

Esophagus

Esophagostomy tube placement

Esophagostomy tube placement is typically recommended in anorectic chelonians, given the difficulty of oral administration of food and/or medication. It may also be indicated in aggressive, chronically ill squamates.

Surgical technique

Curved mosquito hemostats are inserted in the mouth and pushed on the side of the neck. Gentle pressure favors displacement of the jugular vein and carotid artery (**Fig. 4**A). A small skin incision is made over the tip of the mosquito, exposing the external muscular layer of the esophagus (see **Fig. 4**B). The esophageal wall is incised and the tip of the forceps is exposed. The feeding tube is grasped and passed through

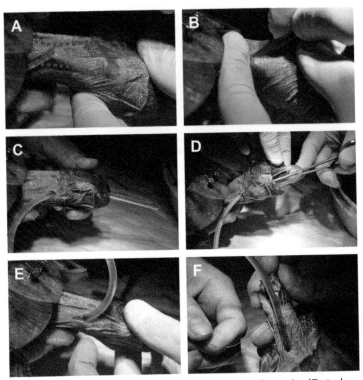

Fig. 4. Placement of an esophagostomy tube in a marginated tortoise (*Testudo marginata*) (*A–E*) and in a Russian tortoise (*Agrionemys horsfieldii*) (*F*). (*A*) Gentle pressure favors displacement of the jugular vein and carotid artery (*dashed lines*). (*B*) A small skin incision is made over the tip of the mosquito hemostats exposing the external muscular layer of the esophagus. The esophageal wall is incised and the tip of the hemostats is exposed. (*C*) The tube is grasped by the hemostats, passed through the incision and directed cranially. (*D*) Once visualized through the mouth, the tube is gently curved and pushed into the esophagus up to the stomach. (*E*) The tube is correctly placed. (*F*) A standard roman sandal suture with a purse-string pattern around the tube is performed. (*Courtesy of* Nicola Di Girolamo, Rome, Italy.)

the incision and directed cranially (see **Fig. 4**C). Once visualized through the mouth, the tube is gently curved (see **Fig. 4**D) and pushed into the esophagus toward the stomach up to the level of the predetermined length of the tube (see **Fig. 4**E). A standard roman sandal suture (synonym, Chinese finger knot) with an optional purse-string pattern around the tube is performed (see **Fig. 4**F). Confirmation of the proper positioning of the tube is usually not necessary, but may be performed by administration of contrast media through the tube.

Esophagotomy
Food items (eg, fishbone), substrates (eg, bark), plant material (eg, grass seed), or fish hooks may all act as esophageal foreign bodies in reptiles.[11,22] Clinical signs in reptiles with esophageal foreign bodies can include regurgitation and open-mouth breathing. Removal should be attempted through the oral cavity, by means of direct or endoscopic visualization.[23] Whenever removal from the oral cavity is not feasible, esophagotomy is performed.[22]

Surgical technique: cervical esophagotomy

With the animal in lateral or dorsal recumbency and the neck extended, the esophageal lumen is accessed laterally or ventrally in proximity of the foreign body. The foreign body is visualized (**Fig. 5**) and removed. In certain instances, the insertion of an endoscope through the incision may assist in the identification of the foreign body. The esophageal incision is closed with simple interrupted sutures. The skin is closed with an interrupted horizontal mattress pattern. In large reptiles, the musculature should be closed in a separate layer.

Surgical technique: supraplastronal esophagotomy

A supraplastronal coelomic approach has been described in a loggerhead sea turtle in which cervical esophagotomy did not allow retrieval of the foreign body.[24] A transverse incision is made at the junction of the cervical skin and the cranial edge of the plastron. The subcutaneous tissues and musculature are retracted to expose the ventral esophagus.[24] Esophagotomy is then performed as described previously.

Thyroid

In snakes and chelonians, there is a single, spherical thyroid gland located ventral to the trachea and cranial to the heart. In lizards, the thyroid is generally bilobed with an isthmus over the trachea, although some species have a single or paired thyroids.[25]

Thyroidectomy

In reptiles, thyroid hormones maintain and stimulate metabolism, playing an important role in shedding and growth. Neoplastic disorders and adenomatous hyperplasia are the main indication for thyroid surgery and are sparsely reported in reptiles.[26,27]

Surgical technique

Consider using diagnostic imaging techniques (eg, high-frequency ultrasonography, scintigraphy) for definitive location of the glands. The patient is positioned in dorsal recumbency and the cervical region is aseptically prepared. A skin incision is performed over the thyroid. The musculature is incised and reflected or bluntly separated so as to expose the thyroid. The blood vessels are ligated by use of absorbable sutures or ligation clips. The thyroid is removed and the muscle layers are closed using absorbable sutures.[26] The skin is closed by standard technique.

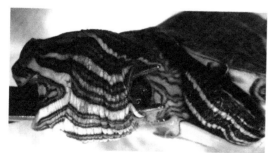

Fig. 5. Esophagotomy for removal of an obstructive esophageal foreign body (fishbone) in a 70-g red-eared slider *(T scripta elegans).* Initial attempts of foreign body removal through the oral cavity were unsuccessful. Curved mosquito hemostats are used for atraumatic dilation of the esophagotomy incision. The incision was closed in 2 layers. (*Courtesy of* Nicola Di Girolamo, Rome, Italy.)

After complete thyroidectomy, oral supplementation with levothyroxine may be required.[27]

COELIOTOMY

Surgical approaches to the coelom greatly vary depending on the species.[11,12] Appropriate preparation of the reptile patient for coeliotomy is mandatory. Sterile scrub brushes may be used to provide effective cleaning of reptiles. Once anesthetized, the patient is instrumented, placed in the recumbency indicated for the surgical procedure (**Fig. 6**), and surgically prepped. In general, the size of the incision will depend on the indications for coeliotomy. During the opening of the coelomic membrane, the surgeon should pay attention for signs of free gas or liquid in the coelom, associated with gastrointestinal (GI) tract and urinary bladder perforation, respectively.[23,28] After entering the coelom, all the organs that are visible should be carefully inspected.

Lizards

In lizards, the 3 main approaches to the coelom include paramedian, median, and flank approach. The paramedian and median approaches are generally indicated in lizards that are dorsally compressed (eg, families Iguanidae, Agamidae, Gekkota). In chameleons and other lizards that are laterally compressed (eg, basilisks), the coelom may be easily approached through the flank.

The paramedian approach is generally preferred over the median approach to avoid the ventral midline abdominal vein, a large vessel that runs just over the linea alba.[18]

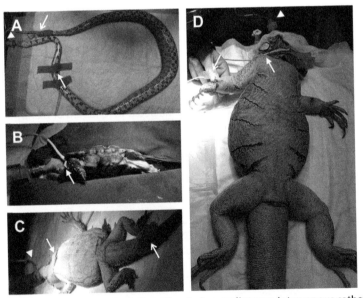

Fig. 6. Positioning and monitoring of reptiles during coeliotomy. Intravenous catheters (*unfilled arrows*), Doppler probe to monitor heart rate (*arrows*), and capnography for measurement of expiratory CO_2 (*arrowheads*) are highlighted. (*A*) Positioning of a corn snake (*Pantherophis guttatus*) in dorsal recumbency for coeliotomy. (*B*) Positioning of a pancake tortoise (*Malacochersus tornieri*) for left prefemoral fossa coeliotomy. (*C, D*) Positioning of a bearded dragon (*P vitticeps*) and a green iguana (*Iguana iguana*) for paramedian coeliotomy. Notice placement of the intravenous catheter in the coccygeal vein (*C*) and in the cephalic vein (*D*). (*Courtesy of* Nicola Di Girolamo, Rome, Italy.)

An incision of the skin is made parallel to the midline (**Fig. 7**A). The incision may be made with a scalpel blade or dissecting devices (eg, lasers, radiosurgical and electro-surgical equipment). In a study conducted on green iguanas, radiosurgery and laser both produced bloodless incisions, but radiosurgery caused significantly less collateral tissue damage in the skin and the muscle.[29]

The distance of the incision from the midline will depend on the size of the lizard. The incision is extended cranially and caudally using scissors, taking care to avoid the ventral abdominal vein. In some instances, the ends of the incision may need to be prolonged at a 90-degree angle, forming a sort of "L" or "H."[11,30] The skin is retracted and the musculature is dissected by use of blunt scissors, cotton-tipped applicators, laser, or electrosurgical equipment. Sharp dissection of the musculature should be avoided to minimize bleeding.

SNAKES

In snakes, a paraventral coeliotomy is indicated for most surgeries. Obviously, a single incision does not permit access to all the organs. Therefore, an incision needs to be made at the level of the organ of interest. The skin is incised between the first and second row of lateral scales (see **Fig. 7**B), and the resulting surgical wound is scalloped. This incision avoids distortion of the ventral scutes once the skin is sutured in an everting pattern.[12]

Closure of the Coelom in Snakes and Lizards

In squamates, the coelomic membrane and muscular wall are fragile and do not hold sutures.[12] Therefore, closure of the coelom relies on the skin sutures. In small to medium-sized squamates, the coelomic membrane, muscularis, and subcutis are

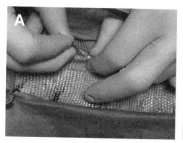
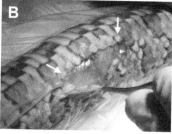
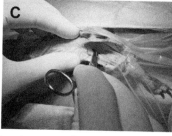

Fig. 7. Soft-tissue approaches to access the coelom. (*A*) Paramedian incision in a green iguana (*I iguana*). The location of the ventral abdominal vein is depicted by the dashed line. (*B*) Paraventral incision in a corn snake (*P guttatus*) in dorsal recumbency. The skin is incised between the first and second row of lateral scales (*arrows*). (*C*) Prefemoral fossa coeliotomy in a Hermann tortoise (*T hermanni*). (*Courtesy of* Nicola Di Girolamo, Rome, Italy.)

sutured together in a simple continuous suture pattern with monofilament absorbable sutures. The skin is sutured with fine monofilament nonabsorbable sutures (eg, nylon) in an everting pattern, as previously discussed (**Fig. 8**A, B, D).[11]

CHELONIANS

In chelonians, the 2 main approaches to the coelom are plastron osteotomy and prefemoral fossa coeliotomy. With the increased availability of laparoscopic and endosurgical equipment, prefemoral fossa coeliotomy has gained popularity due to the reduced invasiveness compared with plastron osteotomy.[1,2,5,31] However, in certain species and for certain surgeries, plastron osteotomy is still required, as it permits a better maneuvering of cranial coelomic organs.[12]

Prefemoral Fossa Coeliotomy

Prefemoral fossa coeliotomy (synonym, prefemoral coeliotomy) is currently considered the surgical access of choice for most reproductive surgeries and for diagnostic endoscopy (see **Fig. 7**C; **Fig. 9**).[1,2,5,32] It should be also considered for urinary bladder and intestinal surgery. This approach is particularly indicated in species with a relative small plastron and in semiaquatic and aquatic species.

The chelonian is placed in ventral, dorsal, or lateral recumbency depending on species, size, and indications for surgery. The skin, subcutaneous tissue, and the transverse and oblique abdominal muscles, and coelomic membrane are transected, and the coelomic cavity accessed (see **Figs. 7**C and **9**). The use of ring retractors is extremely useful to enhance access and visibility.[1] Care should be taken to avoid trauma to the urinary bladder on entering the coelom. Cystocentesis should be performed if the bladder is distended and impairs surgical access to the coelom.

Closure of the body wall should be performed in 2 to 3 layers. It may not always be possible to close the coelomic membrane. Closure of the muscles and skin is routine.

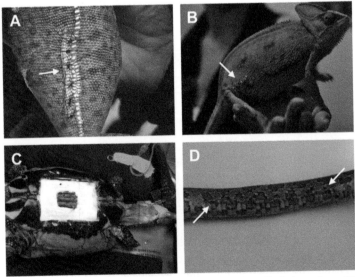

Fig. 8. Appearance of wound closure after coeliotomy (*A*) Veiled chameleon (*Chamaeleo calyptratus*) after paramedian ovariohysterectomy. (*B*) Veiled chameleon after flank ovariohysterectomy. (*C*) Hermann tortoise (*T hermanni*). A waterproof orthopedic epoxy resin is used to stabilize the bony flap. (*D*) Corn snake (*P guttatus*) (*arrows*).

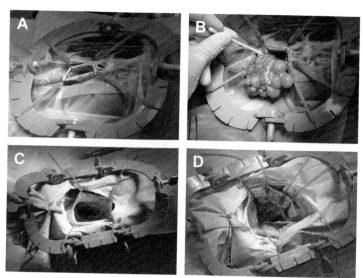

Fig. 9. Prefemoral coeliotomy in chelonians (*A*) red-eared slider *(T scripta elegans)*, (*B*) African spurred tortoise *(Centrochelys sulcata)*. The animals are placed in dorsal recumbency. A ring retractor facilitates the access to the coelom. (*A*) The skin layer is retracted, allowing dissection of the subcutaneous and muscle layer. (*B*) Prefemoral ovariectomy. The ring retractor allows for visualization and access to the coelom. The skin and muscle layers are retracted. (*C*) Skin and muscle layer incised and retracted. (*D*) Same tortoise as in (*C*). The deeper muscle layers are dissected and progressively retracted by adding additional retractor hooks. Note the straight extension pieces of the ring retractor (*C*, *D*), to allow its use in larger animals. (*Courtesy of* Christoph Mans, Madison, WI.)

If substantial amounts of subcutaneous tissue are present, then additional subcutaneous sutures should be considered.

The healing times after prefemoral coeliotomy are substantially shorter than after a plastron osteotomy.[12] Furthermore, in aquatic and semiaquatic chelonia, prefemoral coeliotomy avoids dry-docking. An early return to the aquatic environment is critical to allow normal behavior, food intake, and defecation.

Plastron Osteotomy

The size of the plastron osteotomy (synonym, plastrotomy) is dependent on the indication for surgery (eg, size of eggs, bladder stones, GI foreign bodies) and is limited cranially by the heart and caudally by the pelvic girdle (**Fig. 10**A). The animal is placed in dorsal recumbency. Various instruments (eg, a rotary tool equipped with a cutting circular blade, an oscillating sagittal saw) may be used to create the incision into the plastron (see **Fig. 10**B). Three sides of the flap should be incised at a 45-degree angle to obtain slightly beveled incisions. The fourth side is only partially incised and is used as a hinge (see **Fig. 10**C). A periosteal elevator is used to complete the 3 full-thickness incisions of the plastron and to elevate the flap.[11] The flap is reflected cranially or caudally and covered with moist gauze. The coelomic membrane is visualized and a ventral midline incision is performed, taking care to avoid the ventral abdominal veins.

In chelonians, after plastron osteotomy, the coelomic membrane is gently sutured with a fine monofilament absorbable suture in a simple interrupted or continuous pattern. The lack of suturing of the coelomic membrane has been suggested to be

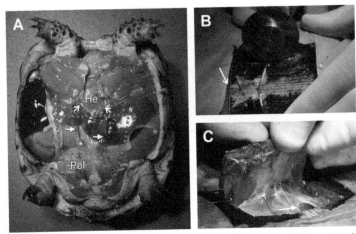

Fig. 10. Plastron osteotomy in chelonians. (*A*) The cadaver of a Horsfield tortoise (*A horsfieldii*) is used to show the anatomic limits of plastron osteotomy. A trapezoidal to squared plastron osteotomy is depicted (*dashed lines*). The plastron osteotomy incisions are limited by the presence of the heart (He) cranially and by the pelvic girdle (Pel) caudally. Particular care should be paid in avoiding incision on the pericardium (*unfilled arrows*). The 2 parallel abdominal vessels are indicated (*arrows*). (*B*) Use of a rotary tool equipped with a cutting circular blade. Sterile water is applied during the incision to minimize thermal damage to the plastron. Medical tape is used to outline the osteotomy area (*unfilled arrow*). (*C*) Three sides of the bony flap are incised. The flap is then reflected caudally and covered with moist gauze. Notice that inadvertent rupture of the coelomic membrane occurred (*arrow*). (*Courtesy of* Nicola Di Girolamo, Rome, Italy.)

associated with increased risk of postoperative adhesions.[11] The bony flap is repositioned and sutured (in young or demineralized chelonians) or stabilized by means of epoxy resins (see **Fig. 8**C), fiberglass mesh, or metal plates and screws (**Fig. 11**).[11,12]

Plastron osteotomy is generally associated with prolonged surgical procedure time and prolonged recovery, and is thought to be significantly more painful compared with

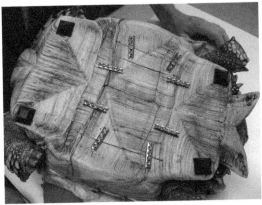

Fig. 11. Plastron osteotomy in an African spurred tortoise *(C sulcata)*. Orthopedic plates and screws are used to stabilize the bone flap, which provides greater stability and reduces the risk of complications, such as infection or dehiscence. (*Courtesy of* School of Veterinary Medicine, University of Wisconsin-Madison, Madison, WI, USA)

the prefemoral soft tissue approach.[1] The plastron flap may become a sequestrum and provide temporary protection to the developing bone. Eventual postsurgical complications are usually serious, require prolonged treatment, and include lack of revascularization of the bone flap and consequent necrosis, infection with consequent coelomitis, and dehiscence of the bone flap margins.

A further limitation of the technique is the need for dry-docking of aquatic turtles. Even with application of fiberglass patch, postoperative leakage may occur, leading to infection. Healing times of the bone flap are variable, but are considered to be approximately 1 to 2 years.[12]

REPRODUCTIVE TRACT SURGERY

Reproductive tract disorders are common indications for surgery in reptiles, and include preovulatory stasis, postovulatory stasis (ie, dystocia), yolk coelomitis, ectopic eggs, and neoplasia, among others.[2] Furthermore, elective surgeries may be performed for population control,[31,33] to limit male aggressiveness,[34] and for preventive care in females with recurrent reproductive disorders.

Ovariectomy, Ovariosalpingectomy, and Salpingotomy

The reproductive tract of female reptiles is generally composed of 2 ovaries and 2 oviducts,[35] although in a few species the left oviduct is vestigial or absent.[36] Ovaries are suspended by a mesovarium and exhibit seasonal changes, with the greatest size reached during the breeding season, that is, before ovulation. Size of the follicles may significantly affect the surgical anatomy and techniques. Ovaries are symmetric in chelonians, whereas in squamates, the right ovary is anterior to the left one.[36] In snakes, this asymmetry is exaggerated, with the right ovary being usually larger and more displaced anteriorly than the left one.[35] Gonadal arteries vascularize the ovaries and oviducts originating from the dorsal aorta. Ovarian veins drain into the postcaval veins.[36]

Indications and preoperative considerations

Clinically, it is often difficult to determine whether a female reptile is undergoing a normal physiologic or a pathologic process. Gestational duration, clutch size, egg size, egg type, and even placentation vary among species of reptiles. Therefore, an in-depth understanding of each species' reproductive cycle is required.[37] Surgery may be indicated when one or more of the following situations occur:

- Follicles neither ovulate nor regress over time and are associated with lethargy and/or anorexia
- Despite proper care, the gravid female suddenly become anorexic and lethargic
- There is evidence that the clutch had been retained for an abnormally long period
- The female laid part of her clutch and retained one or more eggs (or fetus in case of viviparous species)
- There is evidence of a mechanical impediment of oviposition (eg, strictures, cloacal calculi)

In cases of preovulatory stasis, or ovarian neoplasia, ovariectomy (synonym, oophorectomy) is recommended over ovariosalpingectomy.[38] Ovariectomy may be also performed to control reproduction.[31]

Open surgical techniques

Standard access to the coelom is performed. If ovulation has already occurred (ie, the oviducts contain postovulatory follicles or eggs), the oviducts are gently exteriorized before the ovaries (**Fig. 12**A). If ovulation has not occurred (ie, preovulatory stasis),

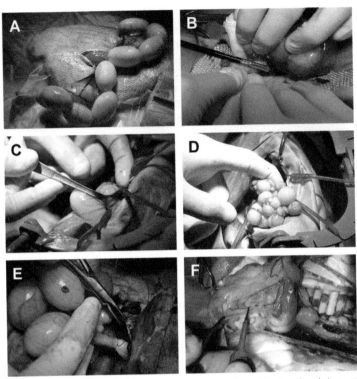

Fig. 12. Ovariectomy and ovariosalpingectomy in reptiles. (*A*) Ovariosalpingectomy in a bearded dragon (*P vitticeps*) with dystocia. (*B*) Ovariectomy in a green iguana diagnosed with preovulatory follicular stasis. Notice the gentle traction on the mesovarium. (*C, D*) Unilateral prefemoral ovariosalpingectomy in a red-eared slider *(T scripta elegans)*. The retained eggs were all located in the left oviduct and were exteriorized using a curved spoon. Note the positioning in lateral recumbency. For bilateral surgery, the turtle is preferably placed in dorsal recumbency. (*E*) Ovariosalpingectomy through plastron osteotomy in a Hermann tortoise. The oviducts are ligated and transected. (*F*) Ovariectomy in a corn snake (*P guttatus*). (*Courtesy of* [*A, B, E, F*] Nicola Di Girolamo; and [*C, D*] Paolo Selleri, Rome, Italy.)

the ovaries are large and several yellowish-to-orange follicles are present (see **Fig. 12**B; **Fig. 13**B) and should be exteriorized first. In small species (eg, chameleons, geckos) the oviducts are thin and fragile, and cotton-tip applicators should be used to minimize trauma during exteriorization (see **Fig. 12**C). Once the oviducts have been exteriorized, the ovaries should be identified and elevated to expose the mesovarium with its vessels (see **Figs. 12**B, D and **13**D). Microsurgical instruments, ligation clips, and radiosurgical and electrosurgical devices facilitate removal of the entire ovaries (see **Fig. 12**B).[38] The vessels that supply the oviduct are carefully ligated using radiosurgery or ligatures (see **Fig. 12**F). The oviduct is ligated distal close to the cloaca and removed (see **Fig. 12**E).

In cases of postovulatory stasis, the goal may be to preserve the reproductive function. In such cases, the eggs may be removed from the oviducts (ie, c-section, salpingotomy). However, eggs often adhere to the oviduct and removal from a single oviductal incision may be difficult. Furthermore, the oviducts are generally fragile and the rims may invert, making closure of the incisions difficult.[39] The incisions are closed with absorbable monofilament suture in an inverting pattern. Alternatively, if

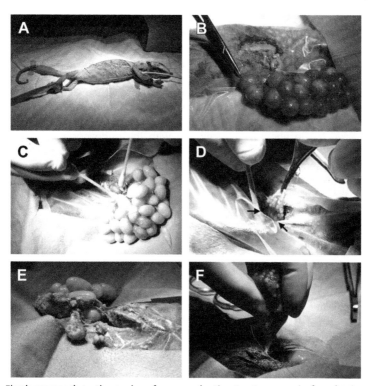

Fig. 13. Flank approach to the coelom for reproductive tract surgery in female chameleons. (*A*) A veiled chameleon (*C calyptratus*) positioned for surgery. Note the ventral coccygeal intravenous catheter, the position of the Doppler, the caudal fixation of the hindlimbs. The *dotted line* indicates the coelomic coeliotomy incision site. (*B*) Surgical resolution of preovulatory follicular stasis in a veiled chameleon through bilateral ovariectomy. Both ovaries are easily accessed through the same unilateral incision. (*C, D*) Surgical resolution of postovulatory stasis (ie, dystocia) in a veiled chameleon through bilateral ovariosalpingectomy. The exteriorization of the eggs is performed with a cotton-tipped applicator to avoid trauma to the oviducts. Once the oviducts have been removed, the ovaries (*D, arrows*) are exteriorized and excised after ligation of the mesovarium. (*E*) Surgical correction of yolk coelomitis in a veiled chameleon. (*F*) Surgical resolution of a large follicular ovarian cyst in a veiled chameleon that had been previously undergone incomplete ovariectomy. (*Courtesy of* Nicola Di Girolamo, Rome, Italy.)

only one oviduct is dystocic, a unilateral ovariosalpingectomy preserves the breeding function. If an oviduct is removed the respective ovary also should be removed. Inadvertent remnants of ovarian tissue may provoke future ovulation into the coelomic cavity (potentially leading to yolk coelomitis),[39] ovarian neoplasia,[38] or ovarian cysts (see **Fig. 13**F).

Endoscopy-assisted prefemoral oophorectomy and salpingectomy
A technique for exteriorization and excision of ovaries and oviducts of chelonians through the prefemoral fossa has been described.[1] The technique relies on the assistance of standard endoscopic equipment (eg, 2.7-mm, rigid endoscope). Depending on species, size, and individual morphology, oophorectomy, salpingectomy, and/or salpingotomy may be performed through the prefemoral approach.[2,40] Chelonians

are preferably placed in dorsal recumbency,[2,40] although ventral or lateral recumbency may be indicated in particular instances (eg, unilateral egg dystocia). A rigid endoscope is introduced into the coelom following through a standard prefemoral coeliotomy approach. The reproductive tract is identified and gently grasped with atraumatic grasping forceps preferably by an avascular connective area of the ovary. Care must be taken to avoid rupture of ovarian follicles. Once all ovarian follicles are exteriorized (see **Figs. 9**B and **12**D) and the mesovarium is visible, the ovarian vasculature in the mesovarium is ligated and transected. Hemostasis and complete excision of the ovarian tissue should be confirmed with the endoscope. If the oviduct is diseased and surgical removal is intended, the ipsilateral oviduct is exteriorized, ligated, and transected through the same prefemoral incision. The procedure is then repeated for the contralateral ovary and oviduct. Often the procedure may be performed for the contralateral ovary via the same prefemoral incision.[1] However, performing salpingectomy or salpingotomy of the contralateral oviduct is usually not possible, and coelomic access is required through the contralateral prefemoral fossa. Retained eggs in the oviduct and ectopic eggs free within the coelom also can be removed using this technique (see **Fig. 12**C).[2]

Orchiectomy

Orchiectomy (synonym, orchidectomy) in reptiles may be performed in an attempt to limit reproduction,[5] control aggression,[34] for physiologic research, and to manage disorders of the testicles.[41] Primary neoplasms of the testes are reported in reptiles,[42] and surgical removal of testicular tumors has been successfully performed.[41,43]

To limit aggression, it is suggested that orchiectomy may be effective if performed before reaching sexual maturity. However, evidence that surgical castration reduces aggressive behaviors in reptiles is still limited. In a controlled trial,[34] 6 juvenile male iguanas were neutered and 6 underwent sham surgery. In the following 30 months, none of the neutered iguanas displayed aggressive behaviors, whereas 4 of 6 intact controls became aggressive. In another study, a surgically castrated Madagascar ground gecko (*Paroedura picta*) showed no aggressive behaviors, whereas the intact controls occasionally showed aggressive behaviors toward other males.[44]

Due to the intracoelomic location of the testicles, orchiectomy is a more invasive procedure in reptiles, in particular in chelonians, as compared with most mammals. Surgical approaches to the testicles in chelonians include the following:

- Prefemoral[45]
- Prefemoral, endoscopic-assisted
- Prefemoral, endoscopic[5]
- Plastron osteotomy

Plastron osteotomy should be avoided for its invasiveness, unless the pathology of the testicles significantly alters their size (eg, neoplasms of large size)[42] and makes prefemoral approaches not feasible.

Open surgical orchiectomy

After standard coeliotomy, the testicles are identified. Testicles have a friable capsule and must be handled carefully. In small species, the testicle may be elevated from the coelomic cavity by placing a suture or a needle through it.[12] In general, full exteriorization is difficult because of the intimate relationship between the testis and major blood vessels (aorta and caudal vena cava). Therefore, ligation of the testicular vessels is facilitated by use of ligation clips and radiosurgical or electrosurgical equipment. While removing the testicles, care should be used to avoid damaging the vena cava and the adrenal glands that are contiguous to them. The vascular pedicles are checked for hemorrhage and the coelom is routinely closed.

Prefemoral fossa orchiectomy in chelonians

Prefemoral endoscopic orchiectomy has been recently described in turtles and tortoises.[5,46] Briefly, the testicle is visualized and grasped, distending the mesorchium. Ligation clips or radiosurgical instruments are used for hemostasis and dissection of the ligaments. The testicle is removed while the epididymis is left in situ.[5]

Orchiectomy also may be performed through the prefemoral fossa approach without endoscopic guidance.[45] An incision is made in the prefemoral fossa and the musculature is dissected. Urinary bladder, intestine, and lungs are manipulated to expose the testicles. The testicle is grasped using a curved hemostat, the spermatic cord is dissected, and ligation clips are placed around the spermatic cord and testicular artery. The spermatic cord and the testicular artery are dissected distal to the ligation clips.[45]

The same technique may be performed under endoscopic assistance with exteriorization of the testicles. The testicle is visualized by prefemoral coelioscopy (**Fig. 14**A, B).

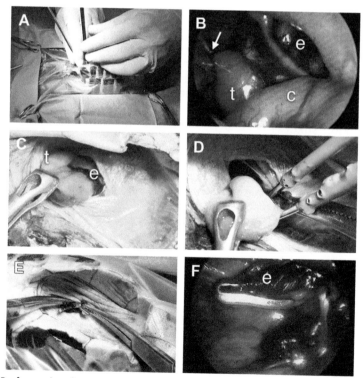

Fig. 14. Prefemoral endoscopic-assisted orchiectomy in Hermann tortoises (*T hermanni*). (*A*) Introduction of a 2.7-mm endoscope with protective sheath and a 5-mm grasping forceps into the coelom. (*B*) The testicle (t) is visualized and grasped (*arrow*). The relationship with epididymis (e), colon (c), and other surrounding tissues is evaluated. (*C*) The testicle is gently exteriorized and the epididymis is clamped with a hemostat. (*D*) Excision of the mesorchium using bipolar radiosurgery. (*E*) Excision of the mesorchium using ligation clips. Ligation clips are positioned around the mesorchium. (*F*) Hemostasis of the following ligation of the epididymis is assessed endoscopically. (*Courtesy of* Nicola Di Girolamo, Rome, Italy.)

The testicle is grasped and exteriorized (see **Fig. 14**C). Ligation clips or radiosurgery is used to excise the mesorchium while preventing bleeding (see **Fig. 14**D, E). The epididymis is evaluated endoscopically for hemorrhage (see **Fig. 14**F). The coelomic access is routinely closed.

Phallectomy

Male snakes and lizards have paired copulatory organs, that is, hemipenes, which lie in respective sacs caudal to the cloaca in the ventral tail. Male chelonians have a single copulatory organ, that is, a penis (synonym, phallus), which lies in the cloaca. Phallectomy is used to resolve penile/hemipenile disorders or for population control, as an alternative to orchiectomy.[33] Corrective surgeries of the penis may be indicated in rare occasions.

Penile or hemipenile prolapse is a very common presentation (**Fig. 15**).[47] If the tissue is already necrotic or the prolapse is recurrent, amputation is required. Amputation is performed in toto, as the penis and hemipenes do not contain the urethra. In squamates, amputation of a single hemipene does not preclude reproduction, whereas in chelonians phallectomy precludes reproduction.[33]

Surgical technique

The reptile is positioned in dorsal recumbency and the penis/hemipene is surgically prepped. In small individuals, 2 transfixing ligatures are placed at the base of the penis/hemipene (see **Fig. 15**B). The tissue is excised distal to the ligatures. In larger chelonians, each half of the phallus may be individually double ligated with encircling absorbable sutures.[48] The penile stump can be closed with a simple continuous or a purse-string suture, in particular in larger species.[33]

URINARY TRACT SURGERY
Kidneys Biopsy

In chelonians, kidneys may be reached by the coelomic or extracoelomic approach. The extracoelomic approach permits visualization of the kidney with the assistance of an endoscope and to obtain endoscopic-guided or open surgical biopsies. Briefly, the prefemoral incision is made slightly more caudal than for standard coelomic access. Advancement of the endoscope in the caudodorsal direction, between the

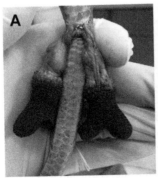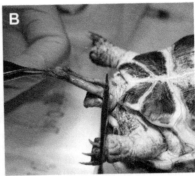

Fig. 15. (A) Bilateral hemipenile prolapse in a snake. Note the engorged size of the hemipenes, making repositioning impossible. Resection of both hemipenes was performed. (B) Phallus amputation in a Russian tortoise (*Testudo horsfieldii*). The base of the phallus is clamped, ligated, and transected. (*Courtesy of* Christoph Mans, Madison, WI.)

coelomic aponeurosis and the broad iliacus muscle, permits visualization of the kidney and obtainment of tissue biopsies (**Fig. 16A**).[49]

In lizards, the kidneys are located dorsally in the pelvic canal, caudal to the gonads. There are 2 main approaches to kidneys in lizards:

- For gross evaluation and surgical biopsy, the lizard is positioned in lateral recumbency, the hindlimb displaced cranially, and an incision is made between the hindlimb and the base of the tail.[50]
- For endoscopic visualization and biopsy, the lizard is positioned in lateral recumbency, the hindlimb displaced caudally, and a vertical incision is made in the left paralumbar region. A rigid endoscope housed in an operating sheath is inserted in the coelomic cavity, which is insufflated with CO_2. Once the kidney is visualized, biopsy forceps are passed through the operative channel and multiple biopsies of representative renal regions are obtained.[51]

In snakes, it is advantageous to mark the exact location of the kidney of interest during an earlier ultrasonographic examination of the coelom. With the snake in lateral recumbency, a standard coeliotomy is performed in proximity of the kidney. Subcutaneous tissue and perirenal fat are bluntly separated. The renal capsule is incised, and, after gross examination of the whole kidney, biopsies are obtained (see **Fig. 16B**).

Nephrectomy

In snakes, neoplasms or degenerative disorders of kidneys are not uncommon, and unilateral nephrectomy is associated with an acceptable prognosis if the remaining kidney is functional.[52] Often, a swelling of the caudal third of the snake is present (**Fig. 17A**).[52] Standard coeliotomy is performed at the level of the affected kidney (see **Fig. 17B**). The contralateral kidney should be grossly inspected (see **Fig. 17C**). The affected kidney is isolated from the surrounding tissue. The renal vein and the renal arteries are ligated (see **Fig. 17D**). The ureter is ligated distal and the kidney removed. A unilateral gonadectomy may need to be performed, as the vas deferens in males and the oviduct in females are in contiguity with the kidney.[52]

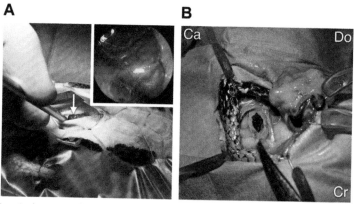

A   **B**

Fig. 16. Surgical approaches for kidney biopsy in reptiles. (*A*) Prefemoral extracoelomic approach, in a Hermann tortoise (*T hermanni*). Notice that renal tissue is visible through the incision (*arrow*). *Inset*: endoscopic visualization of the kidney through the prefemoral extracoelomic approach. (*B*) Open surgical biopsy of the kidney in a red-tailed boa constrictor (*Boa constrictor constrictor*). Ca, caudal; Cr, cranial; Do, dorsal. (*Courtesy of* [A] Nicola Di Girolamo, Rome, Italy; [B] Paolo Selleri, Rome, Italy.)

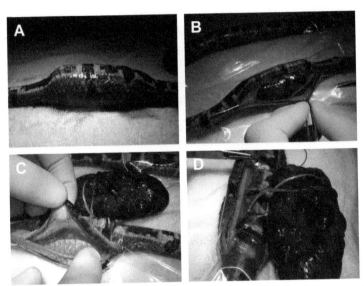

Fig. 17. Nephrectomy in a kingsnake (*Lampropeltis* sp). (*A*) The animal was presented for a swelling of the caudal third of the abdomen. (*B*) Paraventral coeliotomy is performed at the level of the affected kidney. (*C*) The contralateral kidney is grossly evaluated. (*D*) The blood vessels are ligated with absorbable monofilament sutures. (*From* Di Girolamo N, Selleri P. Management of diseased *Lampropeltis* spp. In: Grano M, Cattaneo C, editors. *Lampropeltis*: biology, ethology and breeding. Venice (Italy): Testudo Edizioni. p. 73. [in Italian]; with permission.)

Cystotomy

Cystotomy may be indicated for removal of cystic calculi and ectopic eggs from the urinary bladder.[28,30,53] In recent years, alternative techniques to routine cystotomy, in particular in chelonians, have been reported, which are less invasive. These less-invasive techniques include transurethral endoscopic techniques (cystoscopy) or pre-femoral endoscopy-assisted cystotomy.[28,54–56] However, if such approaches fail, for example, when dealing with cystic calculi of large size,[56] cystotomy may be required. In general, to resolve the presence of cystic calculi or ectopic eggs in the urinary bladder in chelonians, the surgical procedure should be elected in the following order:

- Transurethral endoscopic retrieval, mechanical destruction (eggs), or lithotripsy (calculi)
- Prefemoral fossa coeliotomy and cystotomy
- Standard coeliotomy and cystotomy

Removal of uroliths through a prefemoral fossa approach is not always feasible. In a case series of 10 desert tortoises (*Gopherus agassizii*), good candidates for the prefemoral fossa approach were large tortoises (more than 15 cm in carapace length), with small calculi (less than twice the length of the fossa) that did not have a laminated radiographic appearance.[57]

In rare instances (eg, neoplasms, chronic prolapses of the urinary bladder) partial cystectomy may be indicated.

Surgical technique

Access to the coelom is routinely performed through a paramedian incision in lizards[30] and through plastron osteotomy or prefemoral fossa incision in chelonians.[57] In small to medium species, manipulation and exteriorization of the urinary bladder should be reduced to the minimum, due to the risk of trauma of the thin bladder wall. Stay sutures on the urinary bladder wall and moist gauze around the surgical site minimize urine leakage into the coelom. If prefemoral cystotomy is performed, then the bladder wall should be temporarily marsupialized to the abdominal muscles (**Fig. 18**A, B) or stay sutures placed in the bladder (see **Fig. 18**C) to avoid contamination of the coelom and tearing of the bladder wall during manipulation. In small to medium-sized chelonians undergoing plastron osteotomy, the author uses either a longitudinal incision (**Fig. 19**A) or a transverse incision in the cranio-ventral aspect of the bladder (see **Fig. 19**B). Such incision allows the surgeon to gain a proper access to the urinary bladder, without the need of extending the plastron incision caudally. In lizards, a longitudinal incision is made in the ventral aspect of the bladder.[30] The bladder stones or eggs present in the urinary bladder are removed. Eventually, retrograde use of endoscope may be useful to ascertain the removal of all the material. The urinary bladder wall is closed with a monofilament suture in a single or double inverting layer. A rounded, atraumatic needle and minimal traction are mandatory to avoid rupture of the urinary bladder wall during suture in small to medium-sized reptiles.

GASTROINTESTINAL TRACT SURGERY

Surgery of the GI tract is indicated in reptiles in several situations including, but not limited to the following:

- GI foreign bodies and impaction, due to nonselective feeding habits, active pica, or geophagy, resulting in moderate to severe cases of impaction with need for surgical resolution (**Fig. 20**)[58–60]

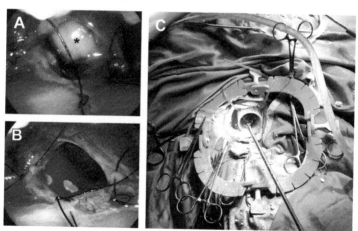

Fig. 18. Prefemoral cystotomy in chelonians. (*A*) Painted turtle (*Chrysemys picta*). The urinary bladder contains an ectopic egg (*asterisk*) and the cystotomy incision in marsupialized to the abdominal muscle at the level of the prefemoral incision. This reduces the risk of contamination of the coelom with bladder content and tearing of the bladder wall during manipulation. (*B*) Same animal after ectopic egg removal from the bladder. Note the sutures are placed for marsupialization. The sutures are removed and the bladder wall closed after egg removal. (*C*) African spurred tortoise (*C sulcata*). Cystotomy was performed for urolith removal. Note the stay sutures placed in the urinary bladder wall to avoid contamination of the coelom. Also note the plastic tube placed through the prefemoral incision into the bladder, to be used as a working channel to aid introduction of instruments and suction into the bladder. (*Courtesy of* Christoph Mans, Madison, WI.)

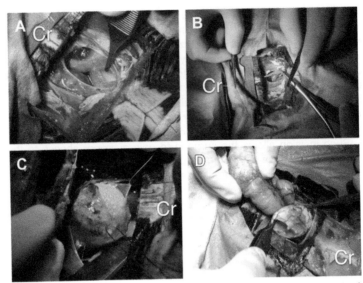

Fig. 19. Ectopic egg retention in chelonians. (*A, B*) Removal of an ectopic egg in the urinary bladder of a Hermann tortoise (*T hermanni*) by plastron osteotomy and cystotomy with a longitudinal incision. After removal of the ectopic egg, the bladder is sutured in a double layer. Note how the assistant maintains the urinary bladder by the 2 stay sutures. Traction on the stay sutures should be avoided to prevent laceration of the urinary bladder wall. (*C*) Cystotomy for removal of an ectopic egg in a Hermann tortoise. In cases in which the urinary bladder is difficult to exteriorize, the author favors a transverse incision on its cranio-ventral aspect. (*D*) Removal of an ectopic egg free in the coelom of a Hermann tortoise. Cr, cranial. (*Courtesy of* Nicola Di Girolamo, Rome, Italy.)

- Fecalomas (synonym, fecalith) may form has a result of dehydration or in carnivores as a consequence of feeding prey too large too frequently[61]
- Gastric or intestinal neoplasia[62]
- Chronic disorders requiring diagnostic biopsies of stomach or intestine[63]
- Intussusceptions,[64] volvulus,[65] and strictures[65]

Minimally invasive surgical techniques are preferred whenever possible. To date, with the availability of endoscopy it is possible to retrieve gastric foreign bodies and obtain gastric biopsies.[23] However, in some instances, endoscopic retrieval of foreign bodies may not be feasible, and endoscopic biopsies of the stomach may not be diagnostic.[62] In such cases, surgical access to the GI tract is required.

Principles of Gastrointestinal Surgery

Basic surgical principles for gastrointestinal surgery in mammals also apply in reptiles.[11,66] Strict adherence to such principles is mandatory, as dehiscence of a wound of the GI tract leads to generalized bacterial coelomitis and potentially death.[64]

A sterile spoon may assist in a delicate exteriorization of the GI tract (see **Fig. 20**A). The exteriorized GI tract should be packed with warm sterile gauze to trap inadvertent leakage and to prevent dehydration of the viscera. After completion of the procedure, copious irrigation with fluids and abdominal lavage are recommended before closure. Apposing or inverting suture patterns are acceptable.[66] Monofilament, absorbable

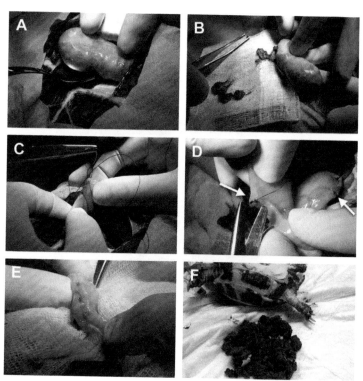

Fig. 20. Gastrotomy and enterotomy in a Horsfield tortoise *(T horsfieldii)* to relieve severe bark impaction. (*A*) The stomach is gently exteriorized with the assistance of a sterile spoon. (*B*) Removal of the abundant foreign material from the stomach. (*C*) The first suture layer is performed with 4 to 0 monofilament in a simple continuous pattern. (*D*) Multiple incisions (*arrows*) in different sections of the gastrointestinal tract were required for removal of the impacted bark. (*E*) Appearance of an enterotomy site after placement of the second suture layer, notice the moderate inversion. (*F*) Removed ingested bark material. (*Courtesy of* Nicola Di Girolamo, Rome, Italy.)

sutures are placed in either continuous or interrupted patterns. Round-bodied or taper-cut needles should be used to prevent tearing of the intestinal wall caused by cutting needles.

Gastrotomy

Standard coeliotomy is performed as previously described. The stomach is identified and stay sutures are applied to maintain the stomach at the level of the surgical site. Traction of stay sutures should be avoided in small to medium-sized reptiles, as the gastric serosa is thin and prone to rupture. A stab incision with a scalpel is performed along the greater curvature. After removal of stomach contents and foreign bodies, the stomach is lavaged and inspected. The stomach is approximated in 2 layers using monofilament absorbable sutures (**Fig. 21**).

In a recent report, a complete gastrectomy was attempted in a diamond python because of gastric adenocarcinoma, but the snake died the night following the procedure.[62]

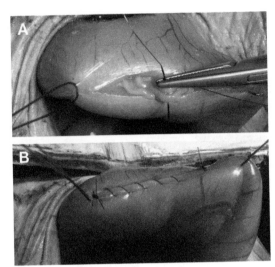

Fig. 21. Closure of the stomach in a leopard tortoise (*Stigmochelys pardalis*) following gastrotomy via the plastron osteotomy approach. (*A*) Note the use of stay sutures to maintain the stomach at the level of the plastron. The mucosa was sutured with a simple continuous suture pattern as a separate layer. (*B*) The second apposing suture layer incorporates the submucosa, serosal, and muscularis layers. (*Courtesy of* Nicola Di Girolamo, Rome, Italy.)

Enterotomy

Standard coeliotomy is performed. In large chelonians, the prefemoral fossa approach also may be used.[67] In snakes, coeliotomy is performed in proximity of the intestinal section of interest. The intestinal wall is inspected and palpated. Possible abnormal findings during intestinal obstructions include a change in color of the affected tract (dark red to violet), vascular stasis, and congestion.[59] The mesentery has a variable length and may prevent exteriorization through the coeliotomy incision. A stab incision is performed between 2 stay sutures and the content of the intestine is evacuated (see **Fig. 20**B; **Fig. 22**A). In cases of intestinal impaction caused by substrate or excessive food intake, difficulties may be encountered when trying to remove all the content from the intestine. Multiple incisions[60] (see **Fig. 20**D) or removal of all the material from a proximal single incision through gently retrograde massage of the bowel (ie, "milking") are viable options. The intestine is lavaged with warm fluids (see **Fig. 22**B). The enterotomy incision is closed using monofilament absorbable suture in a 2-layer simple interrupted or continuous pattern (see **Figs. 20**C, E and **22**C, D). In most cases, before and after radiographs are valuable tools for communication with the owner (see **Fig. 22**E, F).

Enterectomy

End-to-end anastomosis is technically feasible in reptiles and is performed when ischemic, necrotic, neoplastic segments of intestine are present. Although in an experimental study in Burmese pythons (*Python molurus bivittatus*), the middle third of the small intestine was resected without complications in 21 snakes,[68] in general these surgeries carry an uncertain prognosis in clinical cases.[64]

After placement of intestinal occluding forceps, the diseased section of the bowel is transected. Anastomosis of the 2 cut ends is performed with a simple continuous suture on either side of 2 simple interrupted sutures at the dorsal and ventral aspects of

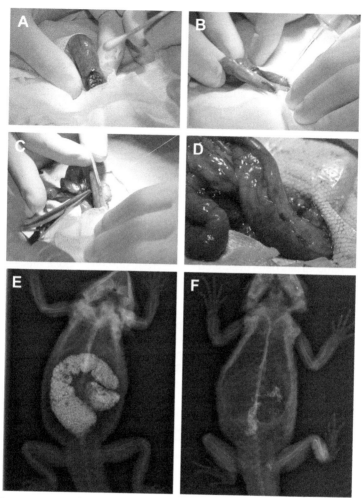

Fig. 22. Enterotomy to relieve intestinal impaction in a bearded dragon (*P vitticeps*) presented for abdominal distension and anorexia. (*A*) Visualization, exteriorization, and enterotomy of a constipated intestine. (*B*) After removal of foreign material, the intestine is lavaged with warm fluids. (*C*) The enterotomy site is sutured in a simple interrupted pattern. (*D*) Close-up view of the intestine after a second layer of sutures was placed in a Cushing pattern. Notice the inverting pattern. (*E*) Dorsoventral radiograph at presentation. Notice severe impaction caused by the litter. (*F*) Dorsoventral radiograph following the surgery. (*Courtesy of* Nicola Di Girolamo, Rome, Italy.)

the intestinal lumen. Standard techniques may be used to resolve differences in bowel diameter of the orad and aborad bowel segments. Usually, disparities can be resolved just by suture spacing techniques. Alternatively, the smaller bowel segment can be cut at a 30° to 45° angle or the larger bowel segment can be partially closed.

If colonic lesions occur near the cloaca, biopsy or resection of masses also had been successfully performed after exteriorization of the colon through the cloaca.[69] Briefly, the cloaca may be partially everted by manual pressure. Once the lesion is localized, the affected area of the bowel is excised and an end-to-end anastomosis is performed.[69]

Enterostomy

If the 2 ends of the intestine cannot be approximated without excessive tension, a permanent enterostomy should be considered.[64] The intestinal mucosa is sutured to the body wall with absorbable monofilament sutures in a simple interrupted pattern. A catheter is placed in the enterostomy site to maintain patency. The aborad segment of the intestine is closed with a purse-string suture. In a pine snake (Pituophis melanoleucus) that underwent enterostomy as a consequence of ileocolic intussusception, dehiscence of the enterostomy site, with leakage of the intestinal contents and a fibrinous peritonitis occurred, with death of the snake at day 30 following surgery.[64]

LIVER AND GALLBLADDER

The surgical approach to the liver and gallbladder is indicated for resection of hepatic masses (eg, neoplasm, granuloma, abscess), for collection of diagnostic samples and for removal of choleliths.[32,70,71] Minimally invasive laparoscopic techniques for liver biopsy have been described in lizards, chelonians, and snakes, which are preferred.[32,72,73]

Cholelith removal has been described in a bearded dragon (Pogona vitticeps).[71] The surgical technique is identical to the one currently used in small animal surgery.

Open Surgical Biopsy/Partial Hepatectomy

In squamates, a standard coeliotomy is performed. In snakes, coeliotomy is performed in their middle third at the level of the liver. If only tissue biopsy is needed, the coelomic access may be extremely small. Adequate visualization of the liver is obtained by dilation with retractors (**Fig. 23**). The connective tissue capsule, Glisson capsule, is incised and liver tissue may be sampled. Ligation clips may be used to provide hemostasis.

For partial hepatectomy, a larger coelomic incision is needed to allow partial exteriorization of the liver. The altered part may be removed by placing loose suture around the liver that crush the tissue as the ligature is tightened (ie, "guillotine technique") or placing ligation clips.[70] Attention should be paid to avoid rupture of the caudal vena cava and the hepatic portal vein, located centrally on the ventral and dorsal surfaces of the liver.[73] The coelom is closed in a standard manner.

CLOACAL PROLAPSES

A variety of organs may prolapse from the cloaca of reptiles, including penis/hemipene, cloacal tissue, oviducts, urinary bladder, and intestine.[47] In a retrospective study, the incidence of prolapses in reptile patients was 1.9%.[47] Prolapses were more frequent in lizards and chelonians than in snakes, and the most common prolapsed organs were the penis/hemipene (35.7% of the prolapses). It is of critical importance to identify the prolapsed tissue because therapeutic approaches depend on the tissue involved.

Treatment of Cloacal Tissue Prolapse

If the tissue is vital, repositioning of the prolapse under sedation, intrathecal anesthesia, or general anesthesia can be attempted. Repositioning is performed by means of gentle pressure with cotton-tipped applicators after the application of hyperosmotic solution or sugar (**Fig. 24**B) on the tissue. Once repositioned, 2 sutures are placed at the side of the vent to reduce the chances of further prolapse (see **Fig. 24**C; **Fig. 25**D, E).[74] The use of purse-string suture, although widely used in the past, is not

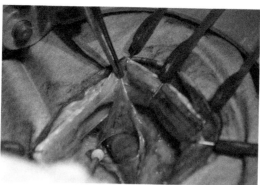

Fig. 23. Open surgical biopsy of the liver in an albino boa constrictor (*Boa constrictor imperator*). The lone star retractor permits to make a relatively small incision on the skin. (*Courtesy of* Paolo Selleri, Rome, Italy.)

recommended because of the risk of damage to the cloacal sphincter. In squamates, percutaneous tagging sutures also can be used if the cloaca itself is prolapsed (**Fig. 25B**). If these techniques fail to prevent reoccurrence of cloacal tissue prolapse, then cloacopexy and/or colonpexy should be considered (see **Fig. 25C–E**).

Resection and Anastomosis

If a hollow organ prolapse (eg, colon, oviduct) and the tissue has suffered consistent trauma, a resection and anastomosis is performed.[75] With the reptile anesthetized in dorsal recumbency (**Fig. 26A**), the prolapsed tissue is cleaned. A cylindrical stent (eg, a syringe case) is placed in the lumen and the tissue is transfixed by orthogonal needles (see **Fig. 26B**). The nonviable tissue is excised (see **Fig. 26C**), and mattress sutures are placed all around the organ (see **Fig. 26D**). With this approach, continuity of the hollow organ is maintained.

If the prolapsed organ was an oviduct, the animal should be monitored carefully for future reproductive disorder. In such instance, a unilateral ovariosalpingectomy should be performed. If the prolapsed tissue was colon, there may be risk of stricture following resection and anastomosis.[75] In such cases, under standard coeliotomy a longitudinal enterotomy incision is performed on the stricture and sutured in a transverse orientation, to increase luminal diameter.

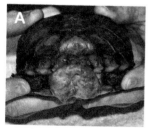
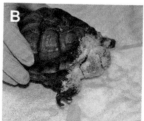
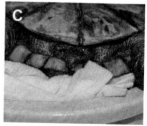

Fig. 24. Cloacal tissue prolapse in a 3-toed box turtle (*Terrapene carolina triunguis*). (*A*) Initial appearance of the prolapse. (*B*) Granulated sugar is applied to reduce the size of the prolapse. (*C*) The prolapsed tissue has been replaced and 2 simple interrupted nylon sutures are temporarily placed through the cloacal opening, to prevent recurrence of the prolapse, while the primary underlying cause was identified and treated. (*Courtesy of* Christoph Mans, Madison, WI.)

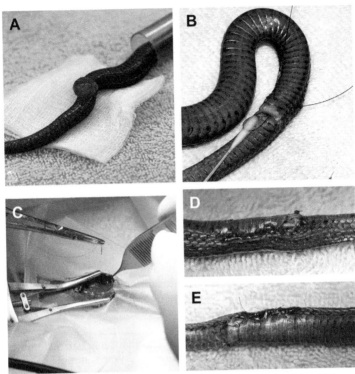

Fig. 25. Cloacal tissue prolapse in a common garter snake (*T sirtalis*). (*A*) Initial presentation. (*B*) After replacement of the prolapsed cloacal tissue, a nonabsorbable suture is placed percutaneously thought the ventral cloacal wall. The suture is passed through the tip of the cotton-tipped applicator to ensure that no additional cloacal tissue is tagged. The suture is freed from the cotton-tipped applicator before tightening of the suture. (*C*) Due to recurrence of the prolapse, a cloacopexy was performed. During coeliotomy the cloacal wall was sutured to the body wall (*D, E*). Completed cloacopexy and skin closure. In addition, 2 simple interrupted sutures have been placed through the cloacal opening. (*Courtesy of* Christoph Mans, Madison, WI.)

PEDIATRIC SURGERY
Omphalectomy

Omphalectomy, that is, removal of the yolk sac, may be indicated in case of the following:

- Lack of yolk sac internalization
- Yolk sac infection
- Retained yolk sac

In case of chronic lack of internalization, the yolk sac and the associated vasculature are surgically prepared and ligated. Ideally, ligation and excision should be made as close to the intestine as possible. After yolk sac removal, the opening of the coelomic cavity is routinely closed. The yolk sac may be removed after internalization, typically in case of infection.[76] A full-thickness incision of the plastron is performed cranially and caudally from the umbilicus. The yolk sac is exteriorized and its attachment to the intestine is ligated with a ligation clip.[76] The yolk sac is excised distal to the clip and the plastron apposed with a horizontal mattress pattern.

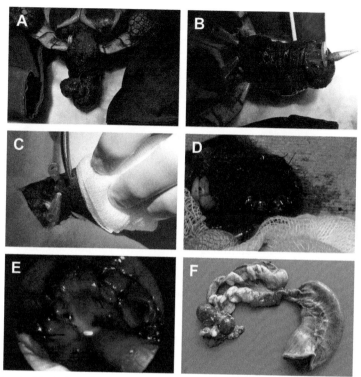

Fig. 26. Surgical technique (resection and anastomosis) for hollow organ prolapse through the cloaca. (*A*) An adult female Hermann tortoise (*T hermanni*) presented with a 48-hour history of tissue prolapse from the cloaca. (*B, C*) A syringe is placed in the lumen and the tissue is transfixed by orthogonal needles. (*C*) The nonviable tissue is excised. (*D*) The 2 layers were anastomosed with 5 to 0 absorbable monofilament synthetic sutures in a simple interrupted pattern. (*E*) The tissue is repositioned in the cloaca under endoscopic visualization. A cotton-tipped applicator is used to apply gentle pressure. (*F*) The excised tissue was the right oviduct and the right ovary. (*Courtesy of* Nicola Di Girolamo, Rome, Italy.)

TAIL AMPUTATION

Amputation of an infected, traumatized or necrotic tail is a common problem in lizards. Surgical amputation of the tail is recommended to achieve primary wound healing following surgical resection of the diseased distal tail and closure of the amputation site. Radiographs should be taken before surgical amputation to evaluate for underlying bone involvement. Amputation of a significant portion of the tail in arboreal lizards (eg, green iguana), has substantial effects on their ability to balance and climb. Therefore, owners should be informed that the enclosure may require adjustment after tail amputation and that changes in locomotion are possible.

Technique

The patient is anesthetized and placed in ventral recumbence. The tail amputation site is surgically prepped and a tourniquet is placed. The location of the hemipenes should be considered in cases of proximal tail amputation. Symmetric wedge incisions of the skin are made on lateral aspects of the tail in lizards with laterally flattened tails (eg, iguanas, **Fig. 27**A) or on the dorsal and ventral aspect in lizards with dorso-ventrally

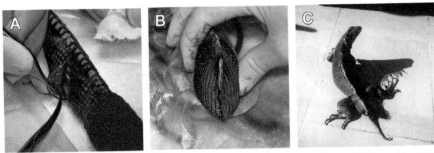

Fig. 27. Tail amputation in a green iguana (*I iguana*). (*A*) Wedge-shaped skin incisions are made on the lateral aspects of the tail. (*B*) Appearance of the amputation site after completion of surgery. Note the laterally flattened shape of the tail. (*C*) Regrowth of a partial tail several months after proximal tail amputation. (*Courtesy of* Christoph Mans, Madison, WI.)

flattened tails (eg, bearded dragons, **Fig. 28**). The skin incision should be made distal enough to allow for tension-free wound closure following amputation, but at the same time be proximal enough to avoid incomplete excision of diseased tissue. The soft tissue and bone are transected (see **Fig. 28**A). The ventral tail vein may require ligation in larger lizards. The amputation site is lavaged and assessed for hemorrhage after release of the tourniquet (see **Fig. 28**B). The muscles should be apposed over the

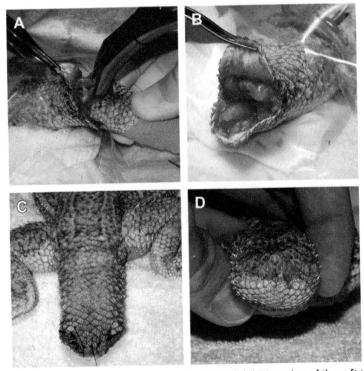

Fig. 28. Tail amputation in a bearded dragon (*P vitticeps*). (*A*) Dissection of the soft tissue and bone. (*B*) Appearance of the amputation site after resection of the distal tail. (*C*) Tail amputation site after closure. (*D*) The healed amputation site after suture removal. (*Courtesy of* Christoph Mans, Madison, WI.)

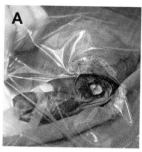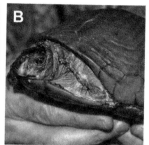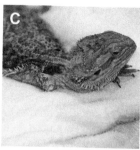

Fig. 29. Forelimb amputation in reptiles. (*A*) Left forelimb amputation through the scapula-humeral joint in a three-toed box turtle (*T carolina triunguis*). (*B*) Appearance of the surgical site after recovery. (*C*) Bearded dragon (*P vitticeps*) after amputation through the scapula-humeral joint. (*Courtesy of* Christoph Mans, Madison, WI.)

vertebrae with simple interrupted sutures. The skin edges are trimmed and closed with horizontal mattress sutures (see **Figs. 27**B and **28**C). The amputation site can be bandaged for the first few days after surgery to aid in absorption of wound discharge. Suture removal is recommended 4 to 6 weeks after amputation (see **Fig. 28**D). Regrowth of the tail is possible after surgical amputation, but not commonly seen (see **Fig. 27**C).

LIMB AMPUTATION

Indications for amputation of limbs in lizards and chelonians are severe trauma or infection, severe joint infections, which are refractory to treatment, as well as nonhealing chronic fractures or neoplasia. In general, chronic infected distal limb wounds and joint infections, in particular with associated osteomyelitis, usually do not respond to medical therapy and wound management, and instead limb amputation should be considered. Amputation of the forelimbs should be performed through the scapulohumeral joint (**Fig. 29**), and amputations of the hindlimbs through the coxofemoral joint. Midshaft amputation of the humerus or femur is not recommended, because it is very likely that the remaining limb stump will be traumatized by attempted ambulation. In female reptiles used for breeding purposes or planned to be released in the wild, amputation of the hindlimb might interfere with successful reproduction, because digging of nesting sites may be impaired. Limb amputation is performed using the same techniques as in mammals. Complications are uncommon.

ACKNOWLEDGMENTS

Dr Paolo Selleri and Dr Tommaso Collarile are kindly acknowledged for suggestions, images and assistance during some of the surgeries described in this article.

REFERENCES

1. Innis CJ, Hernandez-Divers S, Martinez-Jimenez D. Coelioscopic-assisted prefemoral oophorectomy in chelonians. J Am Vet Med Assoc 2007;230:1049–52.
2. Mans C, Sladky KK. Diagnosis and management of oviductal disease in three red-eared slider turtles (*Trachemys scripta elegans*). J Small Anim Pract 2012; 53:234–9.

3. Mans C, Sladky KK. Endoscopically guided removal of cloacal calculi in three African spurred tortoises (Geochelone sulcata). J Am Vet Med Assoc 2012; 240:869–75.

4. Selleri P, Di Girolamo N, Melidone R. Cystoscopic sex identification of posthatch-ling chelonians. J Am Vet Med Assoc 2013;242:1744–50.

5. Innis CJ, Feinsod R, Hanlon J, et al. Coelioscopic orchiectomy can be effectively and safely accomplished in chelonians. Vet Rec 2013;172:526.

6. Stumpel J, Benato L, Eatwell K. Transcutaneous pulmonoscopic removal of intra-pneumonic mucus in a bearded dragon (Pogona vitticeps). Vet Rec 2012;170: 338.

7. Myers DA, Wellehan JF Jr, Isaza R. Saccular lung cannulation in a ball python (Python regius) to treat a tracheal obstruction. J Zoo Wildl Med 2009;40:214–6.

8. Jenicek M. Clinical case reporting in evidence-based medicine. London: Arnold; 2001.

9. Di Girolamo N. Characteristics and limits of effectiveness of intervention studies in veterinary medicine. Proceedings of the 86th SCIVAC international congress. May 31st 2015. Rimini, Italy. p. 467.

10. Schumacher J, Mans C. Anesthesia. In: Mader DR, Divers SJ, editors. Current ther-apy in reptile medicine and surgery. St Louis (MO): W.B. Saunders; 2014. p. 134–53.

11. Frye FL. 2nd edition. Biomedical and surgical aspects of captive reptile husband-ry, vol. II. Melbourne (Australia): Krieger Publishing; 1991.

12. Mader DR, Bennett RA. Surgery: soft tissue, orthopedics and fracture repair. In: Mader DR, editor. Reptile medicine and surgery. 2nd edition. St Louis (MO): Sa-unders Elsevier; 2006. p. 581–612.

13. Smith DA, Barker IK, Allen B. The effect of ambient temperature and type of wound on healing of cutaneous wounds in the common garter snake (Thamno-phis sirtalis). Can J Vet Res 1988;52:120–8.

14. Govett PD, Harms CA, Linder KE, et al. Effect of four different suture materials on the surgical wound healing of loggerhead sea turtles, Caretta caretta. J Herpetol Med Surg 2004;14:6–11.

15. McFadden MS, Bennett RA, Kinsel MJ, et al. Evaluation of the histologic reactions to commonly used suture materials in the skin and musculature of ball pythons (Python regius). Am J Vet Res 2011;72:1397–406.

16. Hannon DE, Garner MM, Reavill DR. Squamous cell carcinomas in inland bearded dragons (Pogona vitticeps). J Herpetol Med Surg 2011;21:101–6.

17. Kroenlein KR, Sleeman JM, Holladay SD, et al. Inability to induce tympanic squamous metaplasia using organochlorine compounds in vitamin A-deficient red-eared sliders (Trachemys scripta elegans). J Wildl Dis 2008;44:664–9.

18. Mans C, Braun J. Update on common nutritional disorders of captive reptiles. Vet Clin North Am Exot Anim Pract 2014;17:369–95.

19. Chen S, Hottinger HA, Antinoff N. Permanent tracheostomy in a red tailed boa with tracheal avulsion. In: Proceedings of the Annual Conference Association of Reptilian and Amphibian Veterinarians. Seattle, WA, August 6–12, 2011. p. 118.

20. Drew ML, Phalen DN, Berridge BR, et al. Partial tracheal obstruction due to chon-dromas in ball pythons (Python regius). J Zoo Wildl Med 1999;30:151–7.

21. Diethelm G, Stauber E, Tillson M, et al. Tracheal resection and anastomosis for an intratracheal chondroma in a ball python. J Am Vet Med Assoc 1996;209:786–8.

22. Hyland RJ. Surgical removal of a fish hook from the oesophagus of a turtle. Aust Vet J 2002;80:54–6.

23. Mans C. Clinical update on diagnosis and management of disorders of the diges-tive system of reptiles. J Exot Pet Med 2013;22:141–62.

24. Jaeger GH, Wosar MA, Harms CA, et al. Use of a supraplastron approach to the coelomic cavity for repair of an esophageal tear in a loggerhead sea turtle. J Am Vet Med Assoc 2003;223:353–5, 311.
25. Lynn WG. The thyroid. In: Gans C, Parson TS, editors. Biology of reptilia. New York: Academic Press; 1970. p. 201–34.
26. Hernandez-Divers SJ, Knott CD, MacDonald J. Diagnosis and surgical treatment of thyroid adenoma-induced hyperthyroidism in a green iguana (*Iguana iguana*). J Zoo Wildl Med 2001;32:465–75.
27. Hadfield CA, Clayton LA, Clancy MM, et al. Proliferative thyroid lesions in three diplodactylid geckos: *Nephrurus amyae, Nephrurus levis,* and *Oedura marmorata.* J Zoo Wildl Med 2012;43:131–40.
28. Di Girolamo N, Selleri P. Clinical applications of cystoscopy in chelonians. Vet Clin North Am 2015;18(3):507–26.
29. Hernández-Divers SJ, Stahl SJ, Rakich PM, et al. Comparison of CO(2) laser and 4.0 MHz radiosurgery for making incisions in the skin and muscles of green iguanas (*Iguana iguana*). Vet Rec 2009;164:13–6.
30. Kwantes LJ. Surgical correction of cystic urolithiasis in an iguana. Can Vet J 1992; 33:752–3.
31. Knafo SE, Divers SJ, Rivera S, et al. Sterilisation of hybrid Galapagos tortoises (*Geochelone nigra*) for island restoration. Part 1: endoscopic oophorectomy of females under ketamine-medetomidine anaesthesia. Vet Rec 2011;168:47.
32. Divers SJ, Stahl SJ, Camus A. Evaluation of diagnostic coelioscopy including liver and kidney biopsy in freshwater turtles (*Trachemys scripta*). J Zoo Wildl Med 2010;41:677–87.
33. Rivera S, Divers SJ, Knafo SE, et al. Sterilisation of hybrid Galapagos tortoises (*Geochelone nigra*) for island restoration. Part 2: phallectomy of males under intrathecal anaesthesia with lidocaine. Vet Rec 2011;168:78.
34. Funk RS. Early neutering of male green iguanas, Iguana iguana—an experiment. In: Proceedings of the Annual Conference Association of Reptilian and Amphibian Veterinarians. Reno, NV, October 17–21, 2000. p. 147–9.
35. Blackburn DG. Structure, function, and evolution of the oviducts of squamate reptiles, with special reference to viviparity and placentation. J Exp Zool 1998;282: 560–617.
36. Fox A. The urinogenital system of reptiles. In: Gans C, Parsons TS, editors. Biology of the reptilia, vol. 6. London: Academic Press; 1977. p. 1–157. Morphology E.
37. Stahl SJ. Veterinary management of snake reproduction. Vet Clin North Am Exot Anim Pract 2002;5:615–36.
38. Cruz Cardona JA, Conley KJ, Wellehan JF, et al. Incomplete ovariosalpingectomy and subsequent malignant granulosa cell tumor in a female green iguana (*Iguana iguana*). J Am Vet Med Assoc 2011;239:237–42.
39. Funk RS. Lizard reproductive medicine and surgery. Vet Clin North Am Exot Anim Pract 2002;5:579–613.
40. Innis CJ. Endoscopy and endosurgery of the chelonian reproductive tract. Vet Clin North Am Exot Anim Pract 2010;13:243–54.
41. Biron K, Heckers K. Removal of a testicular tumor from a veiled chameleon (Chamaeleo calyptratus). In: Proceedings of the Annual Conference Association of Reptilian and Amphibian Veterinarians. South Padre Island, TX, October 23–29, 2010. p. 77–8.
42. Pees M, Ludewig E, Plenz B, et al. Imaging diagnosis–seminoma causing liver compression in a spur-thighed tortoise (*Testudo graeca*). Vet Radiol Ultrasound 2015;56:E21–4.

43. Willuhn J, Hetzel U, Preuss D, et al. Seminoma in a brown housesnake (*Lamprophis fuliginosus fuliginosus*). Tierarztl Prax 2003;3:176–9.
44. Golinski A, Kubička L, John-Alder H, et al. Elevated testosterone is required for male copulatory behavior and aggression in Madagascar ground gecko (*Paroedura picta*). Gen Comp Endocrinol 2014;205:133–41.
45. Kinney ME, Johnson SM, Sladky KK. Behavioral evaluation of red-eared slider turtles (*Trachemys scripta elegans*) administered either morphine or butorphanol following unilateral gonadectomy. J Herpetol Med Surg 2011; 21:54–62.
46. Paries S, Funcke S, Ziegler L, et al. Endoscopic assisted orchiectomy in Herman's tortoises (*Testudo hermanni* sp.). Tierarztl Prax Ausg K Kleintiere Heimtiere 2014;42:383–9.
47. Hedley J, Eatwell K. Cloacal prolapses in reptiles: a retrospective study of 56 cases. J Small Anim Pract 2014;55:265–8.
48. Innis CJ, Boyer TH. Chelonian reproductive disorders. Vet Clin North Am Exot Anim Pract 2002;5:555–78, vi.
49. Hernandez-Divers SJ. Endoscopic renal evaluation and biopsy of Chelonia. Vet Rec 2004;154:73–80.
50. Mader DR. A minimally invasive procedure for renal biopsies in the green iguana, Iguana iguana. In: Proceedings of the Annual Conference Association of Reptilian and Amphibian Veterinarians. Kansas City, MO, 1998. p. 141–2.
51. Hernandez-Divers SJ, Stahl SJ, Stedman NL, et al. Renal evaluation in the healthy green iguana (*Iguana iguana*): assessment of plasma biochemistry, glomerular filtration rate, and endoscopic biopsy. J Zoo Wildl Med 2005;36:155–68.
52. Keck M, Zimmerman DM, Ramsay EC, et al. Renal adenocarcinoma in cape coral snakes (*Aspidelaps lubricus lubricus*). J Herpetol Med Surg 2011;21:5–9.
53. Thomas HL, Willer CJ, Wosar MA, et al. Egg-retention in the urinary bladder of a Florida cooter turtle, *Pseudemys floridana floridana*. J Herpetol Med Surg 2002;12:4–6.
54. Minter LJ, Wood MW, Hill TL, et al. Cystoscopic guided removal of ectopic eggs from the urinary bladder of the Florida cooter turtle (*Pseudemys floridana floridana*). J Zoo Wildl Med 2010;41:503–9.
55. Mans C, Foster JD. Endoscopy-guided ectopic egg removal from the urinary bladder in a leopard tortoise (*Stigmochelys pardalis*). Can Vet J 2014;55:569–72.
56. Nardini G, Bielli M, Nicoli S, et al. Endoscopic lithotripsy in chelonians: two cases. Veterinaria 2014;28:33 [in Italian].
57. Mangone B, Johnson JD. Surgical removal of cystic calculi via the inguinal fossa and other techniques applicable to the approach in the desert tortoises, Gopherus agassizii. In: Proceedings of the Annual Conference Association of Reptilian and Amphibian Veterinarians. Kansas City, MO, 1998. p. 87–8.
58. Skoczylas R. Physiology of the digestive tract. In: Gans C, Gans KA, editors. Biology of the reptilia, vol. 8. London: Academic Press; 1978. p. 589–717. Physiology.
59. Büker M, Foldenauer U, Simova-Curd S, et al. Gastrointestinal obstruction caused by a radiolucent foreign body in a green iguana (*Iguana iguana*). Can Vet J 2010;51:511–4.
60. Rahal SC, Teixeira CR, Castro GB, et al. Intestinal obstruction by stones in a turtle. Can Vet J 1998;39:375–6.
61. Corbit AG, Person C, Hayes WK. Constipation associated with brumation? Intestinal obstruction caused by a fecalith in a wild red diamond rattlesnake (*Crotalus ruber*). J Anim Physiol Anim Nutr (Berl) 2014;98:96–9.

62. Baron HR, Allavena R, Melville LM, et al. Gastric adenocarcinoma in a diamond python (*Morelia spilota spilota*). Aust Vet J 2014;92:405–9.

63. Cerveny SN, Garner MM, D'Agostino JJ, et al. Evaluation of gastroscopic biopsy for diagnosis of *Cryptosporidium* sp. infection in snakes. J Zoo Wildl Med 2012; 43:864–71.

64. Wosar MA, Lewbart GA. Ileocolic intussusception in a pine snake (*Pituophis melanoleucus*). Vet Rec 2006;158:698–9.

65. Helmick KE, Bennett RA, Ginn P, et al. Intestinal volvulus and stricture associated with a leiomyoma in a green turtle (*Chelonia mydas*). J Zoo Wildl Med 2000;31: 221–7.

66. Fossum TW, Hedlund CS. Gastric and intestinal surgery. Vet Clin North Am Small Anim Pract 2003;33:1117–45, viii.

67. Isenbugel E, Barandun G. Surgical removal of a foreign body in a bastard turtle. Vet Med Small Anim Clin 1981;76:1766–8.

68. Secor SM, Whang EE, Lane JS, et al. Luminal and systemic signals trigger intestinal adaptation in the juvenile python. Am J Physiol Gastrointest Liver Physiol 2000;279:G1177–87.

69. Latimer KS, Rich GA. Colonic adenocarcinoma in a corn snake (*Elaphe guttata guttata*). J Zoo Wildl Med 1998;29:344–6.

70. Lawton MPC. Partial hepatectomy in a snake. In: Proceedings of the Annual Conference Association of Reptilian and Amphibian Veterinarians. Kansas City, MO, 1998. p. 127–9.

71. Ritzman TK, Garner MM. Cholelitiasis and surgical cholelith removal in a bearded dragon (Pogona vitticeps). In: Proceedings of the Annual Conference Association of Reptilian and Amphibian Veterinarians. Milwaukee, WI, August 8–15, 2009. p. 117.

72. Hernandez-Divers SJ, Stahl SJ, McBride M, et al. Evaluation of an endoscopic liver biopsy technique in green iguanas. J Am Vet Med Assoc 2007;230(12): 1849–53.

73. Isaza R, Ackerman N, Schumacher J. Ultrasound-guided percutaneous liver biopsy in snakes. Vet Radiol Ultrasound 1993;34:452–4.

74. Divers SJ. Surgery: principles and techniques. In: Girling SJ, Raiti P, editors. BSAVA manual of reptiles. 2nd edition. Gloucester (United Kingdom): British Small Animal Veterinary Association; 2004. p. 147–67.

75. Lloyd CG. Surgical management of colon prolapse and subsequent stricture in a Mediterranean spur thigh tortoise, *Testudo graeca*. J Herpetol Med Surg 2003;13: 10–3.

76. Wright K. Omphalectomy in a Galapagos tortoise, *Geochelone nigra* spp. In: Proceedings of the Annual Conference Association of Reptilian and Amphibian Veterinarians. Kansas City, MO, 1998. p. 100–01.

Avian Soft Tissue Surgery

David Sanchez-Migallon Guzman, LV, MS, DECZM (Avian, Small Mammal), DACZM

KEYWORDS

- Ingluviotomy • Tracheal resection and anastomosis • Celiotomy • Proventriculotomy
- Salpingohysterectomy • Cloacopexy

KEY POINTS

- Soft tissue retractors, microsurgical instrumentation, and magnification with surgical loupes and head-mounted lights are critical to optimize exposure and visualization.
- Hemostasis through appropriate tissue handling and dissection, radiosurgery or electrosurgery, vascular clips, and hemostatic agents are fundamental to decrease the amount of blood loss.
- Celiotomy requires removal of any fluid in the intestinal peritoneal cavity before the procedure as well as special anesthetic considerations.
- Coelomic surgery, like enterotomy or salpingotomy, has a high risk of resulting in peritonitis, airsacculitis, and pneumonia.
- Tracheal surgery could result in postsurgical tracheal stenosis, which can be minimized by near-perfect apposition of the anastomosis site, minimally reactive suture material, applying appropriate suture technique, and reducing tension at the surgical site with tension relief sutures.

INSTRUMENTATION
Microsurgical Instruments

Microsurgical instruments are preferred.[1] They should be a standard length (usually 15–17 cm), have rounded handles, and have small working tips.[2] Many microsurgical instruments are also counterbalanced and shaped to fit the notch between the base of the thumb and the index finger. When performing surgery, the hands rest firmly on the operating table. Both hands are positioned in the same manner as when writing and the instruments are manipulated with the fingers only. The most important instruments in addition to the standard surgical instruments are the microforceps, microscissors, and microneedle holders. Other instruments can be added to the set, such as

Disclosure: The author has nothing to disclose.
Avian and Exotic Pet Medicine and Surgery, School of Veterinary Medicine University of California Davis, One Shields Avenue, 2108 Tupper Hall, Davis, CA 95616, USA
E-mail address: guzman@ucdavis.edu

Vet Clin Exot Anim 19 (2016) 133–157
http://dx.doi.org/10.1016/j.cvex.2015.08.009
1094-9194/16/$ – see front matter © 2016 Elsevier Inc. All rights reserved.

microhemostats and vascular clamps. DeBakey thumb forceps are atraumatic vascular forceps that can be used to handle delicate tissues.

Radiosurgery

Radiosurgery uses high-frequency radio waves to cut with little heat damage to the adjacent tissues.[3] Radiosurgery has been shown to result in less collateral tissue damage than laser CO_2 in the skin of birds.[4] The Surgitron Dual Frequency 120 (Ellman International, Inc, Hewlett, NY) uses 4.0 MHz and offers monopolar/bipolar applications with foot pedal/finger switch control to cut and coagulate. The ground is a plate with an antenna and does not even have to be in contact with the patient. The monopolar cutting needles are mostly used for dissection, whereas the bipolar forceps are used for both dissection and sealing blood vessels (**Fig. 1**). The Harrison bipolar forceps tip have 1 arm of the tip bent at a 45° angle and are used for cutting avian skin. Radiosurgical units should not be used in the presence of flammable material.

Magnification and Illumination

Magnification is recommended to handle small and delicate tissues in small birds.[5] The ideal surgical loupes system would be comfortable; provide magnification of 3 to 5 times; have lenses with a large depth of field so more than 1 plane is in focus; and have a focal distance appropriate to the surgeon's working distance, minimizing stresses on the neck and back (ergonomic) and allowing the surgeon to look around the lenses to accomplish tasks that do not need magnification.[2] SurgiTel System (General Scientific Corporation, Inc, Ann Arbor, MI) provides lenses that meet these

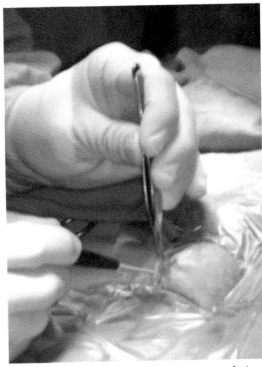

Fig. 1. Monopolar radiosurgery handle and tip used to excise a soft tissue mass. (*Courtesy of* David Sanchez-Migallon Guzman, LV, MS, DECZM (Avian, Small mammal), DACZM, Davis, CA.)

criteria. Illumination with a focal light source is recommended. Head-mounted or lens-mounted lights direct the light where the surgeon needs it, keeping it in the field of view when the head is moved, but focal lights are also available separately from loupes (**Fig. 2**).

Soft Tissue Retractors

The recommended soft tissue retractors are the smallest Balfour and Gelpi retractors for larger patients, and the Bennett avian retractor and the Doolen avian retractor (Sontec Instruments, Inc) for smaller patients.[2] The Lone Star Retractor (Lone Star Medical Products, Inc, Stafford, TX) is available in a variety of configurations and it is likely the most versatile retractor used in avian surgery (**Fig. 3**).

Vascular Clips

Hemostatic clips, such as Hemoclips (Hemoclips and Samuels Hemoclip Applier, RICA Surgical Products, Inc) are made of metal (steel, titanium, or tantalum) and serve the same purpose as ligatures.[2] They are available in various sizes. They are quick and easy to apply. It is recommended that the length of the clip be 2 to 3 times the diameter of the vessel. Right-angled appliers are also available and are especially useful for applications deep in the body cavity of small patients (**Fig. 4**).[2]

Sutures

Polydioxanone suture (Ethicon, Novartis, Somerville NJ), polyglyconate (Maxon, Covidien, Mansfield, MA), and polyglecaprone 25 (Monocryl, Ethicon) are recommended absorbable sutures.[6,7] Polyglactin 910 (Vicryl, Ethicon) causes severe inflammatory response in birds, and it is only recommended for cloacopexy to promote adhesions in the surgical site.[6,7] Polypropylene (Prolene, Ethicon), nylon, and steel are recommended nonabsorbable sutures. The sizes 3-0 to 6-0 are commonly used in avian surgery. The fewest and finest sutures possible should be used and efforts should be made to minimize tissue trauma to decrease the risk of would infection. Birds generally do not traumatize the suture lines, allowing the use of continuous suture patterns in the skin.

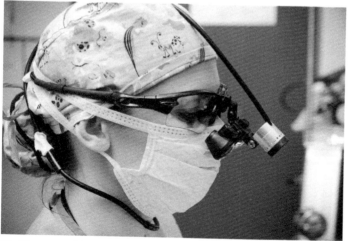

Fig. 2. Surgical loupes and lens-mounted focal light used to improve visualization of soft tissues. (*Courtesy of* David Sanchez-Migallon Guzman, LV, MS, DECZM (Avian, Small mammal), DACZM, Davis, CA.)

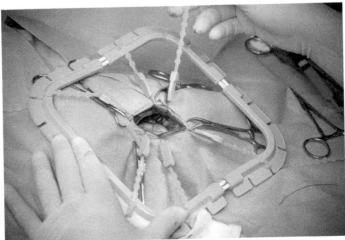

Fig. 3. Soft tissue retractor used to improve exposure of soft tissues. (*Courtesy of* David Sanchez-Migallon Guzman, LV, MS, DECZM (Avian, Small mammal), DACZM, Davis, CA.)

PATIENT PREPARATION

The feathers should be plucked 2 to 3 cm from the surgical site to prepare the skin for surgery. Small feathers can be plucked 3 to 4 at a time, whereas contour and covert feathers should be plucked individually in the direction of their growth to avoid tearing or bruising the skin. Rectrices and remiges should be pulled 1 at a time in the direction of their growth or wrapped with bandage material if possible. Feathers that are plucked regrow quickly (usually nearly regrown in 2 weeks at suture removal); however, cut feathers do not grow back until their normal molt, which can be several

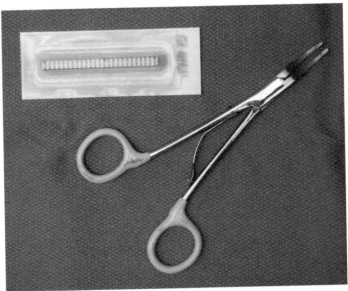

Fig. 4. Vascular clips and applicator use to ligate blood vessels and minimize blood loss. (*Courtesy of* David Sanchez-Migallon Guzman, LV, MS, DECZM (Avian, Small mammal), DACZM, Davis, CA.)

months. The remaining feathers may be retracted from the surgical field with light adhesive tape such as masking tape.

The skin is prepared with routine cleansings with chlorhexidine alternating with sterile saline. The use of excessive amounts of water, alcohol, and chlorhexidine may result in hypothermia. Chlorhexidine is more commonly used because it has residual activity, has a broad spectrum of activity, causes fewer skin reactions, and is not inactivated by organic material. Saline is recommended instead of alcohol because has proved to be as effective in preventing infection when alternated with the disinfectant solution, and because alcohol use results in a greater heat loss.

Clear plastic drapes (Veterinary Transparent Surgical Drape, Veterinary Specialty Products, Inc, Shawnee, KS) allow the patient to be monitored closely; for example, for respiratory rate and character. These drapes are placed in addition to the quarter drapes around the patient and the biggest drape to cover the table.

SURGERY OF THE SKIN
Digit Constriction Repair

Circumferential constriction caused by fibers, scabs, or necrotic tissue may result in avascular necrosis of the digit distal to the constriction. The fiber, scab, or constricting tissue should be removed to reestablish circulation to the digit, preventing circumferential scabs from forming following surgery by using a hydroactive dressing. In neonates, proposed causes for necrosis of digits include low humidity. In the early stages, increasing the environmental humidity, hot moist compresses, and massage therapy may be effective. In more advanced cases, the indented tissue is excised and a circumferential skin anastomosis performed. Following the anastomosis a release incision should be made on the medial and lateral aspects of the digit longitudinally across the anastomosis, and a bandage with hydroactive dressing is applied (**Fig. 5**).[8]

Feather Cyst Excision

Trauma or abnormal development of the follicle may result in the formation of a cyst. Canaries of the Norwich and Gloucester breeds are predisposed. Recurrence is seen following treatment by lancing and curettage. Blade excision of the affected follicle is the recommended treatment. Smaller cysts are easily removed using fusiform excision of a small piece of skin including the cystic feather follicle. Some larger cysts may be

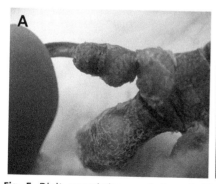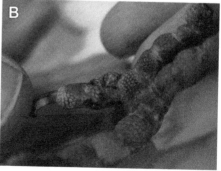

Fig. 5. Digit constriction repair in a Goffin's cockatoo (*Cacatua goffiniana*). (*A*) Severe constriction affecting the medial aspect of the first phalanx in the first digit. (*B*) The indented tissue has been excised and the skin edges are apposed with single interrupted sutures. (*Courtesy of* David Sanchez-Migallon Guzman, LV, MS, DECZM (Avian, Small mammal), DACZM, Davis, CA.)

saved by marsupializing the lining of the follicle cyst to the surrounding skin.[9] An incision is made in the center of the cyst parallel to the direction of the feather's normal growth. The feather debris is removed and the redundant tissue is excised. A simple continuous pattern of monofilament sutures is used to appose the cyst lining to the skin. The growth of the new feather is closely monitored.

Cranial Wound Repair

Trauma to the cranium may result in a degloving wound. Small wounds may be allowed to heal by secondary intention under a hydrophilic dressing. Larger wounds might be closed using a single pedicle advancement flap to cover the defect on a bird's head, preventing the stretching of the facial and upper eyelid skin that would have resulted from simple closure of the wound (**Fig. 6**). Two skin incisions at the lateral aspects of the caudal end of the defect are initiated to create the pedicle flap. Divergence of the lateral incisions creates a wider base that increases blood supply. The pedicle is undermined bluntly and advanced rostrally. Closure is routine.[10]

Sternal Wound Repair

Trauma to the keel may result in a splitting wound affecting the skin and underlying tissues. Small superficial wounds may be allowed to heal by secondary intention. Larger wounds might require surgical debridement of the affected skin, muscle, and bones. The pectoral muscles are sutured together over the keel or anchored to the keel. Smaller defects can be closed by approaching the edges of the wound (**Fig. 7**). Larger defects

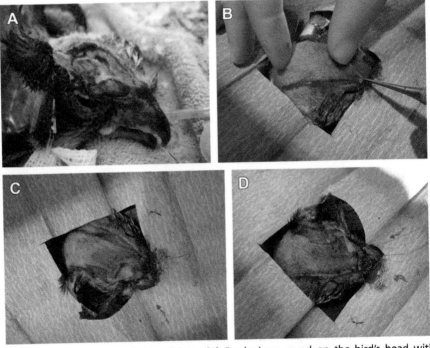

Fig. 6. Cranial would repair in a falcon. (*A*) Degloving wound on the bird's head with feathers removed. (*B*) Incisions at the lateral aspects of the caudal end of the defect creating the flap. (*C*) Advancement of the flap to cover the wound. (*D*) The flap is sutured into place using a single interrupted pattern. (*Courtesy of* Alberto Rodriguez-Barbon, LV, MRCVS.)

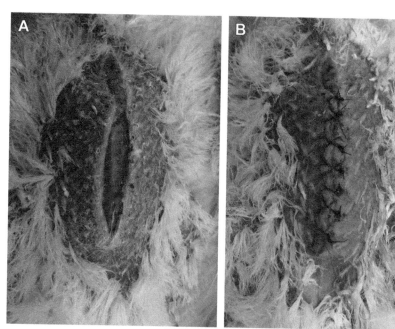

Fig. 7. Sternal wound repair in a Goffin's cockatoo (*Cacatua goffiniana*). (*A*) The skin is split over the keel along its entire length, exposing the subcutaneous tissues. (*B*) The edges of the wound have been removed and cruciate sutures have been placed along the incision. (*Courtesy of* David Sanchez-Migallon Guzman, LV, MS, DECZM (Avian, Small mammal), DACZM, Davis, CA.)

might be closed using a cutaneous axial flap. Two skin incisions on the side of the thorax are initiated. The skin is elevated to ensure that the caudal external thoracic artery and its associated vein were included in the flap at its base. The axial pattern flap is advanced forward with minimal tension to cover. The cranial edge of the flap is sutured to the cranial left corner of the defect. The caudal edge of the flap is sutured to the caudal left corner of the defect in a similar manner. Closure is routine.[11]

Uropygial Gland Excision

Uropygial gland disease (eg, adenoma, adenocarcinoma, and squamous cell carcinoma) may occur requiring surgical excision. The gland is excised, initiating an incision around it. The gland has significant blood supply. The tissue is undermined starting caudally and extending circumferentially and cranially until the gland is removed while bleeding is controlled. Closure is routine. If the defect is too larger to allow primary closure, it may be allow to heal by secondary intention with hydroactive dressing[12] or a skin flap can be used to cover the defect (**Fig. 8**).

SURGERY OF THE GASTROINTESTINAL SYSTEM
Ingluviotomy and Crop Biopsy

Crop impaction or foreign body may require removal via ingluviotomy. Chronic ingluvitis or proventricular dilatation disease may require crop biopsy to confirm the diagnosis. An incision is made through the skin in the thoracic inlet over the left lateral portion of the crop. The skin is bluntly dissected to identify the crop. Stay sutures are placed in both ends of the planned incision of the crop wall. The crop is then

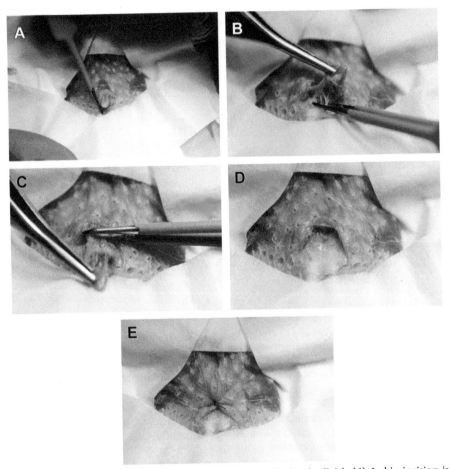

Fig. 8. Uropygial gland excision in a domestic pigeon (*Columba livia*). (*A*) A skin incision is made around the uropygial gland. (*B*) The uropygial gland is undermined, starting caudally. (*C*) The dissection of the uropygial gland extends circumferentially. (*D*) The uropygial gland is removed leaving a defect in the skin and subcutaneous space. (*E*) The defect is closed partially with a cruciate suture. (*Courtesy of* David Sanchez-Migallon Guzman, LV, MS, DECZM (Avian, Small mammal), DACZM, Davis, CA.)

incised at the cranial aspect of the left lateral side of the sac, and a tissue sample from a vascular region is collected if needed for diagnosis of proventricular dilatation disease (**Fig. 9**).[13] The crop is closed using 5-0 or 6-0 monofilament absorbable suture in a continuous pattern, with a second inverting continuous pattern if required to ensure complete closure. Skin closure is routine.[14] Provide small and frequent feedings postoperatively until the incision is healed.

Crop Burn or Laceration Repair

Overheated formula hand-fed to neonates may result in crop burns with or without fistula formation. Trauma to the crop may result in lacerations. Surgery should be delayed 4 to 5 days in the case of a crop burn for declaration of the nonviable tissue. The affected tissue is resected, and closure is routine (**Fig. 10**).

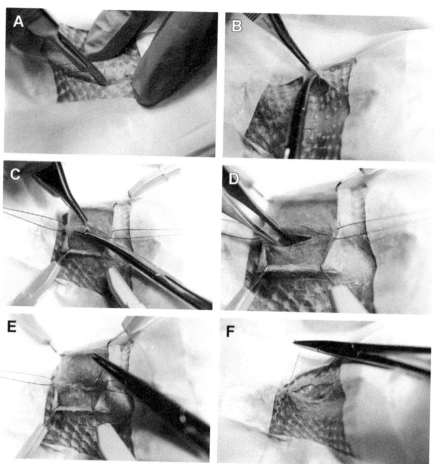

Fig. 9. Ingluviotomy and crop biopsy in a domestic pigeon (*C livia*). (*A*) An incision is made in the skin in the thoracic inlet over the left lateral portion of the crop. (*B*) The skin is bluntly dissected to identify the crop. (*C*) Two stay sutures are placed in both ends of the planned incision of the crop wall and the crop is incised (*D*) The crop is accessed through the incision. (*E*) The crop is closed using monofilament absorbable suture in a continuous pattern. (*F*) The skin is closed routinely. (*Courtesy of* David Sanchez-Migallon Guzman, LV, MS, DECZM (Avian, Small mammal), DACZM, Davis, CA.)

Coeliotomy

There are several surgical approaches to gain access to the gastrointestinal tract, reproductive tract, lower respiratory tract, urinary tract, and other viscera. These approaches include ventral midline, left or right lateral, transverse, or combinations of these (**Fig. 11**).[8] The patient is placed in dorsal recumbency for midline and transverse approaches, or left or right recumbency for right and left approaches respectively. For any approach, the cranial part of the patient should be elevated 30° to 40° to prevent fluids from flowing craniad and entering the lungs. Similarly, patients with ascites should have the fluid removed before celiotomy as a precautionary measure in case the air sacs are penetrated during the procedure, to avoid aspiration of fluid by the lungs. If the air sacs are penetrated, there is also risk of anesthetic gas escape altering the ability to maintain anesthesia.

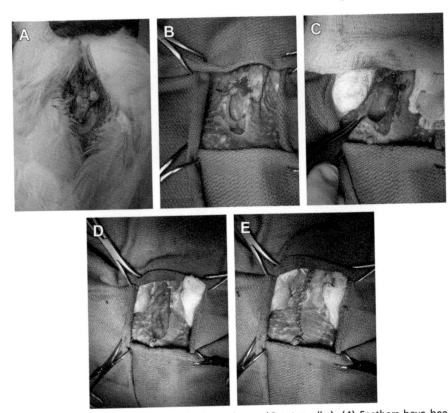

Fig. 10. Crop burn repair in an umbrella cockatoo (*Cacatua alba*). (*A*) Feathers have been separated over the thoracic inlet, exposing the thermal burn affecting the crop and the skin. (*B*) The same area, 5 days later, following removal of the feathers and formation of a crop fistula over the previously affected tissue. (*C*) The edges of the fistula are debrided and the skin and crop are separated by blunt dissection. (*D*) The crop is sutured with a continuous suture pattern. (*E*) The skin is closed with a simple interrupted pattern. (*Courtesy of* David Sanchez-Migallon Guzman, LV, MS, DECZM (Avian, Small mammal), DACZM, Davis, CA.)

Left lateral celiotomy
The left lateral celiotomy provides the best exposure to the proventriculus, ventriculus, and female reproductive tract. The bird is positioned in right lateral recumbency and the left leg may be retracted caudally or cranially to increase exposure of cranial and caudal coelom respectively. The skin is incised over the left paralumbar region from the last rib to the caudal pubic bone. The superficial medial femoral artery and vein over the lumbar fossa should be cauterized. The abdominal muscles (external and internal abdominal oblique and transverse) are incised. The last 2 ribs might be transected to provide adequate exposure to the cranial coelom.[8]

Ventral midline celiotomy
The ventral midline, transverse, or combination celiotomy provides best exposure of both sides of the coelomic cavity. For the midline approach, the skin is incised on the ventral midline from the caudal sternum to the interpubic space. The linea alba is identified, lifted, and incised. Care must be taken to incise only the linea alba, because the duodenum lies directly inside the body wall. The incision can be extended transversally at the sternal border to allow greater exposure.

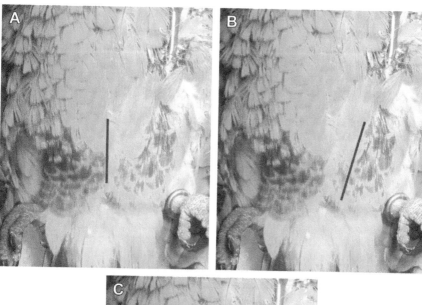

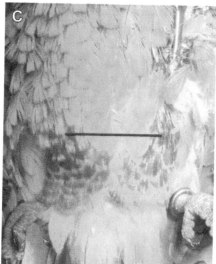

Fig. 11. Celiotomy landmarks in a Hispaniolan Amazon parrot (*Amazona ventralis*). (*A*) Bird in dorsal recumbency showing the landmarks for incision in midline celiotomy over the skin and muscles (*red line*) from the sternum to the interpubic space. (*B*) Bird positioned in dorsal recumbency showing the landmarks for incision in left lateral celiotomy over the skin and muscles (*red line*) from the public bone to the last rib. Note: the preferred position for this approach is with the bird in right lateral recumbency and the leg retracted cranially. (*C*) Bird positioned in dorsal recumbency showing the landmarks for incision in transverse celiotomy over the skin and muscles (*red line*) from side to side. (*Courtesy of* David Sanchez-Migallon Guzman, LV, MS, DECZM (Avian, Small mammal), DACZM, Davis, CA.)

Transverse celiotomy

For the ventral transverse approach a skin incision is made midway between the sternum and the vent. The body wall is lifted and incised. Care must be taken to incise only the body wall. For both approaches, the body wall and skin are closed separately with 4-0 to 6-0 absorbable suture.[8]

Coelomic Hernia and Pseudohernia Repair

Congenital or acquired (eg, hormonal imbalance causing weakening of the abdominal musculature) abdominal hernias (with hernial ring) and pseudohernias (distention and separation of muscle without hernial ring) have been reported. Surgical repair, together with the treatment of the underlying cause, might be required if there is risk for strangulation of the viscera or if the distended skin is traumatized by rubbing on the floor or perch. An incision is made over the distended skin with care not to damage any internal organs. The edge of the abdominal muscles is resected and the abdominal muscles and the skin are close in a standard 2-layer closure with a simple continuous pattern. A complication of pseudohernia repair is recurrence if the underlying cause of the abdominal distension is not treated (**Fig. 12**).

Proventriculotomy and Ventriculotomy

Removal of foreign bodies (eg, hook) or toxic material from the proventriculus or ventriculus may require proventriculotomy or ventriculotomy. The left lateral approach to the coelom is used. The ventral suspensory structures must be dissected bluntly to retract the proventriculus caudally. Stay sutures are placed in the wall of the ventriculus to exteriorize both organs. The proventriculus is fragile and might tear if manipulated with toothed forceps or if stay sutures are placed. The coelomic cavity should be packed with moist laparotomy pads or gauze to prevent contamination. The proventriculotomy is initiated at the isthmus and extended cranially as needed. The ventriculus may be accessed through a proventriculotomy (preferred) or through a ventriculotomy through the caudoventral thin muscle. The proventriculus and ventriculus are accessed through the incision to remove foreign material or sample tissue. The use of collagen[15] or coelomic fat[16] patches to cover the site of ventriculotomy is not recommended. The proventriculus is closed using a simple continuous pattern with a second inverting continuous pattern using a 4-0 to 6-0 absorbable suture. The ventriculus is closed with a simple interrupted pattern using a 3-0 to 5-0 absorbable suture (**Fig. 13**).[14]

Enterotomy or Intestinal Resection and Anastomosis

Removal of foreign bodies, trauma, intussusception, and neoplasia may require enterotomy or intestinal resection and anastomosis. The blood supply to the small intestine is via the celiac artery (to the duodenum) and the cranial mesenteric artery (jejunum and ileum). The surgical approach varies with the location of the intestinal loop of interest. The coelomic cavity should be packed with moist laparotomy pads or gauze to prevent contamination. Following enterotomy or intestinal resection and anastomosis, the intestinal wall is sutured using a 6-0 to10-0 absorbable monofilament suture on a quarter-circle atraumatic needle. Typically 6 to 8 simple interrupted sutures are necessary for end-to-end anastomosis. The surgical site is tested for leakage carefully with a 26-gauge needle catheter and saline solution. Muscle and skin closures are routine.[14] A complication of intestinal resection and anastomosis is postsurgical adhesions between the intestinal anastomosis and the dorsal coelomic wall, resulting in a partial luminal stricture and requiring surgical removal of the adhesions.[17]

Cloacoplasty and Cloacopexy

Minor cloacal prolapses are reduced and held in place with simple interrupted or mattress sutures on both sides of the vent while the underlying cause is treated (**Fig. 14**). Major or recurrent cloacal prolapse may require cloacopexy or colopexy.[18] A ventral midline coeliotomy is performed and the cloaca identified. For cloacopexy,

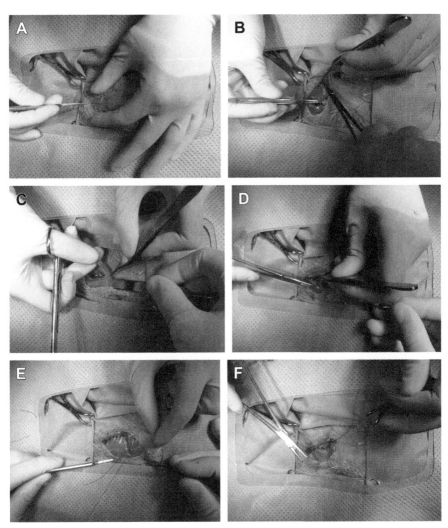

Fig. 12. Herniorrhaphy in a domestic turkey (*Meleagris gallopavo*). (*A*) The feathers have been removed on the skin over the abdominal muscles with the bird positioned in dorsal recumbency, and a midline incision in the skin is made taking care not to damage any internal organs. (*B*) The subcutaneous tissue is dissected to identify and separate the edges of the abdominal muscles from the skin. (*C*) The edges of the abdominal muscles are resected. (*D*) The abdominal muscles are sutured to each other in a single interrupted pattern. (*E*) The abdominal muscles are sutured to the keel with simple horizontal mattress sutures. (*F*) The skin is sutured routinely. (*Courtesy of* David Sanchez-Migallon Guzman, LV, MS, DECZM (Avian, Small mammal), DACZM, Davis, CA.)

the fat on the ventral surface of the cloaca is excised. The cloaca is sutured full thickness or partial thickness with seromucosal incisions created in the ventral body wall. In the first method, the suture passes through one side of the body wall, through the full thickness of the cloaca, and through the other side of the body wall in a simple interrupted pattern. In the second, incisions are created in the seromuscular surface of both the body wall and the cloaca, a few millimeters paramedian from the midline.

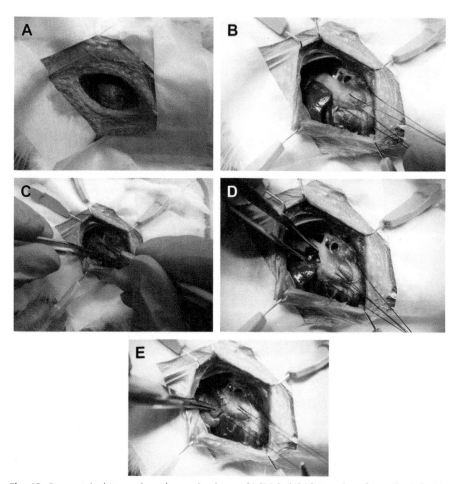

Fig. 13. Proventriculotomy in a domestic pigeon (*C livia*). (*A*) The coelom from the left side with the bird positioned in right lateral recumbency and the left leg retracted cranially, after incising the skin and abdominal muscles with bipolar forceps over the left paralumbar region from the last rib to the caudal pubic bone. (*B*) Two stay sutures are placed in the wall of the ventriculus to exteriorize part of the proventriculus and ventriculus. (*C*) The proventriculotomy is initiated at the isthmus and extended cranially as needed. (*D*) The proventriculus and ventriculus are accessed through the incision to remove foreign material or collect biopsies. (*E*) The proventriculus is closed using a simple continuous pattern with a second inverting continuous pattern using an absorbable suture. (*Courtesy of* David Sanchez-Migallon Guzman, LV, MS, DECZM (Avian, Small mammal), DACZM, Davis, CA.)

Three or 4 simple interrupted or simple continuous sutures of 4-0 to 7-0 nonabsorbable monofilament or polyglactin 910 are used to bring together the dorsal and ventral edges of the seromuscular incision with the corresponding edge of the incision in the abdominal wall (**Fig. 15**).[19] A third surgical technique for incisional and rib cloacopexy, in which a suture is placed around the last rib in each side of the bird and passed through the full thickness of the ventral aspect of the craniolateral extent of the urodeum, has also been reported.[8] Complications associated with rib

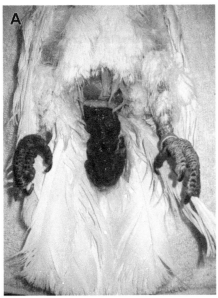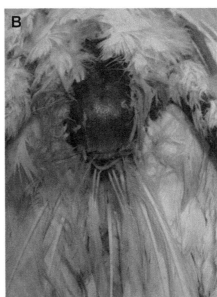

Fig. 14. Oviductal prolapse in an umbrella cockatoo (*C alba*). (*A*) The oviduct is prolapsed through the cloaca. (*B*) The prolapsed tissue has been reintroduced through the cloaca after lavaging and assessing viability, and 2 simple interrupted sutures have been placed on both sides of the vent to prevent reprolapse. (*Courtesy of* David Sanchez-Migallon Guzman, LV, MS, DECZM (Avian, Small mammal), DACZM, Davis, CA.)

cloacopexy include colonic entrapment, which can be avoided with proper tension on the cloaca maintained during rib cloacopexy and elimination of the space between rib and incisional cloacopexies during closure of the celiotomy.[20] Excessive tension in the cloaca could inadvertently create a 180° turn in the colon-cloaca junction that could result in a partial or complete colonic obstruction. For a colopexy, the seromuscular layer of the colon is incised longitudinally at the antimesenteric side. A corresponding incision is made in the craniocaudal direction in the opposing left musculus transversus abdominis while the colon is retracted cranially. The dorsal and ventral edges of the seromuscular incision are sutured to the corresponding edge of the incision in the abdominal wall with simple continuous sutures of 4-0 to 7-0 nonabsorbable monofilament.

SURGERY OF THE RESPIRATORY SYSTEM
Rhinolith Removal

Infection and malnutrition may result in rhinolith formation from desiccated secretions and debris. Mild cases may respond to nasal flushes with saline. Severe cases may require debridement. A stainless steel aural curette may be used to gently elevate and remove the mass from the naris. A lacrimal cannula may be used in smaller avian patients, such as budgerigars and passerines. The nares should be flushed copiously after removal of the bulk of the mass to remove any small pieces or material and to assist in resolution of any pathogens. Samples should be collected for cytology and culture.[8]

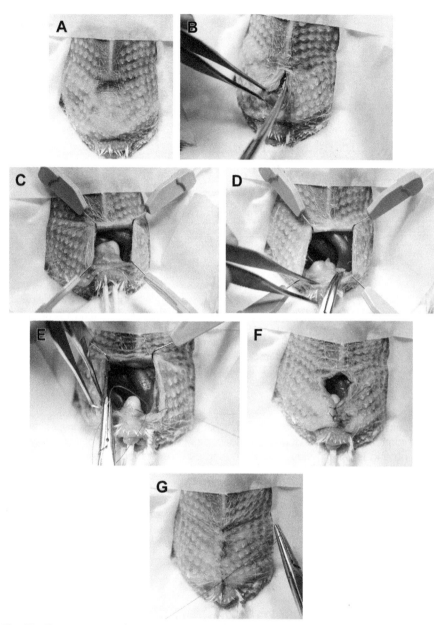

Fig. 15. Cloacopexy in a domestic pigeon (*C livia*). (*A*) The feathers have been removed on the skin over the abdominal muscles with the bird positioned in dorsal recumbency. (*B*) A midline incision in the skin and muscles is performed. (*C*) Soft tissue retractors and cotton-tipped applicators introduced in the cloaca are used to expose the cloaca within the coelomic cavity. (*D*) The fat on the ventral surface of the cloaca is excised. (*E*) The suture passes through 1 side of the body wall, through the full thickness of the cloaca, and through the other side of the body wall in a simple interrupted pattern. (*F*) The abdominal muscles are closed with a simple interrupted pattern. (*G*) The skin is sutured routinely. (*Courtesy of* David Sanchez-Migallon Guzman, LV, MS, DECZM (Avian, Small mammal), DACZM, Davis, CA.)

Sinusotomy

Infection may result in periorbital swelling of the infraorbital sinus. Mild cases might respond to medical management. Severe cases may require sinusotomy. The skin is incised in the ventral aspect below or rostral to the eye, and the material accumulated in the infraorbital sinus is removed. The sinus is flushed copiously and the skin is closed with 4-0 to 5-0 absorbable suture or left open and allowed to heal by secondary intention.

Tracheotomy and Tracheal Resection and Anastomosis

Foreign bodies or masses in the trachea might require tracheotomy, and trauma, infection, or neoplasia may result in tracheal stenosis requiring resection of the affected segment of the trachea. Tracheal surgery requires prior air sac intubation to maintain anesthesia. The bird is positioned in dorsal recumbency. The skin is incised along the ventral midline of the neck or just lateral to the crop. The subcutaneous tissues are dissected to reveal the paired sternothyroideus muscles. The recurrent nerves are identified and avoided. A possible complication is injury to the recurrent nerves resulting from surgical manipulation or radical resection. The recurrent nerve does not innervate the larynx in birds but instead innervates the esophagus, crop, tracheal, and syringeal muscles; thus, damage to the recurrent nerves does not cause laryngeal paralysis but might instead cause a change in voice. The larynx in birds is innervated by the glossopharyngeal nerve. For tracheal resection and anastomosis, a tracheal ring cranial and caudal to the affected segment is bisected circumferentially with a no. 11 scalpel blade (**Fig. 16**). The tracheal ends are approximated by

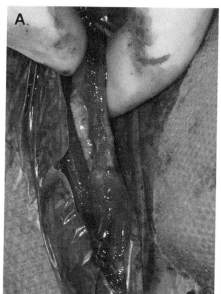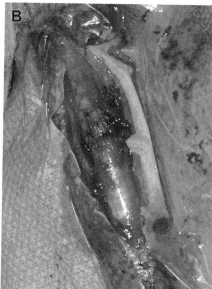

Fig. 16. Tracheal resection and anastomosis in a mallard duck (*Anas platyrhynchos*). (*A*) The collapsed tracheal segment is exposed following incision of the skin and muscles over the ventral aspect of the trachea with the bird positioned in dorsal recumbency. (*B*) The collapsed segment has been resected and the ends of the trachea anastomosed with simple interrupted and tension relief sutures. (*Courtesy of* David Sanchez-Migallon Guzman, LV, MS, DECZM (Avian, Small mammal), DACZM, Davis, CA.)

preplacing simple interrupted sutures of 4-0 to 6-0 polydioxanone on a tapered needle. The sutures are tightened individually with extraluminal knots to appose the tracheal ends. A possible complication is postsurgical tracheal stenosis and efforts should be made to minimize anastomotic stenosis by near-perfect apposition of the anastomosis site, minimally reactive suture material, applying appropriate suture technique, and reducing tension at the surgical site if needed with tension-relieving sutures each encircling a tracheal cartilage proximal and distal to the anastomosis site. Tracheotomies are performed when less invasive approaches, like endoscopy or suction, have failed to resolve the problem. For tracheotomy, a transverse incision over the surgical site of approximately 50% of the tracheal circumference is performed on the ventral tracheal surface. Stay sutures are placed around the tracheal rings adjacent to the tracheotomy site to manipulate the trachea. Foreign material may be grasped and removed, gently debrided, and suctioned, or material cranial to the incision may be pushed cranially to exit through the glottis. Simple interrupted sutures are preplaced to incorporate 1 or 2 tracheal rings on each end of the incision using small, absorbable monofilament sutures[5] (**Fig. 17**). The sternohyoid muscles are apposed over the ventral aspect of the trachea. The skin closure is routine.[21]

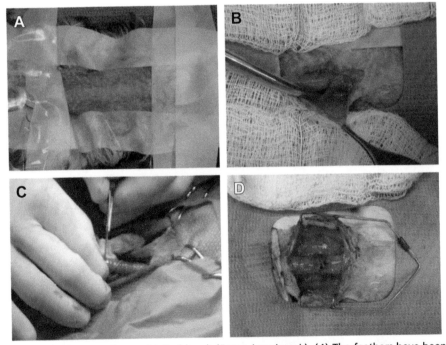

Fig. 17. Tracheotomy in a red-tailed hawk (*Buteo jamaicensis*). (*A*) The feathers have been removed over the skin in the ventral cervical region with the bird positioned in dorsal recumbency. (*B*) The subcutaneous tissues are dissected to reveal the paired sternothyroideus muscles. The recurrent nerves are identified and avoided. (*C*) A transverse incision over the ventral aspect of the trachea is performed with a no. 11 blade. (*D*) Simple interrupted sutures are placed incorporating 1 tracheal ring on each end of the incision using an absorbable monofilament suture. (*Courtesy of* David Sanchez-Migallon Guzman, LV, MS, DECZM (Avian, Small mammal), DACZM, Davis, CA.)

Tracheostomy

Glottal and periglottal lesions can result in upper airway obstruction requiring a tracheostomy. The patient preparation and surgical approach are as described in the tracheotomy. The surgical site is 1 to 2 cm ventral to the mandible, ensuring that the stoma is not obstructed when the bird flexes its neck. A transverse incision between the tracheal rings of approximately one-third the circumference of the trachea is made with a no. 11 blade. A second parallel incision is made in the trachea so that the final stoma length would is approximately 3 times the width. The parallel incisions are connected incising the tracheal rings, resulting in a rectangular-shaped stoma. The skin is sutured to the stoma with 5-0 to 7-0 monofilament absorbable suture material with a cutting or reverse cutting needle in a simple continuous pattern.[22]

Pneumonectomy

Infection or neoplasia may require partial pneumonectomy. The lungs may be approached through the caudal thoracic air sac or the dorsal intercostal spaces following retraction or removal of the ribs. The lung is elevated from the ribs and other structures using a spatula or moistened cotton-tipped applicator. Hemostatic clips are placed on the lung tissue to isolate the portion to be removed. The portion distal to the clips is then removed. The skin is closed routinely.

SURGERY OF THE REPRODUCTIVE SYSTEM
Ovocentesis

If the egg cannot be removed by manual manipulation, ovocentesis may be required. To perform ovocentesis, insert a large-gauge needle (20–18 gauge) into the egg visible through the vent and aspirate the content of the egg while applying gentle finger pressure to collapse the shell. If the egg is not visible through the vent, ovocentesis can be performed percutaneously. The shell fragments are usually passed within a few days. Keep in mind that if significant oviductal disorder is present ovocentesis and collapsing the shell can lead to oviductal rupture. Severe cases of dystocia may require surgical egg removal.[5]

Ovariectomy

Ovarian neoplasia, ovarian granulomas, oophoritis, and ovarian cysts that do not resolve with medical therapy may require ovariectomy. The ovary is tightly adhered to its dorsal attachments, making complete excision of the ovary difficult and posing significant risk of hemorrhage to the patient. The avian ovary is attached to the cranial renal artery by a short stalk and the attachment to the common iliac vein is intimate and extensive. There is a significant risk of damaging the left adrenal gland, significantly altering blood flow through the renal portal system and the cranial renal division, and damaging the overlying kidney and lumbar and/or sacral nerve plexus.[19]

Salpingohysterectomy

Chronic egg laying, dystocia, neoplasia, or infection unresponsive to medical therapy may require salpingohysterectomy. The left coelomic approach is preferred. The avian oviduct is suspended via the dorsal and ventral ligaments within the coelomic cavity. The cranial, middle, and caudal oviductal arteries run through the dorsal mesentery vascular supply to the oviduct. Species variations exist, but in general the cranial oviductal artery arises from the left cranial renal artery, aorta, or external iliac artery. The middle oviductal artery arises from the left internal iliac artery or the pudendal artery. Venous blood from the cranial oviduct enters the caudal vena cava via the

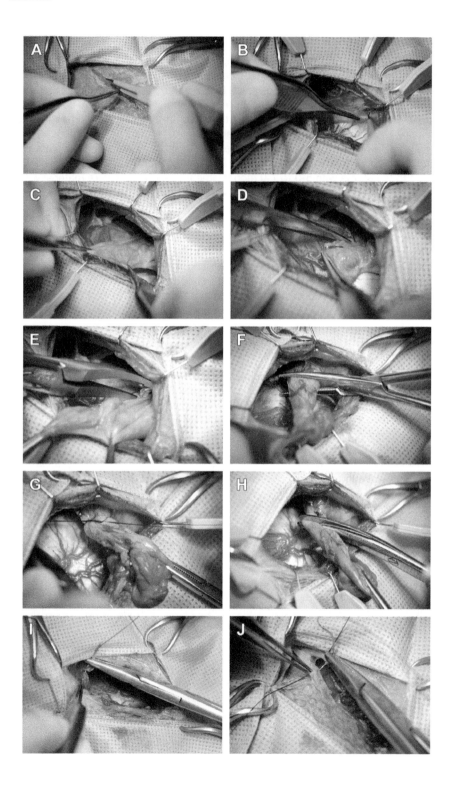

common iliac vein and venous blood from the caudal oviduct enters the renal portal or hepatic system.[5] The ventral ligament is dissected to allow the oviduct to be released and positioned in a linear fashion. The fimbria of the infundibulum lies caudal to the ovary and may be elevated to expose the dorsal ligament. A small blood vessel can be identified coursing from the ovary through the infundibulum and should be coagulated. The remainder of the suspensory ligament may then be dissected. With the infundibulum free, the oviduct is retracted ventrally and caudally exposing the dorsal suspensory ligament and the small vessels perpendicular to the oviduct and uterus. As dissection continues toward the cloaca, the ureter may be identified and must be avoided. The uterus courses along with the terminal colon and enters the cloaca. It is ligated at its junction with the vagina using 1 to 2 clips a short distance from the cloaca. Closure is routine (**Fig. 18**).[19]

Cesarean Section

Birds used for breeding or birds in critical condition that would not tolerate a longer procedure like salpingohysterectomy may require cesarean section to preserve the integrity of the reproductive tract and decrease surgical time. The surgical approach varies with the location of the egg. If located cranially, a left lateral celiotomy is recommended, and, if caudally located, a ventral midline approach with or without a transverse incision provides optimal exposure. The oviduct is incised directly over the egg, avoiding obvious blood vessels, and the egg removed. The oviduct is closed with a simple interrupted or continuous pattern using an absorbable monofilament suture. Closure is routine (**Fig. 19**).[19]

Orchidectomy

Testicular neoplasia, testicular cysts, and infectious and inflammatory conditions of the testicles that are unresponsive to medical therapy may require orchidectomy. Behavioral problems like excessive vocalization or aggression suspected to be associated with increased sexual hormones and unresponsive to medical therapy should be carefully evaluated before surgical treatment is performed because of the risks of treatment failure (eg, incomplete testicular removal) and surgical complications (eg, hemorrhage). The ventral midline approach or lateral approach through one side is preferred. The testicle is gently retracted ventrally and a 90° vascular hemostat or hemostatic clip is

---

Fig. 18. Salpingohysterectomy in a domestic pigeon (*C livia*). (*A*) The skin and abdominal muscles are incised with bipolar forceps over the left paralumbar region from the last rib to the caudal pubic bone, with the bird positioned in right lateral recumbency and the left leg retracted cranially. (*B*) The soft tissue retractors are exposing the coelomic cavity and the air sacs are incised to allow access to the oviduct. (*C*) The ventral ligament is dissected to allow the oviduct to be released and positioned in a linear fashion, and the fimbriae of the infundibulum are elevated to expose the dorsal suspensory ligament. (*D*) Vascular clips are placed over a blood vessel coursing from the ovary through the infundibulum and the dorsal ligament is transected between clips. (*E*) With the infundibulum free, the oviduct is retracted ventrally and caudally, exposing the dorsal suspensory ligament and the small vessels perpendicular to the oviduct, which are ligated in a similar fashion with the vascular clips. Careful dissection of the ligament is needed to prevent damaging the ureters as they enter the cloaca. (*F*) The oviduct is clamped with hemostats cranial to the junction with the cloaca. (*G*) The oviduct is ligated over the previously clamped tissue. (*H*) The oviduct is transected distal to the ligature. (*I*) The abdominal muscles are sutured. (*J*) The skin is sutured routinely. (*Courtesy of* David Sanchez-Migallon Guzman, LV, MS, DECZM (Avian, Small mammal), DACZM, Davis, CA.)

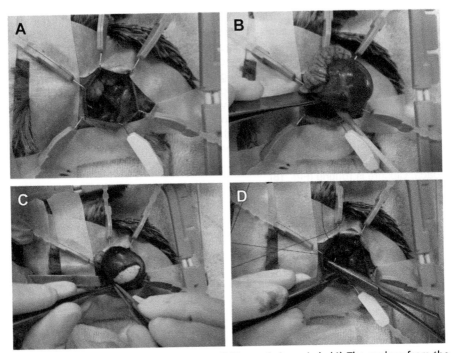

Fig. 19. Cesarean section in a Japanese quail (*Coturnix japonica*). (*A*) The coelom from the left side with the bird positioned in right lateral recumbency, using the approach described for salpingohysterectomy and the soft tissue retractors exposing the cavity. (*B*) The oviduct is gently exteriorized with the help of cotton-tipped applicators. (*C*) An incision is made over the oviduct with bipolar forceps to remove the egg. (*D*) The oviduct is closed using a continuous pattern using an absorbable monofilament suture. (*Courtesy of* David Sanchez-Migallon Guzman, LV, MS, DECZM (Avian, Small mammal), DACZM, Davis, CA.)

applied to the base of one testicle with 90° clip applicators incorporating the vascular supply. The hemostat or clip must be applied parallel to the spine to avoid entrapping the aorta and peripheral nerves. If possible, a second clip is applied just ventral to the first. One clip is applied in a craniocaudal direction and the second clip in a caudocranial direction to incorporate the entire vascular supply. The base of the testicle is incised between the hemostat or clip and the ventrally applied clips with a scalpel blade. Any remaining testicular tissue that protrudes through the hemostatic clip may be ablated with electrocautery or a laser. Residual testicular tissue may result in tissue hyperplasia and produce reproductive hormones. Closure is routine.[19]

Vasectomy

So-called teaser males and control of reproduction may require vasectomy. In the budgerigar, the patient is placed in dorsal recumbency and a 3-mm to 7-mm incision is made lateral to the cloacal sphincter. The fat and abdominal muscles are carefully dissected to enter the coelomic cavity. An operating microscope is used to locate the ductus deferens and a 5-mm section of the ductus deferens is excised. The skin is closed routinely.[23] In the finch, a 3-mm incision is made

5 mm lateral to the cloaca with the use of an operating microscope. The fat and abdominal musculature are incised to access the seminal glomera. The ductus deferens is carefully separated from the ureter and one or more sections excised without ligation. The skin is closed routinely.[24] Vasectomy in larger avian patients

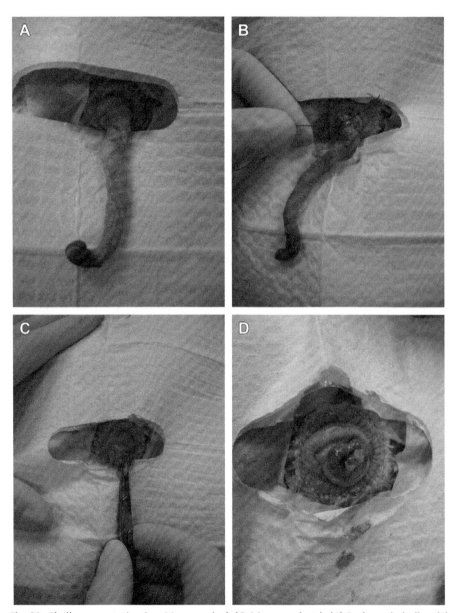

Fig. 20. Phallus amputation in a Muscovy duck (*Cairina moschata*). (*A*) Prolapsed phallus. (*B*) A transfixion suture is placed between the fossa ejaculatoria and the sulcus phalli. (*C*) The phallus is transected distal to the ligature. (*D*) The stump is reintroduced in the cloaca. (*Courtesy of* David Sanchez-Migallon Guzman, LV, MS, DECZM (Avian, Small mammal), DACZM, Davis, CA.)

is performed via transection of the ductus deferens via lateral or transverse celiotomy or laparoscopically.[25]

Phallectomy

Chronic phallus prolapse in male ducks may require amputation. The phallus is penetrated with absorbable 3-0 to 5-0 suture between the fossa ejaculatoria and the sulcus phalli, and sutured with a transfixion suture pattern. The phallus is transected distal to the ligature, and the stump is reintroduced in the cloaca (**Fig. 20**).[26]

ACKNOWLEDGMENTS

The author would like to thank Dr Olivia Petritz, Claire Grosset, Krista Keller, and Miranda Sadar for assisting during these surgical procedures, and to Don Preisler for capturing some of the images used in the article.

REFERENCES

1. Bennett RA, Harrison GJ. Surgical considerations. In: Ritchie BW, Harrison HG, Harrison LR, editors. Avian medicine: principles and application. Lake Worth (FL): Wingers Publishing; 1994. p. 1081–95.
2. Bennett RA. Cold knife or hot laser: instrumentation considerations. Proceedings of the Association of Avian Veterinarians Annual Conference. 2010. p. 221–36.
3. Altman R. Radiosurgery (electrosurgery). In: Altman R, Clubb SL, Dorrestein GM, et al, editors. Avian medicine and surgery. Philadelphia: WB Saunders; 1997. p. 767–72.
4. Hernandez-Divers S, Stahl SJ, Cooper T, et al. Comparison between CO2 laser and 4.0 MHz radiosurgery for incising skin in white Carneau pigeons (*Columba livia*). J Avian Med Surg 2008;22:103–7.
5. Bowles H, Odberg E, Harrison G, et al. Surgical resolution of soft tissue disorders. In: Harrison GJ, Lightfoot LT, editors. Clinical avian medicine volume II. Palm Beach (FL): Spix Publishing; 2006. p. 775–829.
6. Bennett R, Yaeger M, Trapp A, et al. Histologic evaluation of the tissue reaction to five suture materials in the body wall of rock doves (*Columbia livia*). J Avian Med Surg 1997;11:175–82.
7. Pollock C, Wolf K, Wight-Carter M, et al. Comparison of suture material for cloacopexy. Proceedings of the Association of Avian Veterinarians Annual Conference 2006. p. 31–2.
8. Bennett R, Harrison G. Soft tissue surgery. In: Ritchie B, Harrison G, Harrison L, editors. Avian medicine: principles and application. Lake Worth (FL): Wingers Publishing; 1994. p. 1096–136.
9. Harrison G. Microsurgical procedure for feather cyst removal in a citron-crested cockatoo (*Cacatua sulphurea citrinocristata*). J Avian Med Surg 2003;17:86–90.
10. Gentz E, Linn K. Use of a dorsal cervical single pedicle advancement flap in 3 birds with cranial skin defects. J Avian Med Surg 2000;14:31–6.
11. Ferrell ST, De Cock HE, Graham JE, et al. Assessment of a caudal external thoracic artery axial pattern flap for treatment of sternal cutaneous wounds in birds. Am J Vet Res 2004;65:497–502.
12. Wise RD. Surgical removal of uropygial gland tumor in budgerigars. Vet Med Small Anim Clin 1980;75:1601–4.

13. Gregory CR, Latimer KS, Campagnoli RP, et al. Histologic evaluation of the crop for diagnosis of proventricular dilatation syndrome in psittacine birds. J Vet Diagn Invest 1996;8:76–80.

14. Forbes N. Avian gastrointestinal surgery. Semin Avian Exot Pet Med 2002;11: 196–207.

15. Ferrell S, Werner J, Kyles A, et al. Evaluation of a collagen patch as a method of enhancing ventriculotomy healing in Japanese quail (*Coturnix coturnix japonica*). Vet Surg 2003;32:103–12.

16. Simova-Curd S, Foldenauer U, Guerrero T, et al. Comparison of ventriculotomy closure with and without a coelomic fat patch in Japanese quail (*Coturnix coturnix japonica*). J Avian Med Surg 2013;27:7–13.

17. Sabater M, Huynh M, Forbes N. Ileo-ceco-rectal intussusception requiring intestinal resection and anastomosis in a Tawny Eagle (*Aquila rapax*). J Avian Med Surg 2015;29:63–8.

18. van Zeeland YR, Schoemaker NJ, van Sluijs FJ. Incisional colopexy for treatment of chronic, recurrent colocloacal prolapse in a sulphur-crested cockatoo (*Cacatua galerita*). Vet Surg 2014;43:882–7.

19. Echols M. Surgery of the avian reproductive tract. Semin Avian Exot Pet Med 2002;11:177–95.

20. Radlinsky M, Carpenter J, Mison M, et al. Colonic entrapment after cloacopexy in two psittacine birds. J Avian Med Surg 2004;18:175–82.

21. Guzman DS, Mitchell M, Hedlund CS, et al. Tracheal resection and anastomosis in a mallard duck (*Anas platyrhynchos*) with traumatic segmental tracheal collapse. J Avian Med Surg 2007;21:150–7.

22. Lennox AM, Nemetz LP. Tracheostomy in the avian patient. Semin Avian Exot Pet Med 2005;14:131–4.

23. Samour JH, Markham JA. Vasectomy in budgerigars (*Melopsittacus undulatus*). Vet Rec 1987;120:115.

24. Birkhead TR, Pellatt JE. Vasectomy in small passerine birds. Vet Rec 1989;125: 646.

25. Samour J. Vasectomy in birds: a review. J Avian Med Surg 2010;24:169–73.

26. Lierz M. Phallus amputation in pet ducks. Exotic DVM 1999;1.3:51–4.

Rabbit Soft Tissue Surgery

Zoltan Szabo, Dr med vet, DABVP(ECM), GpCert(ExAP), MRCVS[a],*,
Katriona Bradley, BVMS, MRCVS[a], Alane Kosanovich Cahalane, DVM, MA, DACVS-SA[b]

KEYWORDS

- Rabbit • Surgery • Soft tissue • Gastrointestinal • Liver • Neutering • Kidney
- Thymoma

KEY POINTS

- Rabbit surgery is generally considered more challenging than dog or cat surgery due to the physiology and anesthetic risks of the species and because postoperative complications in rabbits are more common.
- Abdominal explorations are performed to treat or diagnose different problems within the abdominal cavity.
- The most common indication for gastrointestinal (GI) surgery is ileus due to foreign objects or masses; gastrotomy, enterotomy, intestinal biopsy, and intestinal resection are performed commonly.
- Surgery of the urinary tract is usually necessary due to urolithiasis or neoplasm. Nephrotomy, pyelolithotomy, nephrectomy, uretronephrectomy, ureterotomy, cystotomy, cystectomy, and urethrotomy are discussed.
- Ovariohysterectomy, ovariectomy, and orchidectomy are the most common surgical sterilization techniques in rabbits.

INTRODUCTION AND PRINCIPLES

Parallel to the increasing popularity of rabbits as pets, owners' demands for state-of-the-art surgical treatments are similarly increasing.[1] Rabbit surgery has some additional challenges compared with dog and cat surgery, due to the specific physiology and anatomy of rabbits. The anesthetic risk of rabbits is higher than that of dogs and cats.[2] The lack of knowledge and experience with the species on the part of owners can also lead to unrealistic expectations and complications. Some clinical signs, like anorexia, are mild in dogs but can indicate a potential life-threatening problem in rabbits. Common diseases, like abscesses or intestinal obstruction, can be straightforward in dogs and cats, but the prognosis is usually worse in rabbits. Postoperative

The authors have nothing to disclose.
[a] Tai Wai Small Animal and Exotic Hospital, 75 Chik Shun Street, Tai Wai, Shatin, New Territories, Hong Kong, China; [b] VSH Hong Kong, 165 Wan Chai Road, Wan Chai, Hong Kong, China
* Corresponding author.
E-mail address: drzoltan@icloud.com

complications, like adhesion formation, ileus, and anorexia, are also more common in rabbits.[1]

Presurgical Considerations

Prior to any surgery or anesthesia, each patient should be examined thoroughly. Urinalysis and blood analysis are recommended.[3–5] The coagulation status of patients should be assessed if significant bleeding is expected during surgery, especially in patients with liver disease or anemia. The blood tests are important because, in the authors' experience, subclinical azotemia and anemia are common in rabbits. Abdominal and thoracic radiographs are recommended, especially in geriatric rabbits (>6 years), because subclinical thoracic masses, kidney stones, or other abnormalities can be frequently diagnosed.[6]

Stabilization of a sick rabbit prior to surgery is essential. Rabbits do not need to be fasted, because they cannot vomit. Therefore, induction of anesthesia does not carry the same risk of aspiration as in dogs or cats. Rabbits are prone to GI stasis, and, therefore, should be syringe-fed if anorexic prior to and after surgery.[7] Monitoring and correcting body temperatures are important because hypothermia is common in debilitated rabbits and rabbits cannot pant or sweat effectively and are, therefore, prone to hyperthermia. Fluid therapy should be initiated prior to surgery. Intravenous (IV) catheters can be placed into the marginal ear vein or into the cephalic or saphenous veins. If IV catheter placement is not possible, fluids can be administered subcutaneously or intraosseously.[8] Perioperative antibiotic therapy for routine, sterile surgeries (eg, neutering and skin mass removals) is not necessary.[9]

Analgesia and Anesthesia

Detailed discussion of sedation, analgesia, and anesthesia of rabbits is beyond the scope of this article, but they are discussed in other articles.[10–12] Because of the fragile nature of rabbits, sedation prior to any stressful intervention is important. In the perioperative period, multimodal anesthesia, using a combination of systemic and local anesthetic drugs that target different steps of the body's pain transmission pathway, is essential. Gas anesthesia delivered via tight-fitting facemasks, laryngeal masks, supraglottic airway devices, or endotracheal tubes is the preferred method to maintain anesthesia in rabbits.[13–15] During the surgery, the physiologic parameters (heart rate, respiratory rate, oxygen saturation, body temperature, blood pressure, and carbon-dioxide concentration in the expiratory gases) should be monitored and maintained.

Surgical Principles

The skin is aseptically prepared prior to surgery. The skin is thin and the fur is dense; therefore, clipping should be performed carefully to prevent skin damage. Gentle and atraumatic skin handling is important to reduce postsurgical pain and self-inflicted wound trauma.[16] Alcohol-based disinfectant should be used sparingly to reduce heat loss.[17] Because of the elasticity of rabbit skin, the skin incision can be much shorter compared with the incision through the abdominal muscle during abdominal surgeries. The organs should be handled gently and examined in situ without unnecessary manipulation. Regular lavage with sterile saline as well as the use of moistened gauze squares helps prevent drying of the abdominal organ surface of the organs.

Wound infection is usually due to self-inflicted wound trauma. It can be prevented with gentle preparation of the surgical site, atraumatic tissue handling, wound closure by apposing edges correctly and with no tension, minimally reactive suture materials, and perioperative local anesthesia.[17]

Postoperative Considerations

Continuous fluid therapy, analgesia, and nutritional support are essential to reduce the chance of postoperative complications. H_2 antagonists (eg, ranitidine) and prokinetics (eg, metoclopramide and cisapride) can be used to reduce the incidence of gastric ulcerations and increase the GI motility.[3,18] The use of Elizabethan collars to prevent self-trauma to surgical wounds may be stressful for rabbits and does prevent caecotropy. Postoperatively, a rabbit's appetite, fecal and urine output, heart rate, respiratory rate, and temperature should be monitored. Excessive handling can be detrimental to the health status of the rabbits, and, therefore, the frequency of monitoring should be adjusted according to the temperament of the patient.[8]

ABDOMINAL EXPLORATION
Introduction, Indications

The purpose of abdominal exploration is to diagnose and potentially treat abdominal disease. In rabbits, most abdominal conditions that require surgical intervention are life-threatening. Abdominal explorations in rabbits are performed for the following reasons[1,7,9]:

- Acute abdominal pain due to GI obstruction, urinary tract blockage, peritonitis, liver lobe, or uterine or bladder torsion
- Chronic abdominal pain and recurring GI stasis due to neoplasia, abscesses, uterine problems, or adhesions
- Abdominal trauma, causing intra-abdominal bleeding or organ rupture
- Suspected or confirmed complications after previous abdominal surgeries, such as bleeding, wound dehiscence, or adhesion formation
- Any case of penetrating abdominal injury, including myasis
- Abdominal effusion due to peritonitis
- Extraluminal gas on abdominal radiographs
- To investigate ovarian remnants or adrenal gland disease, biopsy different organs, and repair hernias

Contraindications

Abdominal exploration may be contraindicated if the patient is not stable. Surgery often cannot be delayed, however, in cases of active bleeding causing life-threatening blood loss or in cases of septic peritonitis. In these patients, every attempt should be made to stabilize cardiovascular parameters prior to and during general anesthesia.[9]

Patient Positioning, Preparation, Instruments

The patient is placed in dorsal recumbency, in 10° to 15° reverse Trendelenburg position. The skin is prepared aseptically for the longest possible incision, from the caudal half of the thorax to the pelvis, including the inguinal area, to allow the extension of the incision in both directions, if necessary. A Lone Star retractor (Cooper Surgical, Pleasanton, California) (**Fig. 1**) is beneficial to improve exposure of the abdomen.[19]

Approach

Usually a ventral midline approach is used because it provides excellent bilateral exposure and an incision through the linea alba is less painful than an incision through muscle. The length of the incision is variable: an incision from xiphisternum (or xiphoid process) to the umbilicus allows for examination of the liver and the stomach. An

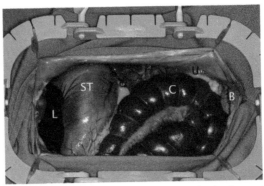

Fig. 1. A retractor is used to expose the abdominal organs during laparotomy. B, bladder; C, cecum; L, liver; SP, spleen; ST, stomach; U, uterus.

incision from the umbilicus to the pelvis is useful to assess the bladder and the reproductive tract. Paramedian, flank, and paracostal approaches are infrequently used, because they do not provide access to the contralateral side.[1]

Technique

- After the skin incision, the cutaneous blood vessels are cauterized and the linea alba is identified.
- The abdominal muscles are tented with forceps away from the viscera and the abdominal cavity is opened through the linea alba with a scalpel blade.
- The interior surface of the linea alba is palpated and adhesions are bluntly broken down if present.
- The initial incision is extended cranially or caudally, as needed, using scissors, while the abdominal wall is kept away from the viscera. Fingers or forceps should be placed between the muscles and the organs to protect the organs.
- Lone Star or Balfour retractor is used to expose the abdominal cavity (see **Fig. 1**).[19]
- The exposed organs should be moistened regularly with warm physiologic saline and covered with wet laparotomy sponges.
- If peritonitis is present or if the abdominal cavity was contaminated during the procedure, the abdomen should be lavaged with copious amounts of warm physiologic saline and then drained.
- Adding antiseptics or antibiotics to the abdominal lavage was recommended historically but they have not shown benefits; moreover, some chemicals can have detrimental effects. The use of free peritoneal additives, including antibiotics, is, therefore, not recommended.[9]
- The abdominal cavity is examined systematically and any necessary interventions are performed.
- The abdominal muscles are closed using simple interrupted or continuous patterns. The authors prefer to use a simple continuous pattern to close abdominal incisions but recommend interrupting the suture line after every 5 bites with an Aberdeen knot to prevent suture insufficiency.[20] This technique is less time-consuming compared with interrupted sutures, without the need for cutting the suture. In addition, if the suture fails anywhere, it acts as an interrupted suture, and, therefore, the failure does not extend along the whole incision.

- For closure of the muscle layer in rabbits, 4-0 or 3-0 monofilament, absorbable suture material is recommended.[21,22] Catgut should never be used in rabbits because of the tissue reaction it causes.[1]
- Because the holding layer of the abdominal wall is mainly the fascia, it should always be incorporated in the sutures. Including the peritoneum in the sutures is controversial. In dogs, suturing the peritoneum could increase the incidence of postoperative intra-abdominal adhesions[9]; however, according to an experiment in rabbits, the closure of the peritoneum results in lower chance of adhesion formation.[23]
- The subcutaneous tissue is closed using continuous or interrupted sutures with 4-0 absorbable suture material.
- The skin is closed with continuous intradermal (or subcuticular) sutures using the same suture material as for the subcutaneous tissue. The use of an Aberdeen knot is recommended for ending the suture and to bury the knot under the skin.[1] The authors do not recommend external skin sutures because the intradermal sutures combined with tissue glue can provide good aesthetic results and adequate comfort with a low chance of interfering with wound healing.

Complications

The common complications after abdominal surgeries are heat loss, anorexia, GI stasis, adhesion formation, inadvertent organ penetration, peritonitis, abscessation, wound infection, seroma development, and abdominal wall dehiscence.[9]

Adhesion formation is common in rabbits and can interfere with gut motility and bladder function, block the ureter, and cause discomfort or pain (**Fig. 2**). Treatment of adhesions is difficult. Surgery breakdown can be attempted; reoccurrence is possible. Therefore, prevention adhesions is critical. The organs should be handled gently using atraumatic methods and they should be kept moist using repeating irrigation and wet surgical sponges. Any form of chemical irritation (powder from gloves, urine contamination, and inappropriate suture materials [eg, catgut]) should be avoided, because it increases the risk of adhesions forming. Sterility of the abdominal cavity should be maintained and any leakage from hollow organs or abscesses should be controlled.

GASTROINTESTINAL SURGERY

For GI surgery, the use of retractors, suction device, magnifying glasses, atraumatic forceps, ophthalmic forceps, and needle holders is recommended. The use of 6-0 monofilament, absorbable suture material with tapering needles is recommended.[19]

Gastrotomy

Indications

In rabbits, gastric surgeries are commonly performed to remove foreign objects (usually hairballs) and less commonly to treat or diagnose gastric neoplasms or ulcerations that are life threatening or nonresponsive to medical treatment.[24,25]

In cases of small intestinal obstruction, the stomach is usually distended and filled with gas and ingesta. If necessary, the gas and the stomach contents can be released via an orogastric tube before the abdominal incision is made.[26]

Generally, gastrotomy is safer and easier to perform than enterotomy due to the small diameter and thin walls of the small intestine in rabbits. Therefore, if possible, small intestinal foreign objects should be carefully milked back to the stomach and removed via gastrotomy.[27] Complications, like peritonitis, stricture, and obstruction, are less common after gastrotomy compared with entrotomy.[1]

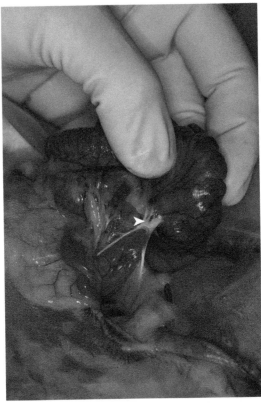

Fig. 2. Adhesion formation (*arrowhead*) between the caecum and the small intestine.

Technique

- Abdominal incision is made from the xiphoid process to the umbilicus.
- Inspect the abdominal organs and locate and identify all foreign objects and other abnormalities before making any incision.
- Inspect the stomach wall and palpate its contents to confirm the location of the foreign object, mass, or ulceration. If the foreign object is in the small intestine, close to the stomach, milk it back to the stomach.[1]
- The stomach is isolated from the abdomen with wet, warm laparotomy sponges (**Fig. 3**A).
- If possible, make the gastric incision at a hypovascular area, between the lesser and greater curvatures of the stomach.
- Stay sutures are placed 1 to 2 cm apart from the ends of the planned incision (see **Fig. 3**A).
- A full-thickness stab incision is made through the stomach wall and the end of the suction tube is placed at the opening, thus occluding it (see **Fig. 3**B).
- The initial stab incision is extended and further suction is used to empty the stomach (see **Fig. 3**C).
- The foreign object is removed, or the mass or ulceration is excised and submitted for histopathology.
- The pylorus is palpated to check its patency.

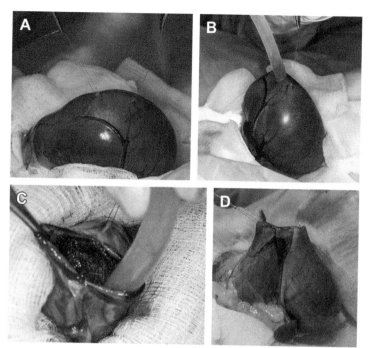

Fig. 3. Gastrotomy. (*A*) Stay sutures are placed in the stomach wall. (*B*) Suction is used to remove fluid from the stomach. (*C*) Larger particles of the stomach content cannot be removed with suction. (*D*) Closure of the stomach wall using an inverting seromuscular pattern.

- The stomach wall is closed in 2 layers, using 3-0 or 4-0 absorbable, monofilament suture material with a tapered needle. Both layers should be closed using an inverting seromuscular pattern. The first layer includes the serosa, the muscularis, and the submucosa but not mucosa. The second layer incorporates the serosal and muscularis layers (see **Fig. 3**D).
- The abdominal cavity is lavaged using warmed sterile physiologic saline.
- Contaminated instruments and gloves are replaced with sterile ones and the abdomen is closed routinely, as described previously.

Complications

- Leakage, dehiscence, perforation, peritonitis, stenosis, ileus, adhesions, shock, and death are possible complications of the GI surgeries.[9]

Postoperative care

Postoperative supportive care, monitoring, analgesia, fluid, and antibiotic and prokinetic therapy should be used. Fasting after GI surgery is not necessary for rabbits. Feeding small amounts of high-fiber herbivore food is recommended 2 hours after recovery to maintain the normal intestinal flora and to encourage normal gut motility.[26]

Enterotomy and Intestinal Biopsy

Indications

The most common indication for enterotomy in rabbits is removal of foreign objects. Intestinal biopsy is performed to collect samples from neoplasms and other intestinal wall abnormalities.[9,28]

Technique

- If an intestinal foreign body is present, try to milk it back to the stomach and perform gastrotomy or try to milk it toward the large intestine. If the object reaches the large intestine, the rabbit usually can pass it without any problem. If the object cannot be moved in either direction, perform an enterotomy to remove it.
- The location of the abnormal intestine (foreign object or neoplasm) is identified and isolated from the abdominal cavity with moistened gauze or surgical sponges.
- The intestinal contents are gently milked away orally and aborally from the identified segment.
- To reduce the chance of contamination, the lumen of the intestine could be occluded temporarily by the fingers of an assistant. Alternatively small and gentle atraumatic clamps can be used. Stay sutures can be used to manipulate the intestine (**Fig. 4**A).
- The intestinal incision is made at the antimesenteric border, through a healthy portion of the intestine, distal to the obstruction. The incision should be long enough to remove the object without tearing the tissue (see **Fig. 4**B).
- Enteric biopsies are performed using a 2-mm biopsy punch or excising a small segment of the intestinal wall.
- After removing the foreign object or successful harvesting of the biopsies, lumen of the intestine is gently cleaned with a swab to reduce the contamination.
- The incision is closed in a simple interrupted or continuous pattern. If possible, to preserve the lumen, a longitudinal incision is closed transversely. If this method is used, 1 simple suture is initially placed at the middle of the wound to transpose the incision to a transverse orientation. The remaining sutures are placed to left and right from the first one.

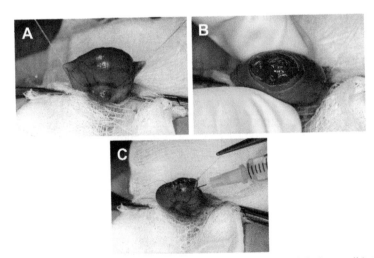

Fig. 4. Enterotomy for treatment of a small intestinal obstruction. (*A*) The small intestine is occluded by a foreign object (hairball). Note the stay sutures. (*B*) Incision of the intestinal wall to exposes the hairball. (*C*) After closure the intestine using simple continuous pattern, the intesintal segment is filled with saline to check for leakage.

- When placing the sutures, the needle is angled slightly so the serosal surface of the intestine is engaged slightly farther from the edge than the mucosa. This method helps to reposition the everting mucosa into the lumen of the intestine.
- The sutures are gently tied to prevent them from cutting through the intestinal layers. The use of crushing sutures is not recommended.
- After closure of the enterotomy, 1 to 2 mL of sterile, warm saline solution is injected into the lumen of the intestine using a 25-gauge or smaller needle, and the seal of the sutures is checked while applying gentle digital pressure. If leakage occurs, additional sutures are placed (see **Fig. 4**C).
- Because of the small size of the omentum in rabbits, omentalization of the surgical site is usually not possible.[1]
- The abdomen is lavaged, the contaminated instruments and gloves are replaced, and the abdomen is closed routinely.

Small Intestinal Resection and Anastomosis

Indications

Intestinal resection is performed to remove an abnormal intestinal segment due to intussusception (**Fig. 5**), stricture, neoplasm, abscess, and ischemia. Any bowel segment of questionable viability should be resected.[9]

Technique

- The diseased intestine is identified, exteriorized, and isolated.
- The viability of the intestine is assessed and the portion that needs to be resected is determined.
- The mesenteric vessels that support the intestinal segment to be removed are ligated and transected.

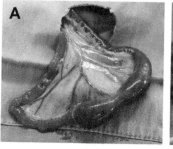
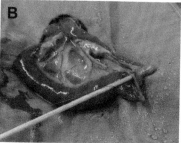
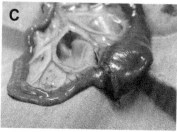

Fig. 5. (*A*) Intussusception in the small intestine. (*B*) A cotton-tipped applicator is placed in the lumen of the thin walled intestine to prevent the opposing intestinal walls being sutured together during anastomosis. (*C*) The anastomosis of the small intestine after closure.

- The intestinal contents are gently milked away orally and aborally from the identified segment.
- Artery forceps can be used to occlude the lumen of the diseased segment because this portion is removed. The lumen of the intestine of the healthy intestine should be occluded with a gentle, atraumatic temporary method, such as by the fingers of an assistant.
- The intestine is transected between the forceps and the fingers of the assistant. To increase the diameter of the lumen, an oblique incision is used.
- If there is a large difference between the lumen diameters of the 2 ends, then use an oblique incision (45°–60°) at the narrow end and a perpendicular incision at the wider. When making the oblique incision, remember the antimesenteric border is shorter than the mesenteric. Using this method, the oblique incision widens the lumen of the smaller segment and reduces the disparity between the 2 ends.
- The anastomosis is closed using 6-0 monofilament, absorbable suture material. The first suture is placed at the mesenteric border; the second one is 180° from this at the antimesenteric border. The sutures are placed through all layers of the intestinal wall and gently tied to appose the edges. The use of crushing sutures is not recommended. To keep the walls of the intestine apart, a sterile cotton-tipped applicator can be placed into the lumen of the intestine during closure (see **Fig. 5**B). After placing the first 2 sutures, the rest of the intestinal walls can be closed using simple interrupted or simple continuous sutures. After closing one side, the intestine is flipped over and the other side is closed in a similar manner (see **Fig. 5**C).
- After closure, the sutures are inspected and the lumen of the intestine is filled with warm saline to test for leakage and lumen patency.
- The mesentery is closed with simple continuous sutures using 6-0 monofilament suture material while taking care not to damage the arcadial vessels around the defect.
- The abdomen is lavaged, the contaminated instruments and gloves are replaced, and the abdomen is closed routinely.

LIVER SURGERY
Indications

Liver biopsy is performed to diagnose abnormalities of the liver, for example, neoplasia, hepatitis, and hepatic lipidosis.[29] The purpose of liver lobectomy is to remove a lesion, such as neoplasia, abscess, or a torsed lobe.

Contraindications

Liver disease often causes coagulation problems and liver biopsies may cause hemorrhage. Therefore, it is essential to assess the coagulation status of the rabbit before surgery and postpone the intervention if the rabbit has coagulopathy.[4] Other contraindications include moderate to severe anemia, moderate to severe thrombocytopenia, decreased renal function, and poor overall health status for general anesthesia. Contraindications for liver lobectomy may include diffuse, disseminated, or metastatic neoplastic disease.[9]

Presurgical Considerations

Liver problems are usually diagnosed by blood biochemical analysis. Rabbits do not have a liver-specific enzyme, but, similar to dogs and cats, measuring the levels of aspartate aminotransferase and γ-glutamyltransferase enzymes and the concentration of bilirubin, bile acids, and total protein can be useful.[4,29] Liver abnormalities can also be diagnosed with imaging methods, such as radiography, ultrasound, CT, MRI, and endoscopy.

Before liver surgery, prophylactic antibiosis against aerobes and anaerobes (eg, enrofloxacin combined with metronidazole) is recommended.[3,8] If hepatic function is compromised, the anesthetic protocol should be adjusted accordingly.

Technique

- For liver surgeries, the rabbit is placed in dorsal recumbency and the skin is surgically prepared for cranial abdominal exploration.
- After a standard midline cranial abdominal incision, retractors are used to expose the abdominal contents and the abdominal organs should be systematically explored.
- The omentum and the stomach are gently reflected and the whole liver is inspected thoroughly.
- The area of interest is identified and isolated. If the abnormality is diffuse through much of the liver, a marginal area is chosen for sampling to reduce the chance of hemorrhage.
- Regardless of the biopsy method, gentle handling of the sample is important.

Punch biopsy

A skin biopsy punch can be used to take small liver samples (see **Fig. 13**). Metzenbaum scissors are used to transect the base of the fragment to avoid trauma to the biopsy fragment itself and then the sample is gently removed (**Fig. 6**). If hemorrhage from the sample is excessive, interrupted capsular sutures can be placed using appropriately sized, monofilament absorbable suture. Alternatively, an absorbable gelatin sponge can be placed at the biopsy site to encourage clot formation.

Guillotine suture biopsy or partial lobectomy

Guillotine suture biopsy is useful to sample or remove peripheral liver lesions. A loop of absorbable suture material is placed around a peripheral segment of liver tissue (**Fig. 7**A) and carefully tightened (see **Fig. 7**B), cutting through the liver tissue and ligating the blood vessels. Once a ligature is placed, the isolated hepatic tissue can be excised.[30]

Excisional wedge biopsy with overlapping guillotine sutures

Full-thickness, overlapping, interrupted mattress sutures are placed in a peripheral region of the liver lobe and ligated, forming a V-shape. The wedge between the rows of sutures is removed using sharp dissection or electrosurgery (see **Fig. 7**C).

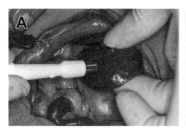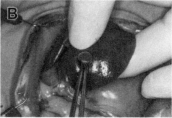

Fig. 6. Liver biopsy. (A) An 8-mm biopsy punch is used to take a sample from the liver. (B) The biopsy sample is gently removed from the liver.

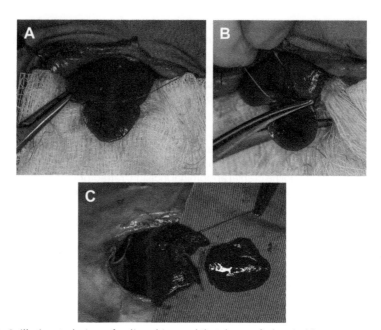

Fig. 7. Guillotine technique for liver biopsy. (*A*) A loop of absorbable suture material is placed around a peripheral segment of a liver lobe and tightened. (*B*) The isolated liver tissue is excised using Metzenbaum scissors. (*C*) The isolated liver tissue is removed after excisional wedge biopsy with overlapping guillotine sutures.

Total lobectomy

Torsion of a liver lobe (usually the caudate or the right lateral lobe) is increasingly diagnosed in rabbits (**Fig. 8**).[31–38] The treatment of the liver lobe torsion is total lobectomy of the affected lobe(s).[34] When performing total lobectomy, the vessels at the base of the lobe are ligated using monofilament, absorbable suture material, vascular clips (eg, Hemoclip, Teleflex, Wayne, Pennsylvania) (see **Fig. 8**), surgical stapling devices, or sealing systems (LigaSure, Covidien, Dublin, Ireland). Because the blood vessels are short and broad, double ligation or stapling is recommended. Once ligatures have been securely placed, the lobe is carefully transected and removed.[30]

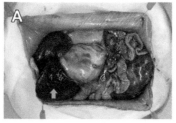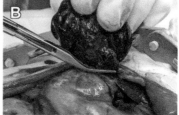

Fig. 8. Liver lobectomy for treatment of liver lobe torsion. (*A*) Abdominal exploration after liver lobe torsion. A torsed liver lobe (*arrow*) is dark and swollen. Bloody, free abdominal fluid is present. (*B*) Vascular clips are used to occlude the blood vessels during lobectomy due to liver lobe torsion.

Complications and Postoperative Care

The most common complication during and after liver surgery is intra-abdominal bleeding. The rabbit is placed in dorsal recumbency immediately after the surgery to let the weight of the liver press the biopsy sites against the abdominal wall and reduce any bleeding. The patient is monitored for signs of bleeding for 24 to 48 hours after the surgery.[31,32]

URINARY TRACT SURGERY

Urinary tract surgery in rabbits is challenging because of the small size of the patients. Urolithiasis is a common occurrence due to the unique calcium metabolism of the rabbits and high calcium excretion in the urine.[39]

Presurgical Consideration

Diagnostic tests should be performed according to the case, including urinalysis and urine bacterial culture.[40] Radiographs are useful to diagnose kidney and bladder stones; both plain and contrast radiographs[41] can be used along with ultrasonography.[42] Cystoscopy and laparoscopy also may be used.[40]

A maintenance fluid rate of 100 mL/kg/d is recommended, with increases as necessary to correct any azotemia or dehydration. Urine production, body weight, and cardiovascular function should be closely monitored to prevent volume overloading, especially at higher fluid rates. IV fluid therapy during surgery at up to 10 mL/kg/h should be used, again with careful monitoring to prevent fluid overload.[1]

Patient Preparation and Instruments

For kidney surgery, a cranial abdominal approach should be used, with a midline incision initially from just caudal to sternum down to umbilicus. For bladder surgery, a caudal laparotomy approach is used, with a midline incision of the caudal third of the abdomen stopping a centimeter or so cranial to the pelvis is advised.

Absorbable, monofilament suture material should be used in kidney, ureter, and bladder surgeries.[1,9]

Postoperative Complications

Complications include bleeding, hematuria, and urine leakage into the abdomen (which may trigger peritonitis). Urine flow blockage may occur due to blood clots, debris, adhesions, and strictures. Fluid diuresis during and after surgery and copious flushing reduce this risk.

Postoperative Care

Prolonged fluid therapy is necessary, especially after kidney surgeries. Antibiotics based on culture results should be considered if bacterial infections are suspected or contamination during surgery has occurred. Monitoring urine output and urinalysis in the postoperative period is important.

Kidney surgeries

The rabbit is placed in dorsal recumbency and the entire ventral abdomen surgically prepared with an initial midline abdominal exploration incision made from sternum to the umbilicus.

Renal Biopsy

Renal biopsy is performed to make a definitive diagnosis of kidney disease and to determine prognosis for nephropathy, kidney masses, and neoplasms. Contraindications include patients with bleeding disorders, large intrarenal cysts, hydronephrosis, perirenal abscesses, and urinary tract obstruction.

Technique

- Both kidneys should be examined in every case and both kidneys should be sampled if bilateral disease is suspected.
- The kidney is bluntly separated from the parietal peritoneum and gently held between 2 fingers while a section of renal tissue is removed by making 2 incisions along the greater curvature of the kidney coming together at a 60° angle, thus removing a wedge of tissue (**Fig. 9**). The sample is gently removed and the incision is closed using 4-0 absorbable suture material.
- For smaller samples, core needle biopsy can be performed using spring-loaded biopsy needles (16–18 G), manual Tru-Cut biopsy needle (CareFusion, San Diego, California), or similar tools. Manual devices are less satisfactory because they may produce fragmented tissue samples. If biopsy needles are used, then collect at least 2 samples, each longer than 1 cm.[9] Bleeding after sampling can be controlled by applying digital pressure or using a cotton-tipped applicator or surgical sponge.

Nephrotomy

The indications of nephrotomy include removal of a kidney stone, masses, or neoplasm from the renal pelvis and exploration of bleeding into the renal pelvis. The main contraindication is that nephrotomy reduces the renal function significantly (30%–40% in dogs and cats); therefore, it is not advisable in cases of impaired renal function.[42]

Technique

- The kidney is bluntly separated from the parietal peritoneum and gently held between 2 fingers while the vessels at the hilus of the kidney are clamped using atraumatic and reversible methods (**Fig. 10**).
- A sagittal incision is made along the midline, and the parenchyma is bluntly dissected to expose the renal pelvis. The urolith (**Fig. 11**), mass, or abscess is removed, and the source of any bleeding is explored.

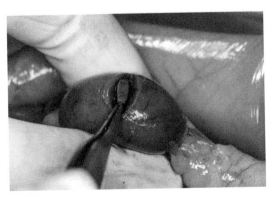

Fig. 9. Kidney wedge biopsy.

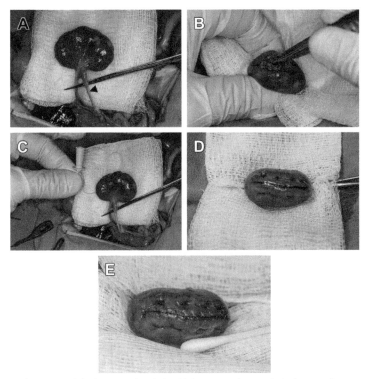

Fig. 10. Nephrotomy. (*A*) The vessels of the kidney are clamped during nephrotomy, while the ureter (*arrowhead*) remained patent to allow for catheterization. (*B*) Removal of the renal calculi. (*C*) A catheter is inserted through into the ureter to check its patency. (*D*) The 2 halves of the renal cortex are apposed using horizontal mattress sutures. (*E*) The kidney capsule is closed using a simple interrupted or continuous suture pattern.

- The pelvis and the parenchyma are sampled for bacterial culture and the exposed tissue and the pelvis are gently flushed with warm, sterile saline to remove any debris or blood clots.
- A 3F (1-mm) size catheter is inserted through the pelvis into the ureter to check its patency, which is only possible if the ureter has not been clamped previously (see **Fig. 10**C).

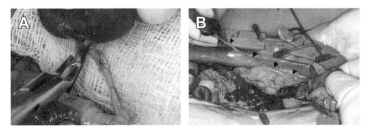

Fig. 11. Nephrectomy and nephroureterectomy. (*A*) The renal artery is ligated using vascular clips. (*B*) During nephroureterectomy, the ureter (*arrowheads*) is followed and detached from the peritoneum along its length and removed with the kidney.

- The surgical incision in the renal cortex is closed using horizontal or cruciate mattress sutures (see **Fig. 10D**).
- The kidney capsule is closed with simple interrupted or continuous suture pattern using 4-0 absorbable suture material (see **Fig. 10E**). The clamps from the vessels of the kidney are removed.
- A lateral approach, caudal to the last rib, has also been described but does not allow inspection of the contralateral kidney.[43]

Pyelolithotomy

Pyelolithotomy is an incision into the renal pelvis and proximal ureter and is indicated when a urolith is found in the extrarenal region of the pelvis of the kidney. This surgery only can be performed if the pelvis is distended due to of obstruction in urine flow through the ureter. The main advantages are that less renal damage is caused compared with nephrectomy because there is no damage to the parenchyma, no need to occlude the renal vessels, and the postsurgical complications are less common.[1]

Technique

- The approach is the same as for nephrotomy.
- A longitudinal incision is made on the distended pelvis over the calculus, and the renal stone is removed. The pelvis is sampled for bacterial culture then gently flushed with warm, sterile saline.
- A 3F (1-mm) size catheter is inserted through the incision into the ureter to check its patency. The incision is closed with simple interrupted or continuous suture pattern using 5-0 absorbable suture material. Transverse closure is recommended to maintain a wider lumen.[1,9]

Nephrectomy

Nephrectomy, the surgical removal of a kidney, is indicated if there is extensive, irreversible renal disease, which could worsen the status of the patient if the kidney is left in place. Examples include severe, irreversible renal trauma, neoplasm, abscess, hydronephrosis,[44] or pyelonephritis that is not responsive to antibiosis or causes uncontrollable pain, urine leakage or hemorrhage.[1,9]

   Contraindications are significantly impaired function of the contralateral kidney. Presurgical diagnostics are aimed at establishing adequate renal function in the contralateral kidney. Biochemistry and urinanalysis in addition to an excretory pyelogram or a glomerular filtration study should be considered.

Technique

- Approach is the same as for nephrotomy.
- The kidney is gently lifted and rotated medially and the hilus, ureter, and renal artery and vein are identified. The renal vessels and the ureters are individually clamped and ligated using 4-0 absorbable suture material or with vascular clips (see **Fig. 11A**).
- Nephroureterectomy (removal of the ureter and the kidney) is performed if the ureter is diseased. The ureter is followed and gently detached from the peritoneum along its length (see **Fig. 11B**). The distal end of the ureter is ligated 1 cm from its insertion into the urinary bladder, transected above the ligature, and removed.

Ureterotomy

Ureterotomy is an incision into the ureter and this procedure is indicated for removal of a urolith from the ureter. It carries a significant risk of postoperative stricture due to the narrow diameter of the ureters in rabbits. An alternative method that reduces this risk is retrograde flushing of the stone to the renal pelvis and removal with pyelolithotomy.

BLADDER SURGERIES
Cystotomy and Cystectomy

Cystotomy is the surgical incision into the urinary bladder and cystolithectomy is the removal of urinary bladder calculi through a cystotomy. Indications for these procedures are removal of large bladder stones, removal of urethral stones that can be flushed back to the bladder, repair of bladder rupture, biopsy or removal of bladder masses, and investigation of chronic, refractory cystitis that is resistant to medical treatment. Small stones and hypercalciuria (bladder sludge) may be removed from the bladder with catheterization and careful, repeated flushing although urethral swelling and blockage may be seen after this method.

Cystectomy is the removal of a portion of the bladder to treat bladder neoplasm, polyps, bladder wall necrosis, and traumatic injuries. It is performed in a similar approach and manner to a cystotomy; 65% to 70% of the bladder wall can be removed without interfering with the function of the bladder if the trigone is left intact and ureters are not damaged.[1,9]

Technique

- A caudal abdominal approach is used, taking care not to inadvertently enter the bladder, if distended. The healthy bladder is thin walled, but bladder wall may be thickened if chronic inflammatory disorders are present.
- The bladder is identified, gently lifted, exteriorized, and moistened and gauze or surgical sponges packed around it. Stay sutures are placed in the bladder wall cranial and caudal to the planned incision. To reduce contamination the urine, the bladder should be drained with a syringe and the needle prior to incision.
- The incision is made through an avascular portion of the bladder wall. A chronically inflamed bladder wall bleeds easily.
- Remove the calculi using a surgical spoon or forceps. Calculi may adhere to the inflamed bladder wall or be buried deep within mucosal fold, and care should be taken not to damage the bladder wall during calculi removal. Calculi may be found deep in the neck of the bladder, far from the incision site.
- If there are calculi lodged in the urethra, retrograde flushing into the bladder from the external urethral orifice, using a urinary catheter, should be performed. If there are multiple small stones and/or urethral stones, it is recommended to place this catheter before surgery.
- Swabs of the bladder wall for bacterial culture and sensitivity testing should be collected, if urine was not collected prior to the incision. Biopsy samples of the bladder wall for aerobic culture and for histopathology may be collected, if indicated.
- The bladder cavity is gently flushed with warm, sterile saline to remove blood clots or debris. The urethra should be gently flushed with saline, either retrograde or normograde, with a sterile catheter inserted through the bladder incision.
- The bladder wall is closed using single or continuous inverting suture pattern (Lembert or Cushing) without the suture material entering the bladder lumen. If

the suture material penetrates the bladder wall, it can act as a nidus of infection and increase the chance calculi recurrence.

- Use 4-0 or 5-0 absorbable, monofilament suture material. If the bladder wall is thin or fragile, a double layer closure is recommended.[45]
- Fibrin sealants are used in human medicine and are a future consideration for bladder wall closure.[46]
- The bladder incision is checked for leakage by filling the bladder with sterile saline.

Complications

Complications include rupture or perforation of the overdistended bladder, especially during the abdominal incision, as well as urine leakage from the bladder incision site. A chronically inflamed bladder may form adhesions to the surrounding intestine or uterus. Iatrogenic damage of the ureters may occur if the incision is made into the dorsocaudal aspect of the bladder. The risk of postsurgical urine leakage can be prevented by checking for leakage after closure of the bladder.

Tube Cystostomy (Prepubic Catheterization)

Tube cystostomy is a temporary solution to alleviate the clinical signs of urethral obstruction or bladder atony, by placing a Foley catheter into the bladder thus bypassing the urethra.[1]

- The approach may be midline, where a small incision caudal to the umbilicus is made, or in the inguinal approach, where a 2-cm to 3-cm oblique inguinal incision is made over the bladder.
- Once the incision is made, locate the bladder, and place stay sutures and a purse-string suture into the bladder wall.
- Place the tip of the Foley catheter into the abdominal cavity through a separate small stab incision. Make a small stab incision into the bladder within the purse-string suture and introduce the Foley catheter into the bladder lumen. Inflate the balloon with saline, and secure the catheter within the lumen by tightening the purse-string suture. Suture the bladder to the body wall with several interrupted absorbable sutures.
- Close the initial incision, and secure the catheter to the skin using a Roman sandal–type suture.

Prescrotal Urethrotomy

Prescrotal urethrotomy is the incision into the urethra of the male rabbit, usually to remove urethral calculi causing blockage of urine flow.[1] Urethral blockage is often initially a medical, not surgical emergency. Hyperkalemia may be present due to post–renal obstruction. Appropriate fluid therapy and bladder drainage may be necessary to correct electrolyte abnormalities, prior to anesthesia.

Technique

- The most common location of the blockage is the distal urethra, and forced, manual expression of the bladder is not recommended because of the risk of bladder rupture.
- In some cases, the urolith can be flushed back to the bladder and cystotomy can performed instead of urethrotomy. Postoperative stricture formation is a common complication after urethrotomy so preference should be given to cystotomy, if possible.

- The pubic area and the hemiscrotal sacs are surgically prepared. And the scrotum is reflected to allow the exposure of the surgical area
- A sterile urinary catheter is placed into the urethra reaching the level of the calculus and measuring the length of the catheter to the skin helps to identify the appropriate location of the skin incision
- A vertical incision is made in the skin on the lateral side of the penis at the level of the calculus, perpendicular to the urethra; then the stone is located in the urethra by digital palpation. Next, a midline longitudinal incision is made into the penis and the urethra directly over the stone and the urolith is removed. The catheter should be further advanced to check the patency of the urethra. Any hemorrhage is controlled by digital pressure.
- The urethra is closed using 5-0 monofilament, absorbable suture material in a continuous suture pattern
- The subcutis and the skin are routinely closed and the catheter is removed.

Complications

Complications include obstruction of the urine flow secondary to tissue swelling, fibrosis, and necrosis. Urine leakage from the wound into the subcutis can lead to infection, irritation, and stricture formation.

OVARIOHYSTERECTOMY AND OVARIECTOMY
Indications

Rabbits have a bicornuate duplex uterus, which lacks a uterine body. The separate uterine horns have each their own cervix and enter into a single long vagina. The indications for ovariohysterectomy are to prevent breeding, prevent uterine and ovarian neoplasms and other diseases, reduce the incidence of mammary gland disease, prevent false pregnancies, and reduce hormonal territorial behavior.[47,48] Uterine adenocarcinoma is the most common tumor in female rabbits.[49] The reported incidence of uterine adenocarcinoma is up to 75% in 7-year-old female rabbits.[50] Surgery is easier once a rabbit has reached puberty because the uterus enlarges and the ligaments become slightly looser (between 6 and 9 months); however, surgery is best not delayed too long because significant fat can be laid down around the uterus and ovaries.[1] Rabbits can be spayed during pregnancy or pseudopregnancy but the surgery should be delayed after giving birth until the babies are weaned at 4 to 5 weeks of age.[1] Ovariectomy can be considered in a doe without evidence of uterine disease. Ovariectomy should be limited to young animals between 6 and 12 months of age.[1,51]

Presurgical Considerations

Diagnostic tests should be performed based on an animal's age and suspected concurrent diseases and may include urinalysis, biochemistry, and hematology. Thoracic radiographs should be taken in animals older because uterine adenocarcinoma readily metastasizes to the lungs.[1] Contraindications include planned future use as a breeding doe, severe systemic disease, and secondary spread of uterine neoplasia.

Patient Positioning, Preparation, and Approach

The rabbit is placed in dorsal recumbency and the caudal half of the abdomen clipped and surgically prepared. For ovariohysterectomy, a midline approach is recommended to the caudal abdomen, with the initial incision made at the level of the last (inguinal) nipples.

Technique

- The initial incision should be approximately 2 to 3 cm, approximately midway between the umbilicus and the pubic symphysis, which often allows for the exteriorization of the uterus while keeping the GI tract within the abdomen. If there is a large amount of fat in the mesometrium around the uterus, the incision may need to be extended. Care must be taken when entering into the abdomen or extending the incision because the bladder and the cecum are in apposition with the body wall.
- The uterine horns are carefully exteriorized, with particular care used to draw the ovaries out because the section between the cranial end of the uterus and the ovary is weak and may tear (**Fig. 12**A).
- The ovary, fallopian tube (or salpinx) and associated fat pads are identified and carefully exteriorized (see **Fig. 12**A). The ovarian ligament can be transected to facilitate the exteriorization (**Fig. 12**B). Two artery forceps are clamped on the ovarian pedicle. Two ligatures are placed between the forceps using 3-0 or 4-0 absorbable suture material or vascular clips (see **Fig. 12**C). The pedicle is transected above the second ligature and checked for hemorrhage before being returned to the abdomen. The ovary should be checked to ensure all ovarian tissue has been removed.
- The same procedure is performed on the contralateral ovary.
- The uterine vessels within the mesometrium are identified and ligated on either side of the uterus using absorbable suture material or vascular clips (see **Fig. 12**D). The fat may be profuse and obscure the vessels.

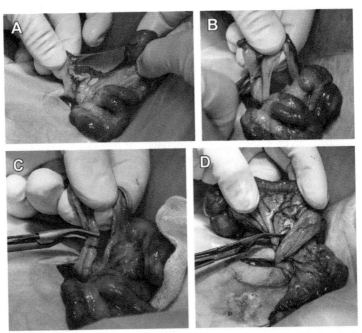

Fig. 12. Ovariohysterectomy. (*A*) Visualization of the female reproductive tract after caudal midline laparotomy. (*B*) The ovarian ligament is transected to help the exteriorization of the ovary. (*C*) Vascular clips are used to ligate the ovarian artery. (*D*) The uterine vessels are ligated using vascular clips. FT, fallopian tube; O, ovary; OA, ovarian artery; OL, ovarian ligament; U, uterine horns; V, vagina.

- The double cervix is clamped and double ligated with 3-0 or 4-0 synthetic absorbable suture and transected above the second ligature. One or both ligatures should be transfixing.
- If the uterine horns or the cervixes appear diseased, all tissue should be removed and the transection performed at the proximal vagina. Because the vagina is not sterile, care should be taken to close the lumen after transection.

Complications

Complications in the immediate postoperative period include GI stasis and wound healing complications and self-inflicted wound trauma. Longer-term problems include adhesion formation.[52] According to Harcourt-Brown and Chitty,[1] transection and ligation of the vagina could result in urine leakage into the abdomen and could cause local peritonitis and adhesions. Good postoperative care is vital to reduce complications. This topic is discussed in the article elsewhere in this issue by Colopy and colleagues.

ORCHIECTOMY (CASTRATION)
Indications and Presurgical Considerations

The indications for castration (or orchiectomy) of male rabbits include prevention of breeding; reduction in aggression, sexual behavior, and urine marking, particularly if done before full sexual development[47]; and prevention of testicular neoplasia.[53–55] Rabbits can be castrated as soon as testicles are palpable within the hemiscrotal sacs, which can be as early as 10 weeks of age.[1] Contraindications include planned future use as a breeding male and systemic disease.

Patient Positioning, Preparation, and Instruments

General anesthesia is induced, the rabbit placed in dorsal recumbency, and the prescrotal area, hemiscrotal sacs, and prepuce are clipped taking care not to traumatize the delicate skin. Local anesthetic can be injected subcutaneously at the incision site and testicular blocks are performed. The surgical site is aseptically prepared.

Approach

The surgical approach may be scrotal, prescrotal, or abdominal.[47,48,56] The scrotal open-to-closed technique has the advantage of short procedure time but it requires 2 incisions; the scrotal skin is easily irritated during surgical preparation; and contamination of the wounds through cage bedding is possible. The prescrotal approach requires only a single incision and sterile preparation of the surgical site is easier compared with the scrotal approach. The procedure time, however, is usually longer. The abdominal approach requires entering the abdominal cavity, is therefore more painful, and should be reserved for repair of inguinal or hemiscrotal herniation or treatment of true cryptorchism.[56]

Orchiectomy in rabbit should always be performed closed or in an open-to-closed manner to prevent herniation of the intestine or urinary bladder through the open inguinal canals.[47,48,56]

Technique

Scrotal approach

- Incise through the scrotal skin on ventral aspect of the testicle (**Fig. 13**A). As the testicle bulges through the incision, gently free and exteriorize it. Gently pull the testicle and tunic caudally exposing the pedicle of the testicle with vessels and

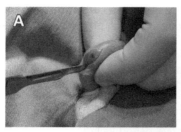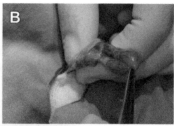

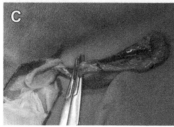

Fig. 13. Scrotal castration technique. (*A*) The skin of the scrotum is incised and the vaginal tunic is exposed. (*B*) The vaginal tunic is opened and the testicle is gently pulled to expose the vessels and vas deferens within the tunic. (*C*) The vaginal tunic is clamped twice with artery forceps at the base of the pedicle. The ligatures will close the tunic and prevent the herniation of the abdominal organs.

vas deferens within the tunic. Opening the vaginal tunic allows removing the fat pad within the tunic and the testicle can be exteriorized easily (see **Fig. 13**B).

- Carefully cut the attachment between the caudal end of the tunica vaginalis and the scrotal skin, allowing the testicle to be exteriorized further.
- Clamp the pedicle of the tunica vaginalis twice with artery forceps toward the base of the pedicle (see **Fig. 13**C).
- Ligate each clamped site firmly in the crushed tissue with 3-0 or 4-0 synthetic absorbable suture, thus ligating the vessels and vas deferens within the tunic and closing the inguinal canal, if the tunic was opened previously.
- If the rabbit is large or obese or if the tunic is abnormally thickened, then a transfixing suture may be used for safety or the vessels should be ligated individually before closing the tunic.
- The vessels, vas deferens, and tunic are transected above the ligature and the testicle is removed; then, the ligatures are checked for hemorrhage.
- No skin sutures are required and are better avoided because they may stimulate self-trauma; tissue glue may be used if necessary.

Prescrotal approach

- A single midline prescrotal incision is made (**Fig. 14**A) and blunt dissection toward the inguinal area is performed.
- The testicular pedicle is grasped and retracted and testicle is drawn up and out (see **Fig. 14**B). The attachment between the caudal end of the tunica vaginalis and the scrotal skin is bluntly separated. The vaginal tunic can be opened to remove the fat fad and to make the pedicle thinner and easier to ligate. The pedicle is then freed from the fascia, crushed, and ligated (as described previously), thus closing the vaginal tunic (see **Fig. 14**C). The tunic distal to the ligation should be resected.
- The skin incision should be closed in 1 or 2 layers.

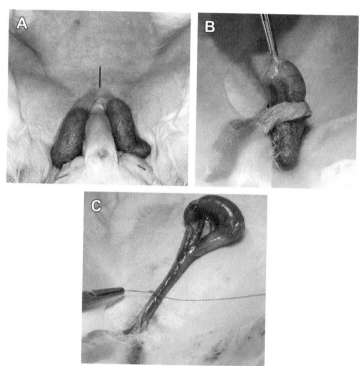

Fig. 14. Prescrotal castration technique. (*A*) A single midline prescrotal incision is made cranial to the base of the scrotum. (*B*) The testicular pedicle is grasped and retracted and the testicle within the vaginal tunic is pulled out. (*C*) The pedicle of the testicle is ligated, which closes the vaginal tunic and prevents the herniation of the abdominal organs.

THORACIC SURGERY
Introduction

In comparison to dogs and cats, the thoracic cavity of rabbit is much smaller in relation to the abdominal cavity, making surgical interventions challenging.[57] Indications for thoracotomy in rabbits include removal of thoracic masses (eg, thymoma), primary lung neoplasms, lung abscesses or foreign objects, and lung lobectomy in cases of lung lobe torsion.

Presurgical Considerations

Routine diagnostics for thoracic and lower respiratory disorders may include diagnostic imaging, bronchoalveolar lavage, tracheoscopsy/bronchoscopy, fine-needle aspiration, cytology, and bacterial culture and susceptibility testing.[58]

Intermediate positive-pressure ventilation (IPPV) is required for thoracotomy procedures. To ventilate the patient during the thoracotomy, an endotracheal tube should be placed[13,14] and sealed and either manual or mechanical ventilation performed.

Thymoma Removal via Median Sternotomy

The thymus is found in the mediastinum, cranioventral to the heart, and in rabbits it does not involute but persists for life.[59] Thymomas are the most common mediastinal tumors in rabbits.[60] On radiographs they appear as a large soft tissue mass in the cranial thorax. They are usually histologically benign and rarely metastasize but they have tendency to recur after incomplete removal. Thymomas are usually not invasive but can be adhered to the pericardium.[1,61] Thymic carcinomas with metastatic tendency in rabbits are rare.[62]

The perioperative mortality rate in rabbits after surgical removal of thymomas has been reported to be high. In 1 case series, 5 of 9 rabbits died within 3 days of surgery; the survival time was 0 to 955 days (median 3 days).[61]

Thymomas are radiosensitive so radiation therapy could be an alternative to surgery, but the proximity of the lung and heart limits the recommended dose of radiation.[63] The short-term survival rate after radiation therapy is 80% to 85%, which is higher than the perioperative survival rate after surgery (40%–50%),[61] but the complications (radiation-induced myocardial failure, pneumonitis, and pulmonary fibrosis) and recurrence are more common compared with surgical excision.[64,65] Andres and colleagues[64] treated 19 rabbits with radiation therapy and 3 rabbits died during the first 14 days; the median survival time of the remaining animals was 727 days. Radiation therapy can be the sole therapy or combined with surgery, if surgical removal is incomplete.[64]

There is limited information regarding the efficacy of chemotherapy in the management of thymomas in rabbits; however, prednisolone can be used postoperatively or after radiation therapy.[65] If cystic lesions are present, draining them can temporarily alleviate the dyspnea and improve quality of life.[61]

Technique

- Midline sternotomy is recommended for thymoma removal to allow access to both sides of the thoracic cavity.[66] The rabbit is placed in dorsal recumbency. The skin is shaved and surgically prepared from the neck to the cranial portion of the abdomen. An intercostal nerve block with bupivacaine (2 mg/kg) should be performed.[9]
- A midline skin incision is made from 2 to 3 cm cranial to the manubrium to the xiphoid process.
- Remaining on midline allows dissection between muscle layers (**Fig. 15A**). If necessary, the sternocephalicus and sternohyoideus muscles are bluntly separated to expose the sternal bone.
- The exposed sternum is cut perpendicular in the midline, with an oscillating saw or diamond cutting disc attached to a rotary tool (see **Fig. 15B**).
- After accessing the thoracic cavity, IPPV is initiated.[13,14] IPPV is performed gently and carefully to prevent the overinflation of the lungs. The inflating pressure should be less than 10 cm H_2O and the lung should not turn pale or expand out from the chest.[1,9]
- After osteotomizing the first few sternebrae, moistened surgical sponges are placed along the edges of the sternotomy site and a retractor (see **Fig. 15C**) is used to stabilize the thorax and facilitate the careful transection of the remaining sternebrae.
- The last 1 or 2 sternebrae should be left intact to stabilize the thorax during recovery. If the goal of the sternotomy is to explore the caudal half of the thorax, then the manubrium should be left intact and the last sternebrae can be cut through.
- The thymic mass is identified and gently and bluntly dissected from the surrounding tissue. Large amounts of fat can be found in the thorax, even in rabbits in normal body condition (see **Fig. 15C**).
- At the thoracic inlet, caution should be exercised when dissecting the mass from the jugular and subclavian veins and from the carotid and subclavian arteries.

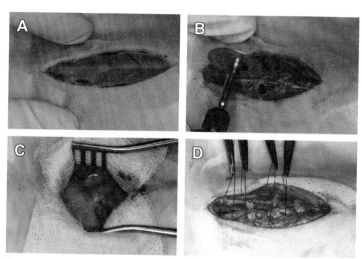

Fig. 15. Thoracotomy via median sternotomy. (*A*) A midline skin incision is made and if necessary the sternocephalicus and sternohyoideus muscles are bluntly separated to expose the sternal bone. (*B*) A rotary tool is used to cut through the sternum midline, perpendicular to the bone. (*C*) Moistened gauze or surgical sponges are placed along the edges of the sternum and a retractor is used to open the thorax. (*D*) Closure of the median sternotomy wound.

- After removing the thymic mass, the thorax is flushed with warm saline and any blood clots and debris are removed. The saline is removed with suction.
- An indwelling thoracic drain is placed if ongoing fluid or air accumulation is expected in the thorax.
- The sternebrae are apposed using preplaced monofilament material, with simple interrupted sutures placed circumferentially around the sternabrae (see **Fig. 15**D).
- The muscle, subcutaneous, and skin layers are closed routinely.
- The excess air from the thoracic cavity is removed and the lungs inflated using the chest drain or a temporary small red rubber tube is left in the chest during closure for immediate postoperative evacuation and then pulled once the lungs are reinflated (**Fig. 16**).

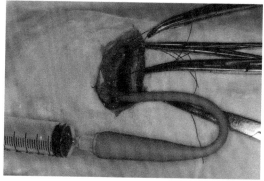

Fig. 16. Closure of a lateral intercostal thoracotomy wound: a small rubber tube is left in the thorax to evacuate the air from the chest after closure and then it is pulled out.

Complications
Most complications occur during and until 10 days after the surgery. The most common complication after thoracotomy is acute perioperative death.[61] This may be related to pain, stress, or anesthetic complications.

Lung Lobectomy via Lateral Intercostal Thoracotomy

Indications
Lateral intercostal thoracotomy is performed to remove thoracic abscesses, a lung lobe after torsion, or primary lung neoplasms. Thoracic abscesses in rabbits are common, probably underdiagnosed, and often asymptomatic. They are caused by a variety of bacteria.[1]

Technique
The rabbit is placed in lateral recumbency, the affected side facing the surgeon, and the patient preparation for surgery is similar to that for medial thoracotomy.

- The skin incision is made at the caudodorsal border of the scapula.
- The latissimus dorsi muscle is incised from ventral to dorsal.
- The thoracic inlet and the first rib are identified by palpation beneath the latissimus dorsi muscle.
- The serratus ventralis muscle is separated and the scalene muscle is transected along the fifth rib.
- The intercostal muscles are transected and the ribs are spread with a retractor.
- Positive pressure ventilation is started immediately after accessing the thoracic cavity.
- The diseased lung lobe is lifted from the thoracic cavity and the short bronchus and vessels are ligated with absorbable suture material or with vascular clips. The lobe is removed and the bronchus is checked for air leakage by filling the thorax chest cavity with warmed sterile saline solution. The saline is thoroughly removed form the thorax using suction.
- The excess air from the thoracic cavity is removed and the lungs inflated using the chest drain or a temporary red rubber tube, similarly to median thoracotomy (see **Fig. 16**).
- The thoracic wall is closed using preplaced absorbable monofilament sutures encircling the ribs cranially and caudally from the wound.
- The closure and postoperative care are similar to those for median sternotomy.

Thoracostomy Tubes (Chest Drain Placement)
A chest drain facilitates the removal of air and fluid from the pleural space, eliminating the need of needle-guided thoracocentesis postoperatively. It can be placed in a closed fashion for air or fluid removal prior to surgical intervention or in an open fashion during any thoracotomy procedure. Advantages to placing thoracostomy tubes intraoperatively include the ability to protect intrathoracic structures as well as guide the thoracostomy tube to its desired location.[1]

Technique
- A stab incision is made at the level of the 10th intercostal space at the dorsal side of the chest.
- The tip of the drain with the trocar is advanced cranially, creating a subcutaneous tunnel to the level of the eighth intercostal space. The trocar is then gently advanced through the eighth intercostal space, perpendicular to the thoracic wall, avoiding the caudal edge of the eighth rib.

- Only a short portion of the trocar is advanced into the thorax to prevent any injuries of intrathoracic organs. The drain on the trocar is pushed forward to cover the sharp end. Both the trochar and the drain are advanced superficially, parallel to the thoracic wall to the level of the second rib. After reaching the desired position, the trocar is pulled back while the drain is held in position.
- The drain is occluded immediately with artery forceps and a connector with a 3-way stopcock. The artery forceps is removed and the excess air is gently drained with a 3–6 mL syringe from the chest. The authors suggest no more than 3 mL negative pressure when using a syringe.
- The 3-way tap is closed and the ports are sealed.
- The chest drain is sutured to the chest wall with Roman sandal tie around the tube, the site of insertion is covered with a dressing, and the tube is bandaged to the chest.

Postoperative care
Gloves should be worn when handling thoracostomy tubes to prevent ascending bacterial infection. The connections are regularly checked to ensure that a closed system is maintained. The bandage is changed daily. An Elizabethan collar could be considered to prevent interference with the tube.[1]

Complications
Complications include infections, pneumothorax if poorly placed and/or managed, lung injury after excessive suction, phrenic nerve irritation, Horner syndrome, or cardiac arrhythmias. Disadvantages of thoracostomy tubes include prolonged surgical time, prolonged hospitalization and increased cost, and intense, regular maintenance required.[1,9]

Postoperative Care After Thoracic Surgeries

After thoracic surgery, the rabbit should receive supplemental oxygen. Radiographs can be taken to assess the condition of the lung and to monitor the presence of air in the thoracic cavity. Bupivacaine (2 mg/kg) can be diluted with saline and instilled into the thoracic cavity every 8 hours through the chest drain for pain control. The chest drain is used for removal of air and fluid after the surgery.[65,66] Antibiotics, fluid therapy, analgesia, and supportive feeding are recommended similarly to abdominal surgeries.

REFERENCES

1. Harcourt-Brown F, Chitty J. BSAVA manual of rabbit surgery, dentistry and imaging. Quedgeley (United Kingdom): British Small Animal Veterinary Association; 2013.
2. Brodbelt DC, Blissitt KJ, Hammond RA, et al. The risk of death: the confidential enquiry into perioperative small animal fatalities. Vet Anaesth Analg 2008;35(5): 365–73.
3. Paul-Murphy J. Critical care of the rabbit. Vet Clin North Am Exot Anim Pract 2007;10(2):437–61.
4. Melillo A. Rabbit clinical pathology. J Exot Pet Med 2007;16(3):135–45.
5. Harcourt-Brown FM, Harcourt-Brown SF. Clinical value of blood glucose measurement in pet rabbits. Vet Rec 2012;170(26):674.
6. Lennox AM. Care of the geriatric rabbit. Vet Clin North Am Exot Anim Pract 2010; 13(1):123–33.
7. Harcourt-Brown F, Harcourt-Brown NH. Textbook of rabbit medicine. Oxford (United Kingdom): Butterworth-Heinemann; 2002.

8. Fisher PG. Standards of care in the 21st century: the rabbit. J Exot Pet Med 2010; 19(1):22–35.

9. Fossum TW. Small animal surgery. 4th edition. St Louis (MO): Elsevier Mosby; 2013.

10. Wenger S. Anesthesia and analgesia in rabbits and rodents. Semin Avian Exot Pet 2012;21(1):7–16.

11. Johnston MS. Clinical approaches to analgesia in ferrets and rabbits. Semin Avian Exot Pet 2005;14:229–35.

12. Barter LS. Rabbit analgesia. Vet Clin North Am Exot Anim Pract 2011;14(1): 93–104.

13. Lennox AM, Capello V. Tracheal intubation in exotic companion mammals. J Exot Pet Med 2008;17(3):221–7.

14. Johnson DH. Endoscopic intubation of exotic companion mammals. Vet Clin North Am Exot Anim Pract 2010;13(2):273–89.

15. Bateman L, Ludders JW, Gleed RD, et al. Comparison between facemask and laryngeal mask airway in rabbits during isoflurane anesthesia. Vet Anaesth Analg 2005;32(5):280–8.

16. Capello V. Common surgical procedures in pet rodents. J Exot Pet Med 2011; 20(4):294–307.

17. Redrobe S. Soft tissue surgery of rabbits and rodents. Semin Avian Exot Pet 2002;11:231–45.

18. Rosen LB. Nasogastric tube placement in rabbits. J Exot Pet Med 2011;20(1): 27–31.

19. Lennox AM. Equipment for exotic mammal and reptile diagnostics and surgery. J Exot Pet Med 2006;15(2):98–105.

20. Singisetti KK, Ashcroft GP. The aberdeen 'continuous interrupted' surgical suturing technique. Ann R Coll Surg Engl 2009;91(4):349.

21. McFadden MS. Suture materials and suture selection for use in exotic pet surgical procedures. J Exot Pet Med 2011;20(3):173–81.

22. Kakoei S, Baghaei F, Dabiri S, et al. A comparative in vivo study of tissue reactions to four suturing materials. Iran Endod J 2010;5(2):69–73.

23. Whitfield RR, Stills HF, Huls HR, et al. Effects of peritoneal closure and suture material on adhesion formation in a rabbit model. Am J Obstet Gynecol 2007;197(6): 644.e1–5. e645.

24. DeCubellis J, Graham J. Gastrointestinal disease in guinea pigs and rabbits. Vet Clin North Am Exot Anim Pract 2013;16(2):421–35.

25. Reusch B. Rabbit gastroenterology. Vet Clin North Am Exot Anim Pract 2005;8(2): 351–75.

26. Harcourt-Brown TR. Management of acute gastric dilation in rabbits. J Exot Pet Med 2007;16(3):168–74.

27. Harcourt-Brown FM. Gastric dilation and intestinal obstruction in 76 rabbits. Vet Rec 2007;161(12):409–14.

28. Pizzi R, Hagen RU, Meredith AL. Intermittent colic and intussusception due to a cecal polyp in a rabbit. J Exot Pet Med 2007;16(2):113–7.

29. Meredith A, Rayment L. Liver disease in rabbits. Semin Avian Exot Pet 2000.

30. Goodman AR, Casale SA. Short-term outcome following partial or complete liver lobectomy with a commercially prepared self-ligating loop in companion animals: 29 cases (2009–2012). J Am Vet Med Assoc 2014;244(6):693–8.

31. Graham J, Basseches J. Liver lobe torsion in pet rabbits: clinical consequences, diagnosis, and treatment. Vet Clin North Am Exot Anim Pract 2014;17(2): 195–202.

32. Graham JE, Orcutt CJ, Casale SA, et al. Liver lobe torsion in rabbits: 16 cases (2007 to 2012). J Exot Pet Med 2014;23(3):258–65.
33. Saunders R, Redrobe S, Barr F, et al. Liver lobe torsion in rabbits. J Small Anim Pract 2009;50(10):562.
34. Stanke NJ, Graham JE, Orcutt CJ, et al. Successful outcome of hepatectomy as treatment for liver lobe torsion in four domestic rabbits. J Am Vet Med Assoc 2011;238(9):1176–83.
35. Taylor HR, Staff CD. Clinical techniques: successful management of liver lobe torsion in a domestic rabbit (Oryctolagus cuniculus) by surgical lobectomy. J Exot Pet Med 2007;16(3):175–8.
36. Weisbroth SH. Torsion of the caudate lobe of the liver in the domestic rabbit (Oryctolagus). Vet Pathol 1975;12(1):13–5.
37. Wenger S, Barrett EL, Pearson GR, et al. Liver lobe torsion in three adult rabbits. J Small Anim Pract 2009;50(6):301–5.
38. Wilson RB, Holscher MA, Sly DL. Liver lobe torsion in a rabbit. Lab Anim Sci 1987;37(4):506–7.
39. Raidal SR, Raidal SL. Comparative renal physiology of exotic species. Vet Clin North Am Exot Anim Pract 2006;9(1):13–31.
40. Harcourt-Brown FM. Diagnosis of renal disease in rabbits. Vet Clin North Am Exot Anim Pract 2013;16(1):145–74.
41. Harcourt-Brown F. Radiographic signs of renal disease in rabbits. Vet Rec 2007;160(23):787–94.
42. Capello V. Diagnosis and treatment of urolithiasis in pet rabbits. Exotic DVM 2004;6(2):15–22.
43. Martorell J, Bailon D, Majó N, et al. Lateral approach to nephrotomy in the management of unilateral renal calculi in a rabbit (Oryctolagus cuniculus). J Am Vet Med Assoc 2012;240(7):863–8.
44. Rhody JL. Unilateral nephrectomy for hydronephrosis in a pet rabbit. Vet Clin North Am Exot Anim Pract 2006;9(3):633–41.
45. Hanke PR, Timm P, Falk G, et al. Behavior of different suture materials in the urinary bladder of the rabbit with special reference to wound healing, epithelization and crystallization. Urol Int 1994;52(1):26–33.
46. Seifman BD, Rubin MA, Williams AL, et al. Use of absorbable cyanoacrylate glue to repair an open cystotomy. J Urol 2002;167(4):1872–5.
47. Richardson C, Flecknell P. Routine neutering of rabbits and rodents. Practice 2006;28(2):70–9.
48. Millis DL, Walshaw R. Elective castrations and ovariohysterectomies in pet rabbits. J Am Anim Hosp Assoc 1992;28(6):491.
49. Walter B, Poth T, Böhmer E, et al. Uterine disorders in 59 rabbits. Vet Rec 2010;166(8):230–3.
50. Greene HS. Uterine adenomata in the rabbit III. Susceptibility as a function of constitutional factors. J Exp Med 1941;73(2):273–92.
51. Divers SJ. Clinical technique: endoscopic oophorectomy in the rabbit (oryctolagus cuniculus): the future of preventative sterilizations. J Exot Pet Med 2010;19(3):231–9.
52. Guzman DS, Graham JE, Keller K, et al. Colonic obstruction following ovariohysterectomy in rabbits: 3 cases. J Exot Pet Med 2015;24(1):112–9.
53. Suzuki M, Ozaki M, Ano N, et al. Testicular gonadoblastoma in two pet domestic rabbits (Oryctolagus cuniculus domesticus). J Vet Diagn Invest 2011;23(5):1028–32.
54. Maratea KA, Ramos-Vara JA, Corriveau LA, et al. Testicular interstitial cell tumor and gynecomastia in a rabbit. Vet Pathol 2007;44(4):513–7.

55. Anderson WI, Car BD, Kenny K, et al. Bilateral testicular seminoma in a New Zealand white rabbit (Oryctolagus cuniculus). Lab Anim Sci 1990;40(4):420–1.

56. Capello V. Surgical techniques for orchiectomy of the pet rabbit. Exotic DVM 2005;7(5):23–31.

57. Johnson-Delaney CA, Orosz SE. Rabbit respiratory system: clinical anatomy, physiology and disease. Vet Clin North Am Exot Anim Pract 2011;14(2):257–66.

58. Quesenberry K, Carpenter JW. Ferrets, rabbits and rodents: clinical medicine and surgery. Philadelphia: Elsevier Health Sciences; 2011.

59. Kostolich M, Panciera RJ. Thymoma in a domestic rabbit. Cornell Vet 1992;82(2):125–9.

60. Pilny AA, Reavill D. Chylothorax and thymic lymphoma in a pet rabbit (Oryctolagus cuniculus). J Exot Pet Med 2008;17(4):295–9.

61. Kunzel F, Hittmair KM, Hassan J, et al. Thymomas in rabbits: clinical evaluation, diagnosis, and treatment. J Am Anim Hosp Assoc 2012;48(2):97–104.

62. Wagner F, Beinecke A, Fehr M, et al. Recurrent bilateral exophthalmos associated with metastatic thymic carcinoma in a pet rabbit. J Small Anim Pract 2005;46(8):393–7.

63. Sanchez-Migallon DG, Mayer J, Gould J, et al. Radiation therapy for the treatment of thymoma in rabbits (Oryctolagus cuniculus). J Exot Pet Med 2006;15(2):138–44.

64. Andres KM, Kent M, Siedlecki CT, et al. The use of megavoltage radiation therapy in the treatment of thymomas in rabbits: 19 cases. Vet Comp Oncol 2012;10(2):82–94.

65. Morrisey JK, McEntee M. Therapeutic options for thymoma in the rabbit. Semin Avian Exot Pet 2005;14:175–81.

66. Clippinger TL, Bennett RA, Alleman AR, et al. Removal of a thymoma via median sternotomy in a rabbit with recurrent appendicular neurofibrosarcoma. J Am Vet Med Assoc 1998;213(8):1140–3, 1131.

Surgical Management of Ear Diseases in Rabbits

Rebecca Csomos, DVM, PhD, Georgia Bosscher, DVM,
Christoph Mans, Dr med vet, DACZM*, Robert Hardie, DVM, DACVS, DECVS*

KEYWORDS

- Rabbit • Ear anatomy • Otitis • Ear canal ablation • Bulla osteotomy

KEY POINTS

- Otitis externa and media are common problems in rabbits, particularly in lop-eared breeds.
- Knowledge of rabbit ear anatomy is essential to understanding the disease processes and treatment strategies.
- Surgical intervention is indicated for cases of otitis externa or media in which clinical signs are recurrent or refractory to medical management.
- A full diagnostic work-up, including otoscopic examination and diagnostic imaging, should be performed before surgical management.
- Significant neurologic complications, such as facial nerve paralysis and, less likely, vestibular disease, can occur with surgical intervention but are usually transient.

INTRODUCTION

Ear disorders are common in rabbits, with otitis externa and media being the most clinically relevant. Medical therapy may aid in controlling clinical signs but rarely resolves otitis externa and media because they are often chronic conditions by the time of diagnosis. The increasing use of surgical intervention is proving to be safe and effective. The surgical techniques are analogous to those used in dogs and cats, with some differences due to variations in anatomy. A complete knowledge of rabbit ear anatomy is essential to understanding the disease processes and treatment strategies.

EAR ANATOMY
External Ear

Rabbit ears are dominated by long pinnae that are used for sound amplification, behavioral communication, and thermoregulation. Large blood vessels course through the

The authors have nothing to disclose.
Department of Surgical Sciences, School of Veterinary Medicine, University of Wisconsin-Madison, 2015 Linden Drive, Madison, WI 53706, USA
* Corresponding authors.
E-mail addresses: cmans@vetmed.wisc.edu; hardier@svm.vetmed.wisc.edu

http://dx.doi.org/10.1016/j.cvex.2015.08.005
1094-9194/16/$ – see front matter
vetexotic.theclinics.com

pinna and provide an extensive blood supply that aids in the release of heat. These vessels are often used for venipuncture and intravenous catheterization (generally the medial or caudal auricular veins) because of their size and accessibility.

The ear canal of rabbits is formed by three interlocking cartilages that provide structure to the ear canal (**Fig. 1**). The most proximal (deep) cartilage is the annular cartilage (synonym: cartilaginous acoustic meatus), which forms a ring and arises from the bony acoustic meatus of the bulla. Distal to the annular cartilage are the auricular and scutiform cartilages that form the distal part of the ear canal and the pinna. The tragus, which is proximal portion of the auricular cartilage, connects to the annular cartilage.[1] The existence of a true horizontal ear canal in rabbits is controversial.[2] The vertical ear canal bends to form a very short section, which is oriented horizontally and attaches to the bony acoustic meatus, just distal to the tympanic membrane (see **Fig. 1**).[2,3]

The vasculature of the ear in rabbits is prominent and can be easily visualized by transillumination. The auricular arteries and veins run along the margins and the center of the pinna (**Fig. 2**).

Breed Differences

In lop-eared breeds, there is a 3–5 mm gap between the cartilaginous acoustic meatus and the tragus of the auricular cartilage. Because of this lack of continuous cartilage, the ear folds over on the soft tissue creating a kink in the ear canal. This kink prevents normal ear secretions (cerumen) from draining properly, resulting in accumulation of cerumen and the increased risk for secondary bacterial or yeast infections of the ear canal. The gradual buildup of cerumen and overgrowth of bacteria or yeast leads to chronic otitis externa that is challenging to manage because of the effective stenosis of the canal that prevents adequate flushing and application of topical therapy.[1] In some cases, the increased accumulation of cerumen escapes through the soft-tissue gap between the annular cartilage and the tragus and forms a diverticulum at the base of the ear.[1] This accumulation of cerumen at the base of the ear is commonly referred to as an ear-base abscess, ear-base empyema or aural diverticulosis, which may or may not be infected.[1] In contrast to upright-eared rabbits, which have a fairly wide and rigid ear canal (**Fig. 3**A, B), the ear canal in lop-eared rabbits is narrower and not rigid (**Fig. 3**D, E), predisposing to accumulation of cerumen and development of otitis externa.

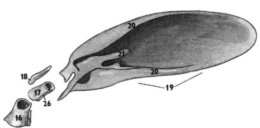

Fig. 1. Cartilages of the ear. The tragus (*21*) interlocks with the annual cartilage (*17*) and scutiform cartilage (*18*) to form the vertical ear canal in rabbits. 16, Bony acoustic meatus; 17, annular cartilage (syn cartilaginous acoustic meatus); 18, scutiform cartilage; 19, auricular cartilage; 20, helix; 21, tragus; 26, cartilaginous incisure of the annular cartilage. (*From* Popesko P, Rajtovà V, Horàk J. Rabbit. In: Popesko P, Rajtovà V, Horàk J, editors. A color atlas of anatomy of small laboratory animals, rabbit and guinea pig, vol. 1. London: Elsevier Saunders; 2002. p. 14–146; with permission.)

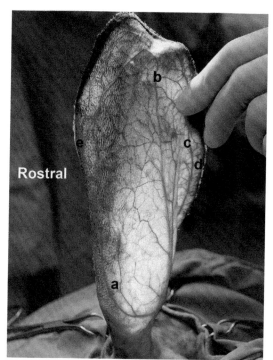

Fig. 2. Vasculature of the pinna in rabbits. Rostral auricular artery (*a*), intermedial branch of the caudal auricular artery (*b*), and caudal auricular artery (*c*). The veins of the pinna are not as prominent in this anesthetized rabbit. The caudal (*d*) and rostral (*e*) marginal veins run along the margins of the pinna.

Middle Ear

The tympanic membrane of rabbits is elliptical and consists of distinct portions, the larger pars tensa located ventrally and the smaller pars flaccida located dorsally (**Fig. 3**B, C).[3,4] It is located just deep to the annular cartilage making it difficult to visualize in upright-eared breeds and impossible in lop-eared breeds, without sedation or general anesthesia. The tympanic bulla is proportionally larger in rabbits compared with dogs and cats. The bone is thicker on the lateral and rostral aspects of the bullae and thinner ventrally.[1]

The facial nerve lies very close to the tympanic bulla.[5] The nerve enters the facial canal on the medial aspect of the bulla and exits the skull immediately caudal to the bulla, through the stylomastoid foramen (**Fig. 4**) coursing along the ventral surface of the tympanic bullae. The facial nerve primarily provides efferent innervation to the facial muscles but also carries some afferent sensory fibers (**Fig. 5**).[5] It also provides parasympathetic innervation to salivary and lacrimal glands. The close proximity of the nerve to the ear canal and bulla can lead to facial nerve paralysis in cases of otitis media.[1]

Diagnostics

A full work-up should start with an otoscopic examination performed on both ears using either a handheld otoscope or preferably videoendoscopy (see **Fig. 3**).[3] A thorough examination of the ear canal and tympanic membrane typically requires heavy sedation or general anesthesia, as the tympanic membrane can be difficult or impossible to

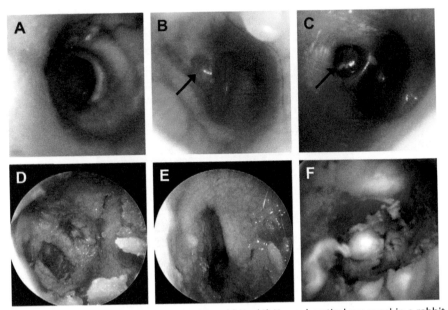

Fig. 3. Otoscopic images of the ear canal in rabbits. (*A*) Normal vertical ear canal in a rabbit with upright ears. (*B, C*) Normal tympanic membranes revealing the two distinct parts. The larger oval is the pars tensa, and the smaller part (*arrow*) is the pars flaccida. (*D*) Accumulation of cerumen and hyperplasia of the epithelial lining of the ear canal in a lop-eared rabbit. (*E*) Ear canal in a lop-eared rabbit. Note the narrowed diameter and partial collapse compared with the ear canal in a rabbit with upright ears (*A*). (*F*) Saline infusion otoscopy in a lop-eared rabbit with severe bacterial otitis externa. Note the presence of purulent debris within the ear canal and severe inflammation of the wall of the ear canal.

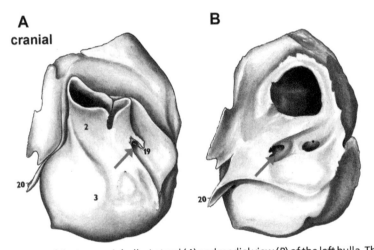

Fig. 4. Anatomy of the tympanic bulla. Lateral (*A*) and medial view (*B*) of the left bulla. The facial nerve exits the cranial cavity through the facial canal (*B, arrow*) and exits the skull through the stylomastoid foramen caudal to the bulla (*A, arrow*). 2, bony acoustic meatus; 3, tympanic bulla; 19, stylomastoid foramen; 20, styloid process. (*From* Popesko P, Rajtovà V, Horàk J. Rabbit. In: Popesko P, Rajtovà V, Horàk J, editors. A color atlas of anatomy of small laboratory animals, rabbit and guinea pig, vol. 1. London: Elsevier Saunders; 2002. p. 14–146; with permission.)

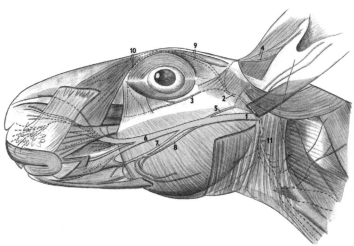

Fig. 5. Anatomy of the facial nerve in rabbits. 1, facial nerve; 2, auriculopalpebral nerve; 3, zygomatic branch; 4, rostral auricular branches; 5, communicating branch with auriculotemporal and facial nerves; 6, dorsal buccal branch; 7, ventral buccal branch; 8, marginal branch; 9, palpebral branch; 10, branches to the nasolabial levator muscle and to the inferior palpebral depressor muscle; 11, branch of the facial nerve to the superficial cutaneous muscle of the neck. (*From* Popesko P, Rajtovà V, Horàk J. Rabbit. In: Popesko P, Rajtovà V, Horàk J, editors. A color atlas of anatomy of small laboratory animals, rabbit and guinea pig, vol. 1. London: Elsevier Saunders; 2002. p. 14–146; with permission.)

visualize in a conscious rabbit. Waxy debris is a common finding and should be distinguished from purulent or caseous material via cytology, if necessary.[1,3] The benefits of videoendoscopy include being able to simultaneously examine the canal while flushing any inflammatory or waxy debris to ensure no abnormalities are missed, as well as guiding in myringotomy, if necessary.[3] Another benefit of endoscopy is the ability to obtain images for documenting disease progress, monitoring treatment, and client education (see **Fig. 3**). Endoscopy is an excellent tool for assessment of the ear canal, but it is of limited use for evaluation of the middle and inner ear.

Skull radiographs may be useful for identifying thickening of the bone or the presence of fluid in the bulla but can be difficult to interpret because of superimposition of structures. Computed tomography (CT) is very useful for diagnosing middle/inner ear disease in rabbits. Cross-sectional imaging provided by CT eliminates problems with superimposition and more clearly shows the anatomy and extent of disease (**Fig. 6**). CT of the head can usually be performed under sedation in rabbits eliminating the need for general anesthesia (see **Fig. 6**A, B).

DISEASES OF THE PINNA
Aural Hematoma/Edema

Vigorous head shaking or ear scratching, especially in lop-eared breeds, can result in aural hematoma or edema formation from trauma caused by the hind feet, nearby cage bars, or simply the centrifugal forces exerted on the thin-walled capillaries of the ear. Hemorrhage from these vessels results in an accumulation of blood trapped within the subcutaneous space between the cartilage and skin of the pinna. Like aural hematomas in dogs and cats, these pockets often require surgical drainage for complete resolution. If left untreated, the pinna may become scarred or deformed, or avascular necrosis may develop, necessitating partial amputation.

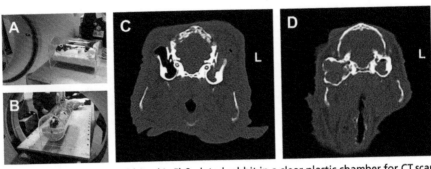

Fig. 6. CT of the head in rabbits. (*A, B*) Sedated rabbit in a clear plastic chamber for CT scan. (*C, D*) Transverse CT images diagnosed with left-sided otitis externa and media (*C*) and bilateral otitis media (*D*). (*D*) Note the expansion and proliferation of the right tympanic bulla.

Clinical signs include a soft to firm fluid-filled swelling on the pinna or base of the ear, which can vary in size and may be warm and/or uncomfortable to the touch (**Fig. 7**A). Other clinical signs may include scratching at the ear or head shaking indicating otitis externa.[1,6]

Treatment of aural hematomas in rabbits is similar to that described for dogs and cats.[7]

- With the rabbit in lateral recumbency, a vertically oriented, partial-thickness incision is made on the surface of the pinna over the length of the hematoma. The incision can be either linear or *S* shaped or multiple smaller incisions can be made (**Fig. 7**B).
- The hematoma is drained, and all clots and fibrinous material are thoroughly lavaged with sterile saline (see **Fig. 7**B).
- Partial- or full-thickness mattress sutures (8–10 mm in length) are placed parallel to the incision leaving a small gap in the incision to allow for continual drainage (**Fig. 7**C, D).
- An ample number of sutures should be placed to prevent reaccumulation of fluid, but caution should be taken to avoid compromising the blood supply or incorporating the auricular vessels. To aid in avoiding the auricular vessels, a light source may be used to transilluminate the ear during suture placement.[1]

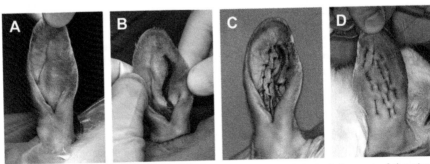

Fig. 7. Surgical treatment of an aural hematoma in a rabbit. (*A*) Medial aspect of the pinna revealing the aural hematoma. (*B*) A vertical *S*-shaped incision made over the hematoma to allow drainage and removal of blood clots and fibrinous material. (*C*) Full-thickness mattress sutures placed parallel to the incision. The incision is left open to allow continued drainage. (*D*) Appearance of the lateral aspect of the pinna after placement of the mattress sutures. (*Courtesy of* Dr Zoltan Szabo, Hong Kong, SAR China.)

As an alternative to surgical drainage and suturing, passive drains or cannulas can be placed and maintained for several weeks. However, this technique can be difficult to maintain because of intolerance and early dislodgement in rabbits.

Lacerations of the Pinna

- Before surgical repair, lacerations should be thoroughly lavaged and cleaned.
- The skin edges should be evaluated for necrosis and debrided where indicated.
- Skin margins should be reapposed if possible with 4–0 or smaller nonabsorbable suture material in a simple-interrupted pattern.
- For flaps of skin separated from the underlying cartilage, reapposition should be achieved with vertical-mattress sutures placed within the center of the flap to reduce dead space and anchor the skin to the cartilage and simple-interrupted sutures placed along the edge of the laceration using nonabsorbable suture material.[7]
- For full-thickness lacerations, the skin on both sides of the ear should be reapposed separately in a simple-interrupted pattern. Alternatively, full-thickness vertical-mattress sutures can be placed on one side incorporating the cartilage and skin and simple-interrupted sutures can be placed on the other side apposing just the skin. In rabbits, the vertical mattress sutures are typically placed on the medial side because the auricular vasculature is less prominent on that side of the ear.[1]

Tumors

Tumors can occur anywhere throughout the ear but are diagnosed most commonly on the pinna. Epithelial tumors are the most common; but other types have been described, including viral-induced Shope fibromas, papillomas, trichoblastomas, and melanomas (**Fig. 8**).[8] Squamous cell carcinoma and lymphoma have also been described but seem to be more common in rabbits bred for laboratory purposes rather than as pets.[9] Malignant trichoepitheliomas have also been described extending into the ear canal.[10]

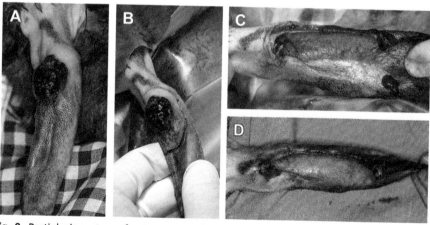

Fig. 8. Partial pinnectomy for treatment of a malignant melanoma in a rabbit. (*A*) Melanoma on the rostral aspect of the pinna. (*B*) A skin incision is made using a monopolar electrosurgery device. (*C*) Following resection of the mass, the edges of the cartilage are trimmed to facilitate apposition of the skin edges. (*D*) Apposition of the skin edges using horizontal mattress sutures. (*Courtesy of* Dr Zoltan Szabo, Hong Kong, SAR China.)

Advanced imaging, biopsy, and histopathology may be required to determine if a tumor is surgically resectable. If the tumor is on the pinna, removal may be achieved with local resection or partial amputation. If the tumor extends within the ear canal, a total ear canal ablation (TECA) and lateral bulla osteotomy (LBO) may be warranted.

Pinnectomy

Surgical management of tumors, avascular necrosis, or trauma to the pinna may involve either partial or complete pinnectomy.

Partial pinnectomy

The affected area of the pinna is identified and resected (see **Fig. 8**).[7] Care should be taken to prevent damage to the caudal and rostral auricular vessels, as damage to these vessels can lead to further pinna edema and potential necrosis (see **Fig. 2**).[1] To achieve proper apposition of the skin edges, the underlying cartilage is resected an additional 1 to 2 mm to minimize tension and allow for direct skin-to-skin apposition (see **Fig. 8**D).[1] If necessary, the skin can be further mobilized by undermining it from the cartilage on both sides of the ear.[7] The skin is sutured over the cartilage edge using 4–0 or smaller nonabsorbable suture material in a simple-interrupted or horizontal mattress pattern (see **Fig. 8**D).

Total pinnectomy

For total pinnectomy, a horizontal incision is made starting cranially at the level of the intertragic incisure and extended circumferentially around the base of the ear.[1] The incision is made through the skin and cartilage; similar to partial pinnectomy, an additional 1 to 2 mm of cartilage is resected to facilitate a tension-free skin closure. In cases where a neoplastic lesion extends into the ear canal, a TECA-LBO should be considered in combination with a pinnectomy.[1] To eliminate any dead space, 4–0 or smaller absorbable sutures may be placed in a simple-interrupted pattern. Similar to a partial pinnectomy, the skin is sutured over the cartilage with 4–0 or smaller nonabsorbable suture material in a simple-interrupted or horizontal mattress pattern.

Postoperative Care

Following pinna surgery, the ear may be lightly bandaged and supported over the head to protect from contamination and trauma, in selected cases. An Elizabethan collar may be indicated in some rabbits if self-trauma is caused by the hind limbs. In addition, general supportive care, including analgesia, antiinflammatory medications, and antibiotic therapy, should be instituted, as necessary.

Complications

Complications include incisional swelling, infection, self-traumatization, or dehiscence caused by excessive tension on the sutures.

DISEASES OF THE EAR CANAL

Otitis Externa

Otitis externa is rare in upright-eared breeds, but when present, may be associated with an ear mite infection, foreign body. In contrast, otitis externa is common in lop-eared breeds due to the abnormal anatomy of the ear canal (see **Fig. 3**D–F) and is difficult to manage medically. Otitis externa can also spread to the middle or inner ear if the tympanic membrane becomes compromised (see **Fig. 6**B, C).

Clinical signs include head shaking, redness and swelling of the outer ear canal, pain, pruritus, and increased malodorous waxy debris or purulent discharge. An ear-base abscess may be present in lop-eared breeds, manifesting as a swelling surrounding the base of the ear canal.[1] The presence of large amounts of cerumen in an ear-base abscess may not necessarily result in clinical signs, if a secondary infection does not develop. Treatment of cases without clinical signs is controversial and rabbits without clinical signs may be best left untreated until clinical signs develop.[11] The presence of waxy cerumen and the narrowed ear canal in lop-eared rabbits make topical treatment unsuccessful in most cases and while temporary improvement may be achieved, relapse is very common.[11] Cleaning of the ear canal should be performed under general anesthesia and preferably using videoendoscopy (see **Fig. 3F**).[3]

Surgery of the Ear Canal

Ear canal surgery is indicated for otitis externa that is refractory to appropriate medical management, as well as, for tumors or trauma not amenable to local resection or reconstruction.[10,12,13] Either partial ear canal ablation (PECA) or TECA, in combination with LBO, should be performed depending on the extent of disease in the distal ear canal.[2,10,12]

Resection of the lateral wall of the ear canal may be useful in select cases of otitis externa, to improve drainage and ventilation. However, case selection is critical and this technique may not resolve clinical signs, if the underlying disease process has not been addressed.[2]

Partial Ear Canal Ablation

A PECA is the preferred surgical procedure for most rabbits with otitis externa with or without otitis media. This procedure is faster, less invasive, carries less risk for complications, and maintains normal ear carriage compared with a TECA.[2] Unless neoplastic or inflammatory disease cannot be adequately resected during a PECA, a TECA should be avoided, if possible.

- The procedure is performed with the animal in lateral recumbency (**Fig. 9**).
- A vertical incision is made over the ear canal, and the canal is isolated from the surrounding tissue using a combination of blunt and sharp dissection (**Fig. 10**A).

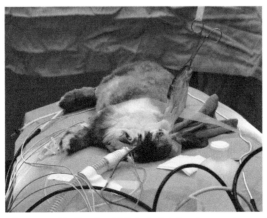

Fig. 9. Positioning of an anesthetized rabbit in left lateral recumbency in preparation for PECA and LBO of the right ear.

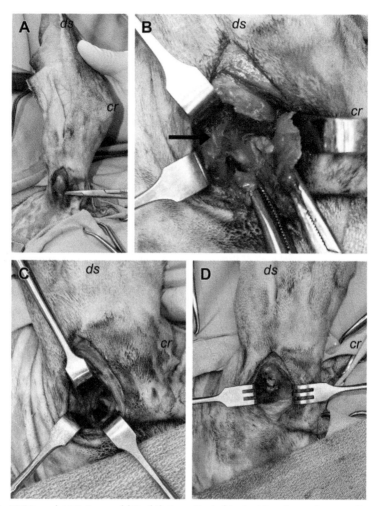

Fig. 10. PECA and LBO in a rabbit. (*A*) A vertical skin incision is made over the middle portion of the vertical ear canal and the ear canal is isolated by blunt and sharp dissection. (*B*) The canal is transected transversely and dissection of the proximal portion is continued to the level of the bony acoustic meatus. Damage of the facial nerve (*arrow*) should be avoided. (*C*) Following excision of the proximal ear canal, a LBO is performed. (*D*) The remaining distal portion of the ear canal is closed in a simple-interrupted pattern using absorbable suture material. cr, cranial; ds, dorsal.

- The canal is transected transversely approximately 2 cm from the external opening and dissection of the proximal portion is continued to the level of the bony acoustic meatus taking care to stay close to the canal to avoid accidentally injuring the facial nerve, which courses caudal and ventral to the base of the ear canal (**Fig. 10**B).
- Once the canal is isolated, it is excised at the level of the bony acoustic meatus.
- Following completion of the PECA, a LBO is performed (see description later) (**Fig. 10**C).
- The site is lavaged with sterile saline. If indicated, the ear canal is also submitted for histopathologic analysis.

- The remaining portion of the ear canal is closed in a simple-interrupted pattern using absorbable suture material (**Fig. 10**D).
- The surgical site is closed in a routine fashion, using 4–0 or smaller absorbable suture material for the subcutaneous tissue and 4–0 or smaller nonabsorbable suture material for the skin (**Fig. 12**A, B).

Total Ear Canal Ablation

In cases of severe otitis externa that extend to the distal portion of the vertical canal, a TECA should be performed to ensure complete removal of diseased tissue not possible with a PECA. Also, a TECA should be considered for tumors of the pinna extending into the ear canal or for tumors originating from the distal portion of the ear canal. The postsurgical complications are considered higher following TECA compared with PECA and include wound dehiscence and vascular compromise of the pinna.

- A TECA is performed with the rabbit in lateral recumbency (see **Fig. 9**).
- A *T*-shaped incision is made over the ear canal. The vertical portion of the incision extends from the midpoint of the horizontal incision down the lateral aspect of the canal (**Fig. 11**A).
- The horizontal incision is continued circumferentially around the ear canal opening and the ear canal is isolated from the surrounding tissue using a combination of blunt and sharp dissection taking care to stay close to the cartilage to avoid accidentally injuring the facial nerve (**Fig. 11**B, C).
- At the level of the bony acoustic meatus, the entire cartilaginous canal is excised.
- Following completion of the TECA, a LBO is performed.
- The surgical site is closed in a routine fashion, using 4–0 or smaller absorbable suture material for the subcutaneous tissue and 4–0 or smaller nonabsorbable suture material for the skin (**Fig. 12**C, D).

Postoperative Care

General supportive care is recommended for rabbits undergoing ear canal surgery, including analgesia, antiinflammatory medications, nutritional supplementation, and

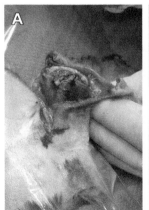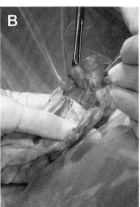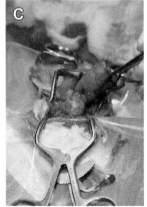

Fig. 11. TECA in a rabbit. Progressive phases of dissection (*A–C*) of the vertical ear canal from the surrounding soft tissues during a TECA and LBO procedure. Note the dilation of the proximal portion of the ear canal in C.

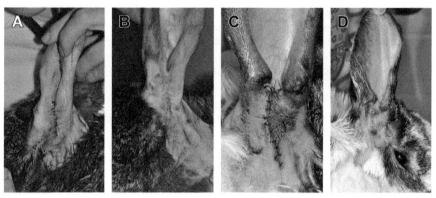

Fig. 12. Postoperative appearance following PECA (*A, B*) and TECA (*C, D*) combined with LBO in rabbits. (*A*) Immediate postoperative appearance of a PECA following closure of the incision using a simple-interrupted pattern. (*B*) Appearance after suture removal. (*C*) Immediate postoperative appearance of a TECA following closure of the incision using a simple-interrupted suture pattern. (*D*) Appearance after suture removal.

appropriate systemic antimicrobial therapy based on culture and susceptibility results. Additional supportive care, such as eye lubrication, should be instituted to reduce the risk of exposure keratitis if facial nerve paralysis is present.[10,13] Suture removal can be performed at 10 to 14 days postoperatively.

Complications

Numerous postoperative complications have been reported following PECA/TECA and LBO. Although the overall complication rate for these procedures in rabbits is unknown, owners should be thoroughly educated about the potential complications and the consequences (ie, exposure keratitis and treatment [application of eye lubricant]). In dogs, vestibular disease (65%), wound dehiscence (15%), and facial nerve deficits (11%) were the most common complications following TECA-LBO.[14] Following PECA/TECA-LBO, temporary or permanent facial nerve paresis or paralysis is common in rabbits. In most cases, facial nerve paralysis (lack of palpebral reflex, ipsilateral drooling, facial drooping) (**Fig. 13**) is temporary and function will return within a few weeks

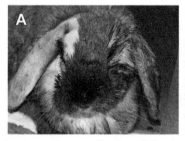
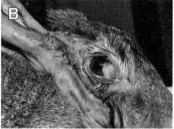

Fig. 13. Postoperative complications following TECA (*A*) and PECA (*B*) combined with LBO. (*A*) Note the right-sided facial asymmetry and droopiness due to acute iatrogenic facial nerve injury following TECA-LBO. (*B*) Postoperative appearance following PECA-LBO. Note the ectropion of the lower eyelid and exposure of the third eyelid due to iatrogenic facial nerve injury. The third eyelid was functional because its muscle is innervated by the abducens nerve.

following surgery. The third eyelid in rabbits is large and movement is not affected by facial nerve paralysis because the associated retractor bulbi muscle receives efferent innervation from the abducent nerve (see **Fig. 13**B).[15] Therefore, the functional third eyelid provides some protection for the cornea in cases of facial nerve paralysis following PECA/TECA-LBO. In addition, incisional dehiscence, infection, and draining tract formation have also been reported.[2,12]

DISEASES OF THE MIDDLE AND INNER EAR
Otitis Media and Interna

Bacterial otitis media and interna may result from hematogenous spread, ascending infection through the Eustachian tube or as an extension of otitis externa following rupture of the tympanic membrane. Lop-eared rabbits with otitis externa are at a higher risk for developing otitis media.[16]

Infection of the middle or inner ear in rabbits is historically associated with *Pasteurella multocida* and has been reported in 33% of rabbits at necropsy.[17,18] However, in pet rabbits, other species of bacteria are often cultured, including *Staphylococcus* spp, *Streptococcus spp*, *Bordetella bronchiseptica, Pseudomonas aeruginosa, Proteus mirabilis*, and *Bacteroides* spp.[19]

Rabbits with otitis media may show no clinical signs. The incidental diagnosis of otitis media was made by CT scan of the head in 27% of rabbits without any related clinical signs.[16] Clinical signs often become apparent if otitis media progresses to otitis interna or externa. Clinical signs can include vestibular signs, including mild to severe torticollis (head tilted toward the affected side), horizontal or rotatory nystagmus, strabismus, ataxia, and falling or circling toward the affected side (**Fig. 14**A). Facial nerve paralysis may result in facial asymmetry, absent or weak palpebral reflex, or corneal ulceration (**Fig. 14**B).[19] Otitis media alone can lead to nonspecific clinical signs, such as anorexia, followed by secondary gastrointestinal stasis, lethargy, altered behavior, or discomfort.

Diagnosis often requires diagnostic imaging to evaluate the extent of disease within the bulla as well as the surrounding soft tissue involvement. Skull radiographs have a low specificity for diagnosis of otitis media because bony changes of the

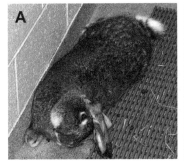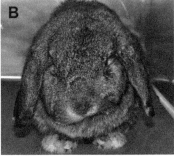

Fig. 14. Clinical appearance of rabbits with otitis media (*A*) and otitis media and interna (*B*). (*A*) Rabbit with left-sided chronic otitis media. Note the asymmetry of the face caused by atrophy of the left facial muscles secondary to chronic facial nerve paralysis. (*B*) Rabbit with peripheral vestibular disease secondary to chronic bacterial otitis media and interna. Note the left-sided head tilt and inability to stand. Also present was a horizontal nystagmus.

bulla may not always be visualized. Therefore, CT of the head is the diagnostic imaging technique of choice (see **Fig. 6**). Medical management of otitis media, which is usually chronic, is frequently unrewarding but is aimed at improving clinical signs and not necessarily eradicating the chronic infection. Response to antibiotic therapy is often disappointing because of the difficulty with penetration to the middle ear. Surgical intervention is the treatment of choice for otitis media and interna, especially if any destruction of the bulla is present on CT.

Surgery of the Middle Ear

Indications for middle ear surgery include otitis media that is nonresponsive to medical management as well as for tumors originating in the bulla.[12] The goal of middle ear surgery is removal of any caseous debris, diagnostic sampling, and local treatment. Concurrent otitis externa will help dictate which surgical procedure should be performed. A ventral bulla osteotomy (VBO) is performed for signs localized to the middle and inner ear only, whereas a LBO is performed in combination with PECA or TECA in cases with disease involving the middle ear and the ear canal.[10,12]

Lateral Bulla Osteotomy

- An LBO is performed in conjunction with either PECA or TECA.
- The soft tissues overlying the bony acoustic meatus and tympanic bulla are bluntly elevated with a Freer periosteal elevator.
- Bulla osteotomy is performed using rongeurs or pneumatic burr. The acoustic meatus is enlarged cranially and ventrally to provide adequate access and drainage of bulla taking care to avoid the facial nerve that exits the stylomastoid foramen immediately caudal to the acoustic meatus.
- Once the osteotomy is completed, the bulla is carefully curetted to remove any debris as well as the epithelium lining the middle ear taking care to avoid the oval and round windows on the dorsal medial aspect of the bulla.
- Samples from the bulla are submitted for bacterial culture and susceptibility and histopathology, as necessary.
- The site is lavaged with sterile saline; antibiotic-impregnated polymethyl methacrylate (PMMA) beads are placed in the surgical field, if necessary, based on previous or anticipated culture and susceptibility results.
- The surgical site is closed in a routine fashion using 4–0 or smaller absorbable suture material for the subcutaneous tissue and 4–0 or smaller nonabsorbable suture material for the skin. Marsupialization of the surgical site and postsurgical flushing or placement of drains does is not recommended in rabbits and has been shown to not improve outcome in dogs that underwent TECA-LBO, when compared with primary closure.[2,14]

Ventral Bulla Osteotomy

- A VBO is performed in dorsal recumbency with the neck fully extended.
- Because of the presence of a prominent semicircular mandibular angle in rabbits, the bulla cannot be directly palpated until the overlying muscles are partially dissected.
- A 4–5 cm skin incision is made parallel and medial to the mandible. The incision is continued through the platysma muscle medial to the mandibular salivary gland.[12]

- The digastricus muscle is dissected from the hyoglossus and styloglossus muscles taking care to avoid the hypoglossal nerve coursing lateral to the hyoglossus muscle.
- Gelpi retractors are used to provide exposure of underlying tissues throughout the procedure.
- The bulla is palpated between the jugular process of the skull and mandibular angle.
- Using a Freer periosteal elevator, blunt dissection is continued until the ventral surface of the bulla is exposed.
- The bulla is entered on the ventral aspect with a Steinmann pin and hand chuck. The osteotomy is extended circumferentially with rongeurs or a pneumatic burr to allow adequate access and drainage.
- The bulla is carefully curetted to remove any debris as well as the epithelium lining the middle ear.
- Samples for culture and susceptibility and histopathology are obtained as necessary and the site lavaged with sterile saline. Antibiotic-impregnated PMMA beads are placed in the surgical field, if necessary, based on previous or anticipated culture and susceptibility results.
- The surgical site is closed in a routine fashion using 4–0 or smaller absorbable suture material for the muscle and subcutaneous tissue and 4–0 or smaller nonabsorbable suture material for the skin.

Postoperative Care

Postoperative care is similar for osteotomy procedures and includes analgesia, anti-inflammatory medications, and antibiotic therapy based on culture results. Suture removal is performed 10 to 14 days postoperatively.

Complications

Facial nerve paralysis, Horner syndrome, vestibular disease, and hypoglossal nerve dysfunction can be observed following bulla osteotomy. Dehiscence, hemorrhage, recurrent infection/abscess, and fistula or draining tracts have also been reported. Although major complications can arise, most are uncommon and transiently observed.[2,10,12]

REFERENCES

1. Chitty J, Raftery A. Ear and sinus surgery. In: Hartcourt-Brown F, Chitty J, editors. BSAVA manual of rabbit surgery, dentistry and imaging. Glouchester (United Kingdom): BSAVA; 2014. p. 212–32.
2. Eatwell K, Mancinelli E, Hedley J, et al. Partial ear canal ablation and lateral bulla osteotomy in rabbits. J Small Anim Pract 2013;54(6):325–30.
3. Jekl V, Hauptman K, Knotek Z. Video otoscopy in exotic companion mammals. Vet Clin North Am Exot Anim Pract 2015;18(3):431–45.
4. Chole RA, Kodama K. Comparative histology of the tympanic membrane and its relationship to cholesteatoma. Ann Otol Rhinol Laryngol 1989;98(10):761–6.
5. Osofsky A, LeCouteur RA, Vernau KM. Functional neuroanatomy of the domestic rabbit (Oryctolagus cuniculus). Vet Clin North Am Exot Anim Pract 2007;10(3): 713–30, v.
6. Manjunatha D, Mahesh V, Ranganath L. Surgical management of aural hematoma in Russian grey giant rabbit (SURGICAL MANAGEMENT OF AURAL HEMATOMA

IN RUSSIAN GREY GIANT RABBIT–A CASE REPORT). Int J Agric Sc Vet Med 2014;2(3):37–8.
7. Fossum TW. Surgery of the ear. In: Fossum TW, editor. Small animal surgery. St Louis (MO): Mosby-Elsevier; 2013. p. 325–55.
8. von Bomhard W, Goldschmidt MH, Shofer FS, et al. Cutaneous neoplasms in pet rabbits: a retrospective study. Vet Pathol 2007;44(5):579–88.
9. Weisbroth SH, Manning PJ, Ringler DH. Neoplastic disease. In: Manning PJ, Ringler DH, Newcomer C, editors. The biology of the laboratory rabbit. San Diego (CA): Academic Press; 1994. p. 259–92.
10. Budgeon C, Mans C, Chamberlin T, et al. Diagnosis and surgical treatment of a malignant trichoepithelioma of the ear canal in a pet rabbit (Oryctolagus cuniculus). J Am Vet Med Assoc 2014;245(2):227–31.
11. Varga M. Chapter 7-skin diseases. In: Varga M, editor. Textbook of rabbit medicine. 2nd edition. Philadelphia: Butterworth-Heinemann; 2014. p. 271–302.
12. Chow EP. Surgical management of rabbit ear disease. J Exot Pet Med 2011;20(3): 182–7.
13. Chow EP, Bennett RA, Whittington JK. Total ear canal ablation and lateral bulla osteotomy for treatment of otitis externa and media in a rabbit. J Am Vet Med Assoc 2011;239(2):228–32.
14. Doyle RS, Skelly C, Bellenger CR. Surgical management of 43 cases of chronic otitis externa in the dog. Ir Vet J 2004;57(1):22–30.
15. Gray TS, McMaster SE, Harvey JA, et al. Localization of retractor bulbi motoneurons in the rabbit. Brain Res 1981;226(1–2):93–106.
16. de Matos R, Ruby J, Van Hatten RA, et al. Computed tomographic features of clinical and subclinical middle ear disease in domestic rabbits (Oryctolagus cuniculus): 88 cases (2007-2014). J Am Vet Med Assoc 2015;246(3):336–43.
17. Fox RR, Norberg RF, Myers DD. The relationship of Pasteurella multocida to otitis media in the domestic rabbit (Oryctolagus cuniculus). Lab Anim Sci 1971;21(1): 45–8.
18. Snyder SB, Fox JG, Soave OA. Subclinical otitis media associated with Pasteurella multocida infections in New Zealand white rabbits (Oryctolagus cuniculus). Lab Anim Sci 1973;23(2):270–2.
19. Campbell-Ward ML. Otitis. In: Donnelly JMM, editor. Clinical veterinary advisor. St Louis (MO): W.B. Saunders; 2013. p. 403–5.

Small Mammals

Common Surgical Procedures of Rodents, Ferrets, Hedgehogs, and Sugar Gliders

Yasutsugu Miwa, DVM, PhD[a],*,
Kurt K. Sladky, MS, DVM, DACZM, DECZM (Herpetology)[b]

KEYWORDS

- Rodent • Ferret • Hedgehog • Guinea pig • Chinchilla • Sugar glider • Surgery
- Anesthesia

KEY POINTS

- Surgical principles developed in dogs and cats can be directly applied to small mammals with some adaptations.
- Maintaining normal body temperature during prolonged procedures and minimizing blood loss are significantly more important in small mammals compared with dogs and cats.
- Key anatomic differences between small mammalian species must be known prior to performing any surgical procedure.
- Small mammal surgery requires knowledge of anesthetic techniques and application of appropriate analgesics.
- Common surgical procedures in small mammals include: integumentary mass and abscess excision, reproductive procedures (orchidectomy, ovariectomy, and ovariohysterectomy), gastrointestinal foreign body removal, prolapsed gastrointestinal tissues, urolith removal, and intra-abdominal mass excision.

INTRODUCTION

Developing skills associated with small mammal surgical procedures is important for clinical practice, whether in private/referral practice, a laboratory animal facility, or a zoologic institution. For quality veterinary care, it is important to understand not only anatomic and behavioral differences between species but also the most common clinical presentations for each small mammal species. This article describes common

The authors have nothing to disclose.
[a] Miwa Exotic Animal Hospital, 1-25-5 Komagome, Toshima-ku, Tokyo 170-0003, Japan;
[b] Department of Surgical Sciences, School of Veterinary Medicine, University of Wisconsin, Madison, WI 53706, USA
* Corresponding author.
E-mail address: miwayasutsugu@hotmail.com

Vet Clin Exot Anim 19 (2016) 205–244
http://dx.doi.org/10.1016/j.cvex.2015.09.001
1094-9194/16/$ – see front matter © 2016 Elsevier Inc. All rights reserved.

surgical techniques in rodents, ferrets, hedgehogs, and sugar gliders. Surgical procedures discussed in this article include integumentary mass and abscess removals, wound management, self-mutilation, management of prolapsed tissues, gastrointestinal and hepatic surgery, reproductive and urinary tract procedures, and endocrine diseases.

PRESURGICAL CONSIDERATIONS
Anesthesia and Analgesia

Anesthesia of small mammals, especially rodents, hedgehogs, and sugar gliders, can be challenging, and although this article is not intended to provide detailed information or protocols for small mammal anesthesia, it is, nevertheless, important to highlight a few important points. There are several premedication and sedation protocols available in the literature for small mammals, but intubation can be difficult for anesthesia maintenance in most small mammal species.[1,2] The exception in this article is the ferret, which is easy to intubate, similar to intubating a small cat or kitten. Most rodent species and hedgehogs, however, require endoscopic intubation due to small oral cavities and obstructed view of the epiglottis.[3] Without access to endoscopic intubation techniques, most clinicians default to using a small facemask for gas anesthetic induction and maintenance. Placement of an intravenous (IV) catheter benefits any animal undergoing a surgical procedure, and this is especially true in small mammals. IV or intraosseous access facilitates fluid administration for maintenance and replacement in the face of blood loss and provides rapid correction of cardiovascular perturbations by use of appropriate cardiopulmonary stimulant drugs.[1,2] Small IV catheters (26 gauge to 23 gauge) can be placed in cephalic or saphenous veins of most small mammals and maintained during the procedure. IO catheters (eg, appropriately sized spinal needles or hypodermic needles) are most commonly placed in the proximal tibia or proximal femur. Appropriate anesthetic monitoring is critical during small mammal surgical procedures by use of a pulse oximeter, capnometer, ECG, and indirect blood pressure units. It is also important to monitor body temperature frequently, because low body temperature can cause markedly delayed, or lack of, postsurgical recovery. Use of circulating water heating pads, microwaveable heating devices, or Bair Huggers (3M, Corporation, St. Paul, MN, USA) for maintaining patient warmth should be considered imperative. Preemptive analgesia, or analgesics administered prior to induction of a painful stimulus, is crucial in small mammals, although the literature is sparse with specifics with respect to analgesic efficacy, dosages, duration, frequency of administration, and safety.[2,4–6] As with most nondomestic species, clinicians tend to extrapolate dosages from domestic mammals and hope there is some efficacy without detrimental side effects.

Surgical Preparation

Once an animal is appropriately anesthetized, maintained on monitors, provided supplemental warmth, and administered presurgical analgesics, and other medications, the hair around the surgical site can be clipped and the site aseptically prepared. Clippers and blades may need to be smaller than those typically used for dogs and cats, and some small mammals have delicate skin that is, easily traumatized by clippers. It is not uncommon for a surgeon to accidently begin an incision with a clippers if not careful. Surgical site preparation is similar to dogs and cats, with chlorhexidine or povidone iodine-based soaps used for cleaning, and alcohol or warm saline used to wipe away excess soap. Excessive removal of hair and application of alcohol contributes to rapid loss in body temperature. It is best to use clear, plastic drapes so that the patient can be easily observed and monitored during the surgical procedure. Gas sterilized cling wrap is useful as a transparent drape for small species during surgery if a plastic drape is not available (**Fig. 1**). Care must be taken when placing towel clamps anchored onto the skin of small mammals, and it may be preferable to anchor the plastic drape to towels underneath the patient to minimize skin trauma. The size of surgical instruments should be small compared with those used in dogs and cats, such as using a mini-instrument pan or ophthalmic instruments for the smallest patients.

POSTSURGICAL CONSIDERATIONS

During recovery, continuing to keep the patient warm is imperative. Recovery in an incubator with constant body temperature monitoring is beneficial. Maintaining an IV catheter for the immediate postoperative period is important, as long as the animal is not attempting to chew at the catheter. Postsurgical analgesic use, including opioids and nonsteroidal anti-inflammatories, should always be anticipated.

COMMON SURGICAL PROCEDURES
Integumentary Surgery

The integumentary system is composed of skin and associated adnexa. Basic elements of the integument are similar across all mammalian species, but a few important, species-specific differences are worth highlighting when evaluated from a surgical perspective. For example, rather than hair, the hedgehog has spines, which must be plucked like bird feathers during presurgical preparation. Some species, such as chinchillas and sugar gliders, have very thin skin, especially in the inguinal or scrotal region; therefore, caution should be implemented when clipping and prepping this area to avoid iatrogenic trauma. On the other hand, the skin associated with the dorsal cervical region of ferrets can be thick and tough, whereas the abdominal skin of ferrets, in particular those with adrenal adenoma/adenocarcinoma, may be very thin. In some small rodent species, in particular hamsters, there is an abundant epidermis and dermis with significant elasticity, which can be of benefit when surgically closing an area with a significant tissue deficit. The skin of Guinea pigs, however, tends to be much less elastic, making it more difficult to close large surgical wounds. Common integumentary surgical procedures in small mammals include trauma (wound closure), epithelial or subcutaneous mass removal, and surgical débridement/excision of abscesses. Additionally, cheek pouch prolapse and diseases associated with scent glands are occasionally observed in hamsters.

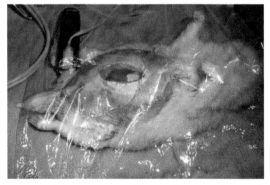

Fig. 1. Veterinary transparent drapes are used for small mammal surgeries. It is also possible to use gas sterilized commercial cling wrap as a transparent drape for small species during surgery.

Traumatic wounds

Trauma is common in small mammals and is associated with intraspecific or interspecific bite wounds (**Fig. 2**), being dropped by a human caretaker, wounds from cage material or cage ornaments, self-mutilation, or other accidental injuries when an animal has free access to their house environment.[7,8] Bite wounds from cage mates are commonly observed in rodents (see **Fig. 2**) and occasionally observed in ferrets. Interspecific bite wounds, especially from cats, frequently lead to fatal septicemia if not treated rapidly and thoroughly. Most traumatized small mammals should be evaluated for hemorrhage and blood loss and signs of infection and the body should be thoroughly examined for less obvious, hidden wounds. Severe hemorrhage resulting from trauma, such as lacerations of major vessels, hematomas, or internal organ damage, is frequently life threatening in small mammals, so immediate hemostasis and supportive care are critical. Sedation or anesthesia is typically necessary for small mammals that need to be evaluated after a traumatic incident. Generally, the hair associated with the skin lesion must be clipped to properly evaluate the wound. Once the hair is clipped, some wounds require suturing, whereas other wounds may heal over time by second intention with intensive bandage changes and wound débridement. Warm disinfectant solutions (eg, dilute povidone iodine or chlorhexidine) and/or saline may be necessary for cleaning large wounds to avoid heat loss. Appropriate use of analgesics, nonsteroidal anti-inflammatories, and antimicrobial drugs should be considered during treatment of traumatic wounds. The basic tenets of small animal (ie, dog and cat) wound management and secondary infection control can be applied to small mammals, except that choice of antimicrobials is based on safety for the species, in addition to microbial culture and sensitivity. Generally, most wounds heal by second intention if secondary infection is controlled, and surgical intervention is only required with open wounds with wide skin margin deflection or with very recent wounds with clean, underlying tissues. As an illustration of excellent second intention wound healing, a ferret was evaluated by one of the authors (YM) for significant inguinal skin sloughing secondary to urolith urethral obstruction and subsequent bacterial infection (**Fig. 3**). In this case, the wounds resolved over time using wet-to-dry bandages, antimicrobials based on bacterial culture and sensitivity, anti-inflammatories, and analgesics.

Abscesses

Abscesses are commonly observed as superficial lumps or masses, especially in rats, guinea pigs and other rodent species. Abscesses in small rodents are most commonly

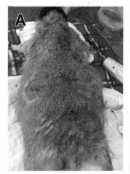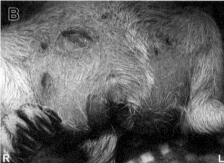

Fig. 2. Intraspecific bite wounds from cage mates in a prairie dog. These wounds were surgically closed after disinfection. (*A*) Dorsal view. (*B*) Ventral view.

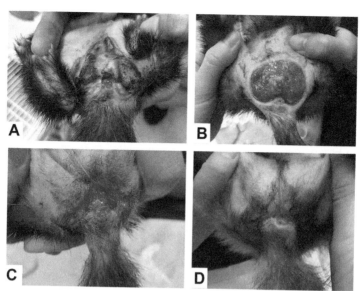

Fig. 3. An example of wound healing by second intention in a ferret. (*A*) First presentation, Day 1. (*B*) Day 9. (*C*) Day 21. (*D*) Day 30. A large area of inguinal skin sloughed secondary to a severe bacterial infection associated with urethral obstruction with urolithiasis in a ferret. The lesion healed by second intention with disinfection of the lesions and replacement of wet-to-dry bandages.

the result of bite wounds from cage mates.[9] Subcutaneous abscesses in rats are common and must be distinguished from mammary adenomas (**Fig. 4**). Initially, differentiating between a soft tissue mass and abscess is important through use of a fine-needle aspirate (FNA) and cytologic examination. Confirmed abscesses are typically obvious once the needle is inserted and purulent material is expressed from the needle insertion site. There are cases of neoplastic lesions, however, with purulent, necrotic cores that can be misdiagnosed as a pure abscess. With abscesses, collecting a sample for aerobic and anaerobic bacterial culture and antimicrobial sensitivity is an important next step. Managing abscesses can occur using 2 methods. First the animal must be sedated or anesthetized and the hair associated with the abscess clipped and the site aseptically prepared. One approach is to lance the abscess using a scalpel blade (#11 or #15); drain the purulent material; irrigate the abscess using warm, sterile saline, dilute chlorhexidine, or povidone iodine; and leave the incision open to heal by

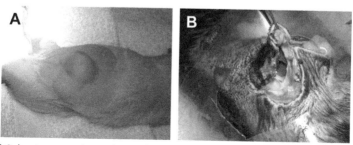

Fig. 4. (*A*) Subcutaneous abscess located on the ventrum of a rat. This was associated with a cage mate bite. (*B*) The abscess capsule and purulent material contained within are visible.

second intention. Administering appropriate antimicrobials is normal standard of practice in these cases. This approach to abscess management is usually curative in ferrets, sugar gliders, and hedgehogs. In other rodents (eg, Guinea pigs, chinchillas, hamsters, rats, and mice), however, recurrence is common if the abscess is not fully excised, without rupturing the capsule, because the abscess capsule remains a constant nidus of infection (**Fig. 5**).[9] Therefore, in rodents, the clinician should always consider surgical excision of the abscess, using an elliptical incision around the abscess and treating it is though it was a soft tissue mass. The skin can be closed using either suture material or staples but with awareness that many rodents, without placement of an Elizabethan-collar (E-collar), vigorously attempt to chew and scratch at their incision. Staples can help slow down the process of having a determined rodent open the surgical wound, and proper E-collar placement prevents access to the surgical site.

Pododermatitis
Pododermatitis is occasionally observed in Guinea pigs, chinchillas, rats, hamsters, hedgehogs, and rats (**Fig. 6**). Generally, surgical intervention is not necessary for mild to moderate lesions, and medical therapy includes the following approach: (1) soaking lesions with dilute chlorhexidine or povidone iodine solutions; (2) applying antimicrobial ointments/creams (eg, silver sulfadiazine) with overlying bandages and regular, repeated bandage changes (see **Fig. 6**); (3) maintaining the animals on soft substrates; and (4) administering appropriate antimicrobials, anti-inflammatories and analgesics. In severe cases of pododermatitis, particularly with radiographic evidence of osteomyelitis, surgical débridement and/or amputation of the affected limb may be necessary. With limb amputation of small mammals, it is usually best to amputate the entire limb, otherwise trauma to the remaining limb stump is a chronic, recurrent medical issue. Limb amputation in small mammals is identical to procedures described in dogs and cats, with an extra focus on hemostasis, analgesia, and warmth. Remarkably, rodents adjust rapidly to loss of a limb, except some Guinea pigs have a difficult time holding their body off the ground with 3 limbs, especially with loss of a forelimb. This can result in dragging of the body and trauma to the ventrum, so this must be considered prior to amputating Guinea pig forelimbs.

Self-mutilation
Self-mutilation is commonly observed in sugar gliders, and it is most common for them to self-mutilate the penis, inguinal region, and base of tail (**Fig. 7**). Although

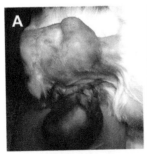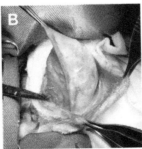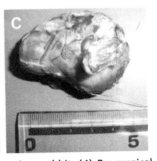

Fig. 5. This is an example of complete excision of an abscess in a rabbit. (*A*) Pre-surgical appearance of the mandibular abscess. (*B & C*) Recurrence is fairly common if the abscess is not excised without rupturing the capsule in rabbits and rodents because the abscess capsule continues to be a nidus of chronic infection and abscessation.

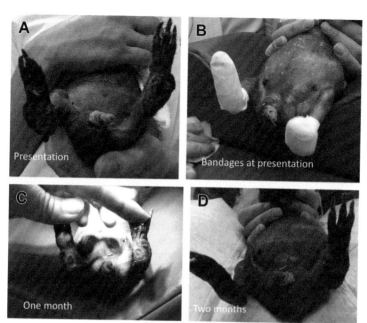

Fig. 6. Severe pododermatitis in a guinea pig. Lesions (*A*) are treated by soaking with dilute chlorhexidine or povidone iodine, applying silver sulfadiazine cream, and bandages (*B*) that are replaced once to twice weekly depending on how clean and dry the bandages are maintained. Appropriate oral antibiotics based on bacterial culture and antibiotic sensitivity, and anti-inflammatory drugs are administered. Bandaging with only elastic adhesive tape is difficult to keep clean, so latex or nitrile glove finger parts or duct tape are used to cover the outside of the bandage to keep clean and dry (*B*). These lesions were resolved within approximately 2 months by second intention healing (*C, D*).

understanding of behavioral mechanisms underlying this condition in sugar gliders is limited, hypotheses include, boredom, lack of appropriate conspecific social or sexual interactions, owner neglect, inappropriate environment and husbandry, and death or recent separation of cage mates.[10] Excessive chewing and self-mutilation of the

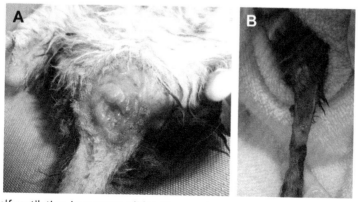

Fig. 7. Self-mutilation in a sugar glider. The most common sugar glider self-mutilation lesions are (*A*) inguinal areas and (*B*) the base of the tail.

perineal-cloacal region may be caused by pericloacal gland impaction/infection or penile prolapse.[10] In cases of tissue necrosis or severe tissue destruction, surgical repair is frequently necessary (**Fig. 8**), but most mild to moderate self-mutilation wounds heal by second intention along with appropriate antimicrobial and anti-inflammatory administration. When the penis is affected, amputation may be necessary (**Fig. 9**). Sugar gliders have a biforcated penis and urinate from the penile base, so amputation at the forked end of the penis does not interfere with urination (see **Fig. 9**). Early castration of sugar glider males is often recommended because sexual frustration may be a factor associated with self-mutilation (discussed later). In most cases, initial treatment involves hair clipping, disinfection of wounds with dilute povi-done iodine or chlorhexidine, the use of antimicrobials and analgesics, and correction of the underlying causes, such as improper socialization, husbandry, nutrition, and so forth. Modified E-collars or Velcro (Velcro Industries, Manchester, NH, USA) and fleece straightjackets are usually necessary to prevent further mutilation during treatment (**Fig. 10**). It is important not to remove the E-collar or straightjacket too soon in the healing process; typically, the authors maintain the protective E-collar/jacket for a minimum of 2 weeks after the wound has completely healed and keep the animal in the hospital to watch for recurrence of self-mutilation for 3 to 6 hours after removing the E-collar/jacket. If this process is not properly maintained and monitored, recurrence of self-mutilation can be so severe that euthanasia or death of the sugar glider is the outcome.

Tail slip

Slip, or traumatic degloving of the tail skin, is occasionally observed in long-tailed rodents, such as degus, gerbils, and chinchillas (**Fig. 11**).[9,11,12] In these species, the skin of the tail is thin and can easily be torn from the underlying tissues by overzealous grasping of the tail or lifting the weight of the animal by the tail. Rather than grasping the tail, the individual should be manually restrained over the dorsal cervical region and the rest of the body supported with the other hand. In cases of tail skin degloving, surgical amputation of the remaining degloved tail is recommended.[9,11,12] Amputation

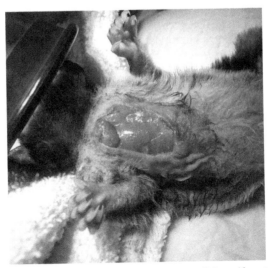

Fig. 8. Severe self-mutilation in a sugar glider. Most sugar glider self-mutilation wounds are small so that surgical intervention is not necessary, but large wounds require surgical intervention.

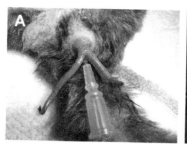
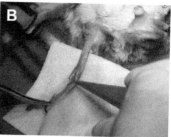

Fig. 9. Penile amputation in a sugar glider. (*A*) The urethral opening is at the bifurcation and this image shows a 24-gauge catheter inserted into the urethra. (*B*) Amputation of the bifurcated penis using bipolar cautery. Amputation at the forked end of the penis does not interfere with urination.

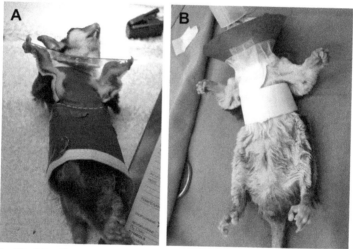

Fig. 10. Modified E-collar and 2 versions of the straightjacket used to prevent access to surgical sites in sugar gliders. Normal E-collars are easy to slip off. The connection of collar with jacket prevents this problem. (*A*) An E-collar modified into a straight jacket. (*B*) Using surgical tape as a bellyband.

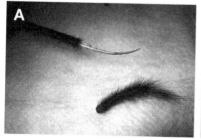
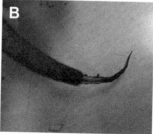

Fig. 11. Tail slip or degloving of the tail skin in (*A*) a degu and (*B*) a rat. This is common in chinchillas, gerbils, degus, and sometime rats and mice when a human grasps the tail and lifts the animal suspending the body weight by the tail. Degloving of the tail skin requires distal tail amputation.

is performed just proximal to the remaining skin margin. The hair associated with the amputation site is clipped, the distal tail is wrapped with aseptic gauze, and the amputation site aseptically prepared for surgery. A tourniquet placed at the very base of the tail aids with perioperative hemostasis. The procedure is nearly identical to that used for dog tail amputation. Once the site is prepped and draped, a local anesthetic, such as lidocaine, is administered around the planned skin incision site. A double V-shaped skin incision is made on right and left lateral aspects of the tail, just distal to the desired intervertebral transection site. Orient the double V-shaped incision to create dorsal and ventral skin flaps that are longer than the desired tail length; start the incision just distal to the desired intervertebral space. Bipolar cautery is useful for hemostatsis, and is critical in such a small working space. Muscles and subcutaneous tissue are bluntly dissected from the vertebrae caudal to the intervertebral transection site using small hemostats, and the distal tail is disarticulated with a scalpel blade (#11 or #15) by incising through the desired intervertebral space. Prior to closure, release the tourniquet at the base of the tail and observe the surgical site for hemorrhage. Use bipolar cautery if necessary to control remaining hemorrhage. Using 5-0 absorbable, monofilament suture material, appose subcutaneous tissues and muscles over the exposed vertebra with a simple continuous suture pattern. To close the skin layer, use 4-0 or 5-0 nonabsorbable, monofilament suture material in a simple continuous or simple interrupted pattern, making sure that there is enough skin to provide good apposition without tension. To protect the surgical site, it is best to place a light, pressure bandage over the incision and maintain the bandage in place for 24 to 48 hours. An E-collar may be necessary to prevent damage to the surgical site.

Tumors of the integument
A variety of skin and subcuticular neoplasms have been reported in small mammal species.[13–16] Based on the authors' experiences, skin and subcuticular neoplasms are common in hedgehogs, rats, ferrets, and hamsters and less common in guinea pigs and mice. Although integumentary neoplasms are uncommon in sugar gliders, with the exception of mammary gland tumors (**Fig. 12**), as sugar glider husbandry improves and captive age increases, it is likely that there will be an increased incidence of integumentary tumors. Of particular importance with respect to integumentary neoplasm incidence, squamous cell carcinomas are common in hedgehogs,[13] benign

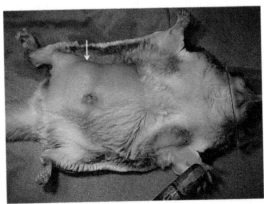

Fig. 12. Mammary gland tumor in a sugar glider. Integumentary neoplasms are common in hedgehogs, ferrets, and hamsters but less common in sugar gliders. Arrow shows a mammary gland carcinoma in a sugar glider.

neoplasms of basal cell origin are the most common in ferrets,[13] and atypical fibromas are the most common in Djungarian (ie, dwarf) hamsters.[15] Djungarian hamsters show a high prevalence of neoplastic disease (5 times greater than Syrian hamsters), and most tumors are integumentary.[15] Neoplastic diseases are rare in chinchillas.[16] Mammary gland tumors, most commonly adenomas, are the most common subcutaneous tumor in rats and mice,[13,14] and the distribution of mammary tissue is extensive so the tumors can occur anywhere from head and neck to perineal region in both males and females (**Fig. 13**).[13] Diagnostic and surgical approaches with small mammal integumentary tumors are similar to those of dogs and cats; however, consideration of self-trauma is important after FNA of masses in some rodent species and sugar gliders. Additionally, hematoma-like lesions are occasionally observed in Djungarian hamsters, and appear as a flaccid, superficial mass (**Fig. 14**). These lesions can lead to life-threatening hemorrhage after FNA, so aspiration should be stopped immediately when blood is aspirated, and surgical removal of the lesion should be considered. The treatment of choice for integumentary tumors is complete surgical excision with histopathologic evaluation. Once the patient is prepped and draped, a scalpel blade or cautery device can be used to make an elliptical incision around the mass, or in cases of rat mammary masses, the incision is commonly made directly over the mass. Generally, little to no hemorrhage is observed if using a bipolar cautery forceps to incise the skin. Using a cautery device requires great caution to prevent ignition with oxygen used simultaneously during anesthesia. Additionally, application of other hemostatic aids, such as LigaSure (Covidien Surgical Solutions, Dublin, Ireland) laparoscopic instruments, contributes to reduction of operative time and minimizes hemorrhage. Making the elliptical incision to include appropriate surgical margins is important in any species, although large surgical margins may make closure more difficult due to the tension created during closure of the skin and subcutaneous tissues. When large epithelial defects are expected, the extent of the incisional line should be decided based on the anticipated skin tension and location of subdermal vascular plexus to avoid circulatory compromise after wound closure. These considerations are especially important for guinea pigs, because their skin is thick and less elastic compared with other rodent species, and Guinea pig integumentary tissues tend to develop a significant inflammatory reaction to excessive suture materials and skin tension compared with other small mammal species. Therefore, surgical wounds may be more likely to either dehisce or develop abscessation with tension

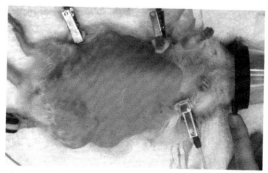

Fig. 13. Mammary adenoma in a rat. Mammary gland tumors are the most common subcutaneous tumor in rats. The distribution of the mammary tissue is extensive so the tumors can occur anywhere from neck to inguinal region in rats and affect both males and females.

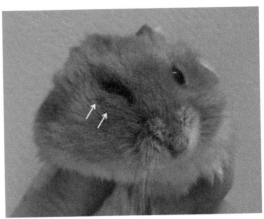

Fig. 14. Hematoma-like lesion in a Djungarian (dwarf) hamster. Hematoma-like lesions (*arrows*) are occasionally observed in Djungarian hamsters as a flaccid superficial mass, and these lesions may lead to severe hemorrhage after FNA, so care should be taken when aspirating such masses.

or excessive suture material. For any small mammal species, such skin tension can be relieved by undermining skin adjacent to the surgical wound through blunt dissection, with care to preserve the subdermal plexus and direct cutaneous vessels that run parallel to the skin surface. If these methods do not allow primary skin apposition, the remaining surgical wound may be allowed to heal by second intention, or reconstructive surgical procedures, using skin flaps or grafts, can be completed with approaches as those used in dogs and cats. For rat mammary tumors, once the incision is made directly over the mass, the subcutaneous tissues can be undermined and bluntly dissected away from the mass using hemostats. Mammary masses in rats are well vascularized, so be careful not to incise the mass. Most typically, the mass can be freed from the subcutaneous layers, and the primary vascular supply can be for at the deep base of the mass. Ligatures or Hemoclips (WECK Hemoclip Plus, Teleflex Medical, Research Triangle Park, NC, USA) can be used to clamp the vessels supplying the tumor and the mass can be removed. Once any integumentary mass is removed from a small mammal, routine closure techniques are similar to those used in dogs and cats, closing the subcutaneous tissues with 3-0 to 5-0, monofilament, absorbable suture materials, and 3-0 to 4-0 monofilament, nonabsorbable suture material for closing the skin layer. Alternatively, skin staples may help in those species most likely to chew their incision, and are easy to apply and faster to apply than sutures. In Guinea pigs, skin staples can reduce the amount of foreign suture material, which is inflammatory in this species. Rat mammary tumors are likely to recur, so this should be part of the client communication.

Male and female Guinea pigs have an equal prevalence of mammary gland tumors, unlike most other species.[13,16] Guinea pigs have 2 mammary glands located just cranial to the inguinal region. Affected mammary glands expand in a solid or cystic manner and often secrete fluid, which has a plasma-like appearance. In these cases of mammary tumors, unilateral mammary resection is most common, because the right and left mammary glands are not physically associated with each other. It can be difficult to remove the entire mass or masses with clean margins, and postsurgical dehiscence is common. Resection of large masses requires deep subcutaneous sutures to minimize dead space and to limit incisional tension.

Cheek pouch eversion in hamsters

Many small mammal species have cheek pouches, which may be located internally within the caudal oral cavity, and may be large and expansile for storing food, or externally in some rodent species. Cheek pouch eversion is occasionally observed in hamsters, especially Djungarian hamsters.[9] Causes of hamster cheek eversion include inflammation associated with a food item or foreign material, and microbial infection or abscessation. Clinically, the prolapsed cheek pouch is visibly hanging outside of the oral cavity and may appear swollen, erythematous, and edematous, with necrosis associated with prolonged cheek pouch tissue prolapse (**Fig. 15**). In acute cases, without severe edema or necrosis, management includes sedation, removal of food or foreign materials from the pouch, and replacement to its normal anatomic conformation using moistened cotton-tipped applicators. If there is concern about reproplasing, a single, full-thickness, percutaneous mattress suture, using 4-0 or 5-0 monofilament, nonabsorbable suture material can be placed into and through the cheek pouch. In this case, the suture can remain in place for several days to 1 week, at which time the suture should be removed. If the prolapsed cheek pouch is moderately to severely edematous, 50% dextrose solution can be applied directly to the tissue, with the hope that the sugar solution will contribute to tissue contraction, allowing the cheek pouch to be replaced with moistened cotton-tipped applicators. If the prolapsed cheek pouch is severely inflamed or discolored or the mucosal tissue appears necrotic, the necrotic tissue should be surgically excised (see **Fig. 15**). Two stay sutures, using 4-0 or 5-0 monofilament, absorbable material can be placed proximal to the planned incision line. The tissue can be transected, circumferentially, just proximal to the necrotic tissue, and the excised tissue placed in buffered formalin for histopathologic analysis and a second piece used for bacterial culture if necessary. Care should be taken if placing

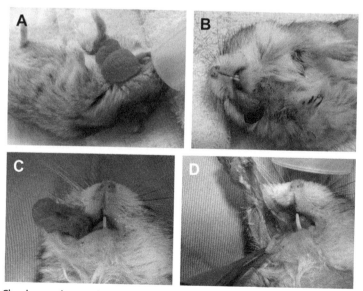

Fig. 15. Cheek pouch eversion in Djungarian hamsters. Typically, the prolapsed cheek pouch is (A) edematous, (C) inflamed, and (B) necrotic. (D) The necrotic portion of the everted cheek pouch can be surgically removed, sutured, and placed back in normal position.

hemostats or using forceps for firm manipulation of prolapsed cheek pouch tissue, because this can cause additional damage to remaining healthy tissue. The incision can be sutured using 5-0 or 6-0 monofilament, nonabsorbable suture material in a simple continuous pattern. Have bipolar or unipolar cautery instruments ready in anticipation of hemorrhage. Postoperatively, it is important to counsel the owner about avoiding food (eg, cooked pasta or rice) and bedding (eg, Kleenex) materials that are likely to adhere to the suture line and contribute to further problems. Additionally, the owner should be instructed to withhold the normal diet, and, instead, syringe-feed a fine-grind feeding formula for 3 to 5 days, and to remove all bedding materials that the patient may attempt to pack into the pouch, which can result in incisional dehiscence.[9] Appropriate antimicrobials and nonsteroidal anti-inflammatory drugs are administered for 5 to 7 days, postoperatively.

Intra-abdominal surgical procedures
Common, nonreproductive, intrabdominal surgical procedures of small animals include gastric or intestinal foreign bodies, hepatocystic diseases, proliferative lesions in abdomen (neoplasms, abscesses, granulomas, and so forth), urologic diseases (eg, uroliths), and rectal prolapses in hamsters and ferrets.

Gastrointestinal tract surgery
The most common surgical procedure of gastrointestinal system is removal of gastrointestinal foreign bodies in small mammals, especially ferrets.[17] Occasionally, it is necessary to collect small intestinal biopsy samples to diagnose underlying causes of chronic diarrhea in ferrets, or surgically excise intestinal tumors and repair intestinal intussusceptions. Preoperative imaging is critical for localizing lesions. During gastrointestinal surgical procedures, the surgeon should consider wearing magnifying surgical loupes. The surgical approach to all gastrointestinal procedures in small mammals is via a ventral midline incision.

Gastrointestinal foreign bodies
Gastrointestinal foreign bodies are occasionally observed in ferrets but are less common in rodents, hedgehogs, and sugar gliders. In a case of one of the authors (YM), an enterolith in a chinchilla was treated by, but this is rare. In ferrets, foreign bodies are most commonly ingested objects from the environment, but there are cases of trichobezoars in ferrets as well. Ingested foreign bodies tend to occur most commonly in younger ferrets, because they are inquisitive and like to chew on various objects, in particular rubber or sponge products (**Fig. 16**).[17–19] In contrast, trichobezoars tend to occur in older ferrets.[17] In cases of trichobezoars, there is usually 1 hairball, which is a comma-shaped, but sometimes 2 or multiple hairballs are found in the stomach and/or small intestine. The clinical presentation of ferrets with partially or completely obstructive foreign bodies includes regurgitation, anorexia, dehydration, lethargy, and melena. Diagnosis of gastrointestinal foreign bodies is based on history, physical examination, and imaging using radiography, CT, or ultrasound. Careful palpation of the ferret abdomen is important, because many gastrointestinal foreign bodies are palpable, and palpation commonly elicits a painful response, such as rapid hunching or vocalization. Abnormal radiographic abdominal findings include segmental ileus, gaseous distention of the stomach, and, occasionally, a visible foreign body. Gastrointestinal contrast studies can be conducted and may be useful in determining the location of the foreign body. Only 30% of foreign bodies, however, were detectable in a study evaluating contrast radiography in ferrets.[19] Supportive care and stabilization of debilitated ferrets with fluid therapy, analgesics, and proton pump inhibitors (eg, omeprazole) or H_2-receptor antagonists (eg, famotidine or ranitidine) may be

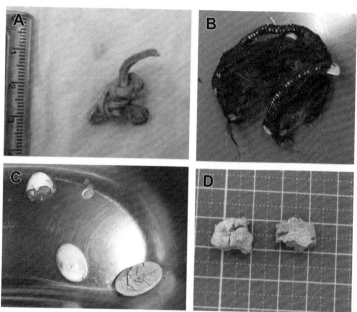

Fig. 16. A variety of foreign materials removed from ferret gastrointestinal systems. (*A*) Rubber band. (*B*) Hair elastic band. (*C*) Rubber toy. (*D*) Pieces of an eraser. Young ferrets tend to chew and swallow objects, especially those with rubber or soft foam.

useful to prevent gastritis and enteritis during anorectic perioperative period. Gastrointestinal foreign bodies can be removed surgically or by endoscopy. Small foreign materials in the stomach can be removed using a flexible endoscope of appropriate diameter, but larger foreign materials, and most trichobezoars, need surgical intervention. An advantage to using a surgical approach is that concurrent diseases associated with other abdominal organs, such as the pancreas, liver, intestines, and adrenal glands, can also be grossly evaluated during the procedure. Surgical procedures are similar to those of dogs and cats, except the authors avoid using hemostats to manipulate tissues, thereby avoiding iatrogenic trauma of delicate small mammal stomachs and/or intestines (**Fig. 17**). Once the location within the gastrointestinal tract is determined, a midline abdominal incision is made, which should be closely associated with the site of the lesion. The organ (stomach or small intestine) involved can be manipulated into the incision and 2 stay sutures can be placed in the serosal surface. Once the lesion, foreign body, or biopsy site is isolated outside of the abdomen, gauze moistened with sterile saline can be used to pack off the abdomen to prevent gastrointestinal content leakage. The stomach or intestine can be incised, biopsied, or resected and anastomosed using identical techniques in dogs and cats. Once the mass, foreign body, or biopsy tissue has been removed, single enterotomy or gastrotomy incisions should be closed in 2 layers, using 4-0 to 6-0 monofilament, absorbable suture material in an inverting pattern (eg, Cushing-Connell or Cushing-Lambert). Anastomoses can be closed in 2 layers, using 4-0 to 6-0 monofilament, absorbable suture material in an inverting pattern as well. The muscle layer is closed using 3-0 to 4-0 monofilament, absorbable suture material in a simple continuous pattern. The skin can be closed using an absorbable suture material in a subcuticular pattern or a nonabsorbable suture material for placing simple interrupted sutures. Skin staples are an alternative and are particularly useful if a clinician is aware that the patient

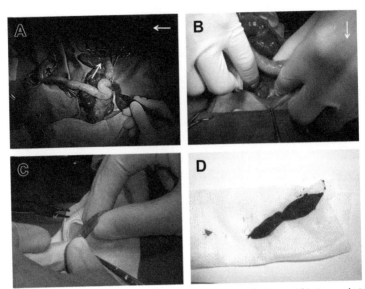

Fig. 17. Surgical removal of a trichobezoar in a chinchilla (*A*). To avoid iatrogenic trauma by using hemostats, the authors prefer to have an assistant hold the intestines of small mammals during enterotomy surgery (*B, C*). A trichobezoar was removed (*D*). *Arrow* indicates craniad.

chews at its incision site postsurgery. In most cases, recovery is rapid after gastrointestinal foreign body removal, and ferrets are able to eat soft foods within one or 2 days after surgery.

Proliferative abdominal lesions in (neoplasms, abscesses, and granulomas)

Neoplasms, abscesses, and granulomas can be found as proliferative lesions in the abdomen of small mammals and associated with 1 or multiple organ systems.[9,16,17,19] Intra-abdominal neoplastic diseases include uterine neoplasms in rodents and hedgehogs; adrenal adenoma/adenocarcinoma and lymphoma and pancreatic beta cell tumors (ie, insulinoma) in ferrets; neoplasms of liver and small intestines, which are occasionally observed in ferrets; uterine and kidney tumors in hamsters; and female reproductive tumors in guinea pigs; among others. Surgical procedures are similar to those performed in dogs and cats, with a ventral midline approach (as discussed previously). Attention must be paid, however, to shorter surgical times, hemostasis, maintenance of body temperature, and gentle tissue handling in small mammals.

Intra-abdominal abscesses are occasionally observed in ferrets and Djungarian hamsters. The cause of many of these abscesses is normally undiagnosed, except for those cases in which foreign material (eg, hay wood fibers) penetration of the gastrointestinal tract is observed. Complete surgical excision of the abscess with capsule is the most effective, but it is occasionally difficult due to development of significant tissue adhesions. In these cases, incise the capsule of abscess and remove as much purulent material as possible and irrigate with dilute antimicrobial solutions, followed by resection of as much of the abscess capsule as possible. The abscess capsule should be submitted for aerobic and anaerobic bacterial culture and cytology, and broad-spectrum antibiotics should be administered until receiving the bacterial culture and sensitivity results.

Intra-abdominal granulomas are occasionally observed in ferrets.[18,19] Treatment includes complete or partial excision or biopsies of the granuloma, followed by submission for cytology, histopathology, and or bacterial and fungal culture. In the authors' experiences, most intra-abdominal granulomas in ferrets are associated coronavirus or mycobacterial infection. In ferrets infected with coronavirus, granulomas are commonly found at the mesenteric lymph node (**Fig. 18**) but can also be disseminated in multiple organ systems (see **Fig. 18**).

Rectal prolapse

Although rectal prolapses can be observed in many small mammal species (**Fig. 19**), the incidence is greatest in ferrets and hamsters.[9,17–19] Young ferrets with chronic diarrhea are especially prone to rectal prolapses, which are generally superficial and typically resolve with treatment of the underlying cause of diarrhea. Prolapses in hamsters are also common but tend to be more severe and may include the rectum and large and small intestines. Additionally, in hamsters, intestinal prolapse can be accompanied by intestinal intussusception. Treatment of rectal prolapses in small mammals depends on severity and integrity of exposed tissues. In ferrets, treatment generally includes sedation or anesthesia, lubrication, and gentle replacement of the prolapsed tissue using cotton-tipped applicators, followed by placement of 2 transanal sutures using 3-0 to 4-0 nonabsorbable, monofilament suture material (**Fig. 20**), making sure that the animal is able to defecate normally. If the prolapsed lesion is severely edematous, 50% dextrose or Preparation H (Pfizer, Inc., Kings Mountain, NC, USA) can be applied to the prolapsed tissues prior to attempted replacement, as discussed previously. The underlying cause of the diarrhea must be addressed immediately as well, and the sutures can remain in place for 3 to 7 days. In cases of multiple rectal prolapse recurrence after addressing the underlying condition, a colopexy can be performed (**Fig. 21**). If the rectal mucosa is significantly and chronically everted and no

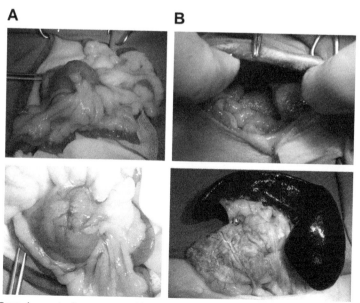

Fig. 18. Granulomas in ferrets caused by coronavirus infection. (*A*) Most ferret granulomatous diseases are associated with a single granuloma, (*B*) but a disseminated granulomatous pattern is occasionally observed.

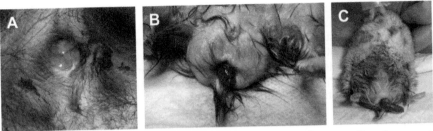

Fig. 19. Appearance of rectal prolapses in (*A*) a ferret and (*B, C*) hamsters. Ferrets are more commonly prone to rectal mucosal prolapses, whereas hamsters are more commonly prone to large intestinal prolapses; (*B*) hamster with a rectal prolapse, and (*C*) hamster with a colonic prolapse.

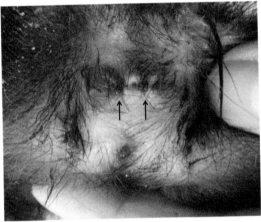

Fig. 20. Treatment of acute rectal prolapse in ferrets. Lubricate and gently replace the mucosa into its normal location using a moistened, cotton-tipped swab, then place 2 transanal sutures (*arrows*). The sutures should close the anus enough to maintain the reduced prolapse without interfering with passage of stool. These sutures can be removed after 3 to 7 days.

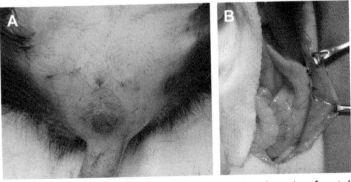

Fig. 21. Colopexy as a treatment of chronic, recurrent rectal prolapse in a ferret. (*A*) Presurgical appearance of the lesion and (*B*) intraoperative image of a colopexy.

longer reducible, the prolapsed tissue can be resected and the rectum sutured to the anus (**Fig. 22**). This procedure, however, may cause permanent anal sphincter atony. In hamsters, rectal prolapses tend to be more significant than those of ferrets (see **Fig. 19**) and include tissues proximal to the rectum, with some cases accompanied by intestinal intussusception (**Fig. 23**). Tissue discoloration and necrosis begin within several hours of the prolapsed tissue, and the affected hamster may be systemically compromised and require intensive supportive care along with urgent surgical repair. With necrosis, the tissue must be excised and the viable tissues anastomosed using 5-0 to 7-0 monofilament, absorbable suture material. An exploratory celiotomy is usually indicated if an intestinal intussusception is diagnosed, although the prognosis for these cases is poor. A routine, ventral midline abdominal celiotomy is performed, and the intussusception identified. Resection and anastomosis of the intestine is the typical approach, although there is evidence that if the intestinal tissues are viable, the intussusception can be reduced manually. With resection and anastomosis, use 5-0 to 6-0 monofilament, absorbable suture material to suture the proximal and distal ends of the intestine as in dogs and cats.

Hepatic Surgery

A surgical approach to the liver of small mammals is indicated for performing liver and gall bladder biopsies and surgically excising primary neoplastic masses and other hepatic diseases. Surgery of the extrahepatic biliary system is uncommon, but one of the authors (YM) has surgically managed several cases of extrahepatic biliary system obstruction in ferrets (**Fig. 24**). Surgical procedures associated with the liver are common in ferrets (**Figs. 25** and **26**) and prairie dogs, primarily for biopsies or tumor

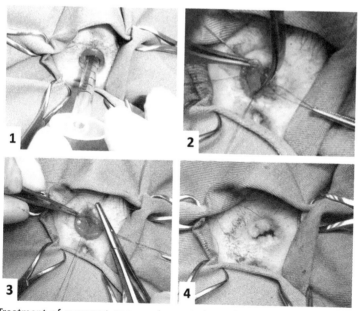

Fig. 22. Treatment of recurrent or severely everted rectal prolapse in ferrets: (*1*) prolapse reduction can be facilitated using a 1-mL syringe or moist swab, with confirmation of the excessive mucosa; (*2*) place 3 to 4 stay sutures in the rectal wall and resect the excess mucosa; (*3*) appose the edges with a continuous suture pattern using 6-0 monofilament absorbable suture material; and (*4*) postoperative appearance.

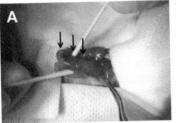
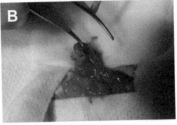

Fig. 23. Intestinal intussusception accompanied by rectal prolapse in a Syrian hamster. (*A*) Intraoperative image, region of intestinal intussusception area (*arrows*); (*B*) confirmation of the distal and proximal ends of the resected intestine.

excision, and less common in rodent species. Clinical signs associated with hepatic disorders are typically nonspecific until the disease process has advanced, and this may exacerbate the risk of anesthesia, because there may be impaired drug metabolism and excretion and prolonged duration of action of anesthetic drugs. These risks are more profound when injectable agents are administered, so a thorough presurgical evaluation of blood parameters and imaging techniques is imperative if severe hepatic dysfunction is suspected. Therefore, inhalational anesthetic agents are preferred for maintaining anesthesia in patients undergoing hepatic surgery, because isoflurane and sevoflurane have not been associated with postoperative hepatic dysfunction.[20] Hypoalbuminemia, or albumin levels less than 2.0 g/dL, may contribute to delayed wound healing and decreased synthesis of clotting factors may contribute

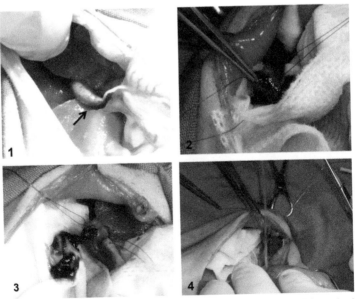

Fig. 24. Surgery for extrahepatic biliary system obstruction in a ferret: (*1*) markedly dilated common bile duct (*arrow*) with biliary sludge; (*2*) place stay sutures in the bile duct then make an incision in the duct wall; (*3*) remove the bile duct contents; and (*4*) confirm no obstruction using catheter and saline flush, and suture the incisional line with 5-0 to 6-0 absorbable suture material.

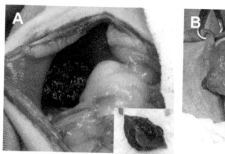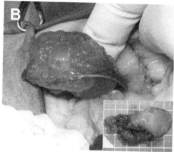

Fig. 25. Cystic hepatic lesions in ferrets. (*A*) Liver cyst and (*B*) biliary cystadenoma. Liver cystic lesions are occasionally observed in ferrets and can be surgically removed as shown.

to coagulopathies.[20] In these patients, preoperative blood transfusions and vitamin K should be considered.

The general approach for any hepatic surgery in small mammals is similar to techniques in dogs and cats, that is, make a cranioventral, midline abdominal incision, identify the section of liver of concern, and biopsy or excise the lesions. Cautery and absorbable hemostatic materials, such as Gelfoam (Pfizer, New York, NY, USA) and Surgicel (Ethicon), are also useful when performing hepatic surgery. Suturing of the abdominal muscles and skin is discussed in previously.

Hepatic Biopsy

Biopsy of the liver is indicated for prolonged liver enzyme elevation, observed ultrasonographic lesions, previous nondiagnostic cytology, diffuse hepatic diseases, and nonresectable, large hepatic tumors.[21] There are multiple techniques for collecting biopsy samples of hepatic tissues, loop guillotine suture (**Fig. 27**), punch biopsy, or stapling methods and partial lobectomy. The guillotine method is adequate for sampling the outer margin of the liver, whereas a skin punch biopsy is ideal for collecting a sample from a local lesion within the central portions of the liver. As with liver biopsies in

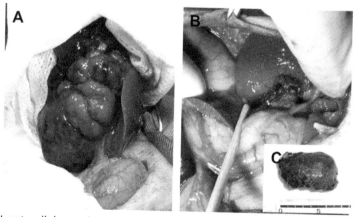

Fig. 26. Hepatocellular carcinoma in a ferret. (*A*) The mass was localized to 1 liver lobe. (*B, C*) Treatment of a solitary tumor is partial or complete liver lobectomy using a thoracoabdominal stapler.

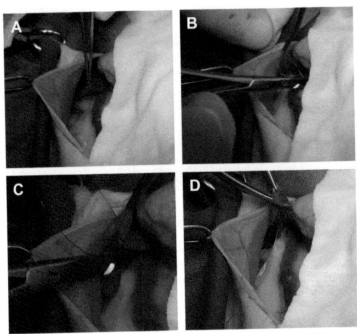

Fig. 27. Guillotine method for liver biopsy: (*A*) hold the tip of a liver lobe; (*B*) place a loop of suture around the protruding margin of a liver lobe; (*C*) ligate using suture to crush the hepatic parenchyma; and (*D*) cut the hepatic tissue distal to the ligature.

dogs and cats, at least 2 to 3 samples should be obtained from separate liver lobes, including both peripheral and central locations as well as grossly normal and abnormal-appearing tissue.[21] This approach may be difficult to impossible, however, for smaller species. Therefore, the authors recommend obtaining 1 to 2 samples, attempting to include both grossly normal and abnormal-appearing tissue. Once the biopsies are collected, rapid hemostasis using Gelfoam or Surgicel is critical. Decreased clotting factors may contribute to difficulty stopping the hemorrhage associated with a biopsy site.

Hepatic Lobectomy for Mass Removal

Liver neoplasms may be primary or secondary metastatic lesions and are occasionally observed in older ferrets and prairie dogs, and most patients present with or without overt clinical signs. Surgical treatment of a solitary tumor is partial or complete liver lobectomy, and liver biopsy or tumor debulking surgery for diffuse neoplastic diseases. Again, hemostasis is extremely critical in small mammal patients.

Surgery of the Spleen

The spleen is located in the left cranial abdominal quadrant of all small mammals, and it varies in size and shape among species. Surgical conditions of the spleen include laceration, torsion, neoplasia (primary and metastatic), and hematoma. For small mammals, however, splenic diseases, especially neoplastic masses, are primarily observed in ferrets. Generalized splenomegaly is common in ferrets, and many clinicians, wrongfully, decide to collect an FNA or biopsy only to receive a diagnosis of extramedullary hematopoiesis.[18,22] In most ferrets with generalized splenomegaly, biopsy and surgery are not indicated, except with severe splenic enlargement that interferes with abdominal visceral function or a ferret's activity (**Fig. 28**). Other causes of ferret splenic enlargement, such as cardiomyopathy, Aleutian disease, and eosinophilic gastritis, have been reported.[22] Additionally, isoflurane anesthesia causes splenic sequestration of red blood cells and the reduction of hematocrit by up to 35% in ferrets.[23] Thus, ferrets with splenomegaly should always be evaluated for underlying disease conditions, and splenectomy should only be considered with ultrasonographic or CT evidence of splenic surface or parenchymal irregularities. The most common indications for considering a splenectomy include, neoplastic diseases (primary or metastatic), and traumatic laceration of the splenic capsule in ferrets. In ferrets, lymphoma is the most common primary splenic neoplastic disease, and hemangiosarcoma, mast cell tumor, and liposarcoma are occasionally observed as primary splenic neoplasia. Metastatic diseases are most commonly associated with adrenal neoplasia or pancreatic beta cell tumors (ie, insulinoma). Laceration of the splenic capsule is a possible sequela to abdominal trauma or hematoma, and many affected ferrets require a blood transfusion (**Fig. 29**). Two primary surgical techniques are used for splenic surgery: partial splenectomy and total splenectomy. Total splenectomy is the most common, an easier procedure to perform, whereas partial splenectomy is rarely indicated. The surgical procedure in ferrets is identical to that performed in dogs and cats.[22] A vascular sealing instrument, such as a LigaSure device, is useful and contributes to a reduction in the surgical time. Because the spleen is a major site of erythropoiesis in ferrets, the consequences associated with a total splenectomy to a patient should be carefully considered prior to undertaking the surgery.[22]

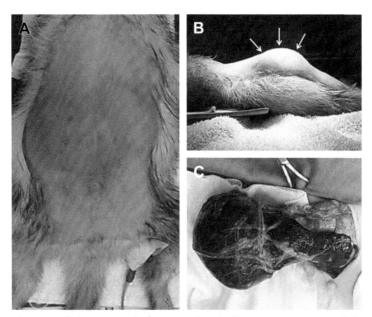

Fig. 28. Splenomegaly is common in ferrets and typically represents extramedullary hematopoiesis, which is not surgical. (*A, B*) Appearance of the enlarged spleen (*arrows*) and (*C*) intraoperative splenomegaly. Surgery for enlarged spleen may be indicated when there is interference with abdominal visceral function.

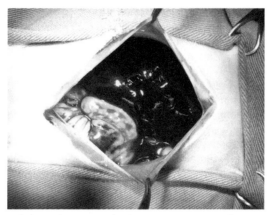

Fig. 29. Laceration of the splenic capsule due to trauma in a ferret. An enlarged ferret spleen may be ruptured by falling or other trauma. In these cases, blood transfusion is commonly recommended.

Urinary Tract Surgery

Urolithiasis

Urolithiasis is a disease manifestation in which a single urinary calculus or multiple calculi are found anywhere in the urinary system. Urolithiasis is common in Guinea pigs and chinchillas but less common in ferrets and other rodent species. Most cases in Guinea pigs and chinchillas were cystoliths and a few renoliths. The overall prevalence of uroliths in ferrets has decreased during the past 10 years due to higher-quality diets, although the authors have observed a recent spike in the incidence of cysteine uroliths, which has been anecdotally attributed to feeding a commercial grain-free diet.[24,25] Prior to the recent increase in cysteine uroliths in ferrets, the most common urinary calculus was magnesium ammonium phosphate (struvite), and inappropriate diets causing alkaline urine were linked to the disease.[25] In one author's (YM) experience, dietary management and subsequent reduction of urine pH contributed to resolution of struvite calculi in the urinary bladder of a ferret after converting the diet to a commercial ferret kibble from a vegetable-based diet (**Fig. 30**). In Guinea pigs, calcium

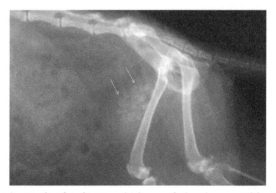

Fig. 30. Lateral radiograph of a ferret, which was fed only vegetables for several years. Many struvite calculi (*arrows*) were observed in the urinary bladder. These calculi were completely dissolved by converting to a proper ferret diet.

is the major constituent of urinary calculi. In all small mammals, the most common clinical signs include hematuria, stranguria, dysuria, anorexia, hunched posture, and vocalization during straining to urinate. Diagnosis is based on imaging via radiographs, CT, or ultrasound. It is important to include the entire urinary system, including the distal penis, when taking radiographs. In male Guinea pigs, ultrasound is beneficial to evaluate the location of calculi, because some calculi are rarely located in the seminal vesicles (**Fig. 31**). Because the urinary pH of herbivorous small mammals is normally alkaline, the use of the urinary acidifiers is contraindicated, and prevention or medical treatment is unrewarding.[26] Therefore, surgical removal of uroliths is the treatment of choice in herbivorous small mammals.

A cystotomy procedure in small mammals is the same technique used in dogs and cats. A ventral midline incision is performed through the skin and muscle layers and the urinary bladder exposed. Two stay sutures are placed on each side of the urinary bladder and sterile, saline-soaked gauze sponges are used to pack around the bladder to maintain tissue moisture and prevent urine contamination back into the patient's abdomen. It is useful to insert a small gauge hypodermic needle into the bladder to empty it of urine prior to making the incision. The urinary bladder is incised approximately along the ventral midline from cranial to caudal and the uroliths removed. Some uroliths are adhered to the urinary bladder mucosa, and care must be taken to peel them from the bladder wall, because hemorrhage is common. To ensure patency of the urethra, a red rubber tube can be passed from the bladder through the urethra and exteriorized. Any remaining small calculi can be flushed using sterile saline. The urinary bladder is closed in 2 inverting layers (eg, Cushing-Connell) using 3-0 to 5-0 monofilament, absorbable suture material. The body wall can be closed using 3-0 or 4-0 monofilament, absorbable suture material in a simple continuous pattern and the skin can be closed using 3-0 or 4-0 monofilament, absorbable suture material

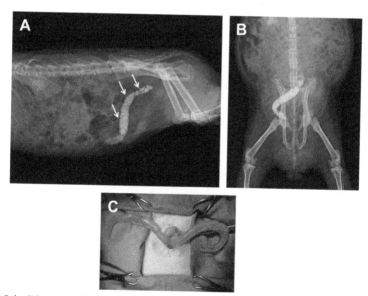

Fig. 31. Calculi locate in the seminal vesicles in a male guinea pig. (*A*) Lateral radiograph (*B*) and ventrodorosal radiograph. (*C*) Normal intraoperative appearance of Guinea pig seminal vesicles. Ultrasound is necessary to evaluate the location of calculi (*arrows*) in male guinea pigs because some calculi are located in the seminal vesicles rather than the urinary tract.

in a subcuticular, continuous suture pattern or simple interrupted skin suture. Skin staples can also be used and may help prevent the patient chewing through skin sutures. After the surgical removal, it is important to submit the calculi for chemical analysis so that preventative dietary changes can be implemented.

Urethral calculi are more common in males than females of most small mammal species, and many urethral stones can be palpated during the physical examination. Confirm the location of the urethral stone by palpation and imaging. Once the location is identified, incise over the stone, dissect the skin and subcutaneous tissue, and identify the urethral wall. Incise the urethral wall and remove the stone, and be careful removing if the urolith is adhered to the urethral mucosa (**Fig. 32**). To close the urethra, suture the urethral wall in 1 layer using 5-0 or 6-0 monofilament, absorbable suture material in a simple continuous pattern, then close the skin using a subcuticular or simple interrupted skin closure. In some cases in which a urethral stone cannot be palpated, a urethral catheter and an attached syringe filled with sterile saline can be used to retropulse the stone into the urinary bladder for removal via cystotomy.

Ureteral calcului are rare in small mammals but frequently cause complete ureteral obstruction and require prompt surgical removal. Clinical signs may vary, depending on whether or not the stone has caused a complete obstruction. Unilateral ureteral calculi with complete obstruction result in hydronephrosis and hydroureter and may present without subsequent renal failure, but bilateral, obstructive ureteral calculi contribute to renal failure. Imaging modalities can help with diagnosing ureteroliths, hydroureter, and hydronephrosis. The authors have experienced bilateral ureterolithiasis in Guinea pigs (**Fig. 33**), which can be resolved with prompt surgical removal of stones and intensive supportive care. The surgical procedure is similar to that performed in dogs and cats, but the monofilament, absorbable suture material needs to be small depending on the species: 5-0 to 8-0. Renal calculi or renal mineralization is occasionally diagnosed radiographically, concurrent with ureteral stones. Whether all renal or ureteral stones should be removed is controversial, and recurrence is expected.

Reproductive Tract Surgery

Reproductive tract surgery in rodents, ferrets, and hedgehogs can be an elective procedure for removal of ovaries and uterus, or testicles, to prevent pregnancy and future diseases associated with reproductively intact animals (eg, uterine and mammary neoplasia, ovarian cysts, and testicular neoplasia).[7,9] In some cases, early testicular and ovarian removal may alter certain gender-specific behaviors. Alternatively,

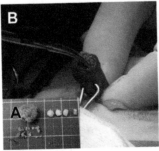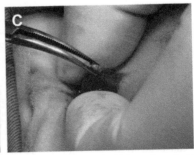

Fig. 32. Surgical removal of urinary bladder and urethral calculi in a ferret. (*A*) Cystine calculi were removed from (*B*) bladder and (*C*) urethra. The surgical procedure is similar to that in dogs and cats.

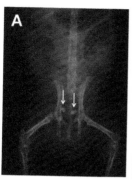
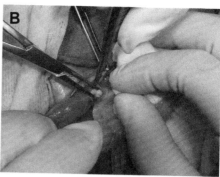

Fig. 33. Bilateral ureteral calculi in a guinea pig. (*A*) Radiograph of the abdomen; (*B*) intra-operative image. Results of the radiograph demonstrates 2 ureteral calculi (*arrows*). The ureteral calculi, located in both ureters, were surgically removed and analyzed to reveal composition of calcium carbonate.

reproductive surgery may be therapeutic in cases of reproductive tract diseases. Most ferrets in North America and Japan are routinely spayed or neutered and undergo simultaneous anal sacculectomies at a young age. Therefore, it is uncommon for clinicians to perform such procedures in many countries. This is not true in European countries, however, in which elective ferret orchiectomy and ovariohysterectomy are more common.

Elective Orchiectomy and Ovariectomy or Ovariohysterectomy

Orchiectomy

Although the surgical techniques associated with orchiectomy in small mammals is not significantly different from techniques used in dogs and cats, there are a few differences worth highlighting. In most rodent species, especially Guinea pigs and chinchillas, the inguinal canal is large diameter, and the testicles move freely from the abdominal cavity into the scrotum.[7] This open inguinal canal is important with respect to the chosen procedure for orchiectomy. There are 2 primary surgical approaches to castrating rodents: bilateral scrotal incisions, with open or closed castration, or a single, prescrotal incision, in which both testicles are excised from the same incision with either an open or closed procedure.[7] The prescrotal approach can be more efficient with 1 less incision, but care must be taken with hedgehogs, chinchillas, and Guinea pigs because the penis is comparatively large and frequently directly in the surgical field. Although many clinicians profess one procedure better than the other, the authors have performed many open and closed orchiectomies through 1 or 2 incisions and have not observed significant complications from any of the chosen surgical procedures. Once the patient is anesthetized and surgically prepared, bupivacaine (2 mg/kg) or lidocaine (4 mg/kg) with 50% of the total dose administered directly into each testicle as a local nerve block (**Fig. 34**). Either bilateral cranial scrotal (**Fig. 35**) or single, prescrotal incisions are made. The general procedure is similar as that used in dogs. Whether using an open or closed technique, it is important to leave as much nontesticular tissue in the distal inguinal canal (eg, the vaginal tunic and epididymal fat pad) to prevent herniation of abdominal organs into the inguinal canal. Application of Hemoclips for ligating vessels can decrease surgical time compared with tying ligatures. Once the testicles are removed, it may be beneficial to use a sterile cotton-tipped applicator to place remaining tissues back into the inguinal canal. In

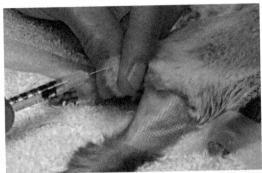

Fig. 34. Intratesticular administration of a local anesthetic, bupivacaine (2 mg/kg) or lido-caine (4 mg/kg), with 50% of the total dose administered directly into each testicle, as a local analgesic. This technique can be used in all male small mammals.

cases in which the tissues are difficult to push cranially into the inguinal canal, it may be helpful for an assistant to hold the tissues within the canal and place a deep sub-cutaneous suture line to close the canal and prevent further herniation into the scrotum. Minimize quantity of suture material in Guinea pigs, however, due to potential for inflammation and abscessation. The prescrotal or scrotal skin incisions can be closed using a subcuticular pattern (3–0 or 4–0 absorbable, monofilament suture ma-terial), nonabsorbable skin sutures or skin staples.

In male sugar gliders, the testicles are located in a pendulous scrotum that is sus-pended from the ventral midline, midway between the sternum and pubis. The most effective and efficient surgical approach, with the least likelihood for postsurgical self-mutilation by the patient, is by use of a CO_2 laser (**Fig. 36**).[27] The scrotal stalk is shaved and aseptically prepared and bupivacaine (2 mg/kg) or lidocaine (4 mg/kg)

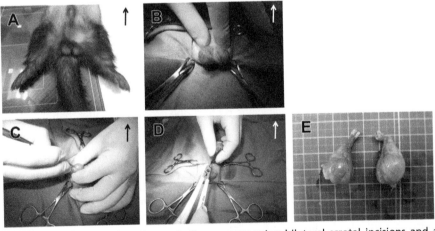

Fig. 35. Male ferret undergoing castration surgery using bilateral scrotal incisions and a closed technique. (*A*) Appearance of perineal region of an intact male ferret. (*B*) Presurgical preparation of male ferret scrotum. (*C*) Skin incision of scrotum to expose the testicle. (*D*) Spermatic cord ligated; E: Surgically removed testicles of male ferret. *Arrows* indicate craniad.

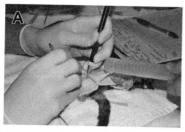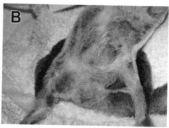

Fig. 36. Male sugar glider undergoing a castration procedure using a CO_2 laser technique. (A) Application of CO_2 laser cutting the scotal stalk skin and spermatic cords in a single motion. (B) Immediate post-operative image of small surgical wound. (*Courtesy of* C. Mans, DVM, DACZM, Madison, WI, USA.)

with 50% of the total dose administered directly into each testicle. Frequently, the size of the testicle limits the volume of local anesthetic instilled in each testicle; for example, it is difficult to administer much more than 0.2 mL in a typical rat testicle or 0.05 mL in a sugar glider testicle. A tongue depressor is placed between the glider's body and the scrotal stalk, and the laser is applied to the stalk cutting rapidly in transverse section, close to the body wall, so as not to leave excess tissue. The laser cuts and cauterizes instantly (see **Fig. 36**). One consequence of using the CO_2 laser is that the skin of the sugar glider skin appears to puff up during laser application, and this can be alarming to a first time user. Also, be careful with a cavalier approach to laser application, because significant, collateral tissue damage may be a consequence. In the authors' experience, there is no postsurgical self-mutilation of the surgical site after use of the laser, whereas self-mutilation is common if using a traditional, scalpel-based surgical approach with sutures.

Ovariectomy/Ovariohysterectomy

As discussed previously, elective ovariectomy and ovariohysterectomy surgical procedures used in small mammals are similar to those used in dogs and cats, with a few notable exceptions. A flank approach to ovariectomies in rodents is, currently, more commonly used than 5 years ago.[7] Laparoscopic ovariectomies are commonly performed in academic veterinary hospitals on dogs and cats, but this approach is not used routinely in small mammals. Other differences include varies and uteri are smaller and tend to be more friable in small mammals, especially rodents, compared with dog and cat tissues. Two surgical approaches are used for ovariectomies and ovariohyterectomies in rodents, ferrets, and hedgehogs.[7] Elective ovariectomy or ovariohysterectomy of sugar gliders is uncommon due to the significant likelihood of postsurgical self-mutilation. The traditional, ventral midline approach to ovariectomy/ovariohysterectomy is identical to the same approach in dogs and cats, although tissues in small mammals are smaller and more friable. In addition, female Guinea pigs have less elastic ovarian suspensory ligaments, which makes ovarian visualization and exposure much more difficult. Application of Hemoclips or use of a LigaSure device can be useful for ligating vessels and hemostasis, because suture ligatures are time consuming and may be difficult in species in which the ovaries are not easily exposed. The uterus can be clamped and ligated at the level of the cervix in most species. The alternative surgical approach for elective ovariectomy is through flank incisions.[7] The primary advantages of this approach include, a shorter procedure, less visceral organ manipulation, faster recovery time, and less postsurgical pain. It is easiest to make 2 flank incisions, 1 in each flank region. The primary disadvantage is lack of access to the uterus, which is most problematic if the surgical procedure is conducted because of pathology. The skin incisions are made, one at a time, in the paralumbar region, from the last rib to the lateral processes of the lumbar vertebrae. The muscle layer is incised and the tissues bluntly dissected. Bipolar cautery can be used for hemostasis. The ovary can be gently manipulated and exposed and a hemostat placed across the ovarian vessels. Hemoclips or suture ligatures can be applied to the ovarian pedicle and the ovary excised. A standard, 2-layer closure of the muscle layer and skin can be performed using suture material and/or staples for the skin layer. The opposite ovary is approached in the same manner.

For nonelective reproductive tract procedures, the primary reproductive diseases associated with ferrets, rodents, and hedgehogs includes Guinea pig ovarian cysts and caesarian sections, pyometra, or mucometra in various species. Ovarian cysts are commonly observed in female Guinea pigs and frequently require surgical intervention.[27–30] Typical clinical signs include bilaterally symmetric and nonpruritic alopecia and abdominal distention associated with enlarging ovarian cysts (**Fig. 37**). Diagnosis is suspected based on typical clinical signs and palpation and confirmed using abdominal ultrasonography or CT. As discussed previously, normal ovaries of guinea pigs have short ovarian ligaments and tend to be located in a more dorsal position compared with rabbits, which can make access to the ovaries more difficult when a ventral midline incision is used. Therefore, some surgeons prefer a dorsal flank approach to the Guinea pigs ovaries.[7] On the other hand, the ovarian cysts are frequently large and easily manipulated through a ventral midline incision, and both authors typically use this approach for ovarian cysts (**Fig. 38**). Once the incision is made, be careful with excessive manipulation of other abdominal organs, especially the gastrointestinal organs, because Guinea pigs tend to have a more dramatic inflammatory reaction to organ manipulation that other small mammal species. It is best to protect the other abdominal organs with moist gauze and minimize traction of the uterus and ovaries. In cases in which the ovarian ligaments are flaccid and stretched by the enlarged ovaries, providing good access to the ovarian pedicle, monofilament, absorbable suture material can be used to place ligatures (**Fig. 39**), or a LigaSure device can be used to ligate the ovarian vessels. For those cases in which the ovarian ligaments are not elastic and extraction of ovaries is difficult, Hemoclips can be useful for ligating the ovarian vessels. A bilateral ovariohysterectomy is most commonly used by the authors, but when only 1 ovary is cystic and approaching

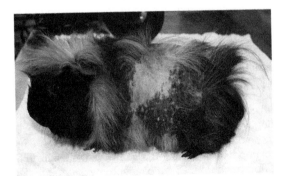

Fig. 37. Female guinea pig with typical clinical signs associated with ovarian cysts. These include bilaterally symmetric and nonpruritic alopecia and abdominal distention.

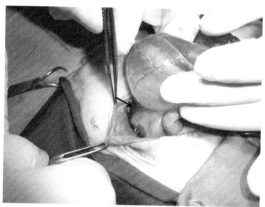

Fig. 38. Ovarian cyst with the ovarian ligament of a female guinea pig. Ovarian ligaments (*black arrow*) of guinea pigs are shorter and less elastic than ovarian ligaments of most other small mammals.

the other side via a ventral midline incision is difficult, a unilateral ovariectomy may be elected.

For uterine or vaginal lesions, including neoplastic diseases and pyometra, the appropriate reproductive organs are surgically removed using a ventral midline approach. With uterine or vaginal pathologic lesions, an ovariohysterectomy is most commonly performed. Because the ovaries of Guinea pigs can be difficult to access through a midline incision, discussed previously, one of the authors (YM) surgically removes uterine or vaginal lesions and leaves the ovaries intact if there is no concurrent ovarian pathology. Large vaginal masses are sometimes observed in female Guinea pigs and may appear unresectable based on ultrasound or exploratory laparotomy results. From the authors' experiences, however, these masses are easy to remove due to minimal adhesions, despite the size of the mass. In such cases, a ventral midline approach is used and the ovaries and uterus are surgically removed. The vagina is incised, the mass is peeled away from the mucosa, and bipolar cautery

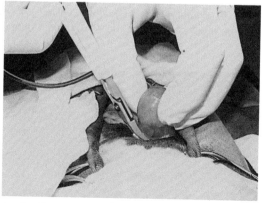

Fig. 39. When the ovarian ligaments are flaccid and stretched enough by the enlargement of the ovaries, use vessel sealing system, such as LigaSure or absorbable suture, for ligation.

is used for hemostasis. The vagina can be closed using 3-0 to 4-0 monofilament, absorbable suture in a 2-layer inverting pattern, and the muscle layer and skin closed as previously described.

Intact female Guinea pigs allowed access to males become pregnant and commonly experience dystocia, which requires caesarian section.[7,9] If female Guinea pigs experience their first parturition prior to 8 months of age, there is dehiscence of the tuberculum pubicum and parturition is smooth. Without an early parturition, however, female Guinea pigs develop a very small pubic opening, leading to dystocia. With pregnancy, the pubic symphysis of all females should be examined radiographically and a caesarian section performed when necessary. The procedure is identical to that of a dog or cat, using a ventral midline approach (**Fig. 40**). The uterus incision should be closed in 2 inverting layers.

In hedgehogs, neoplastic diseases are common, and mammary gland tumors tend to have the highest published incidence.[31] Based on the authors' experience, however, the most common reproductive organ affected by neoplasia is the uterus. Uterine masses are commonly diagnosed in middle-aged and older (greater than 2 years) hedgehogs and present with hematuria, and hemorrhagic discharge from vulva (**Fig. 41**). With sedation or anesthesia, uterine masses are usually palpable in the caudal abdomen and can be confirmed using CT or ultrasonography. Ovariohysterectomy is usually curative if the tumor is contained within the uterus. The hedgehog is placed in dorsal recumbency, and an approximate 2-cm midline incision is made from the umbilicus caudally. The swollen, discolored uterus is detected and is lifted through the incision with Babcock forceps (**Fig. 42**). The uterine horns are coiled and broad ligament of the uterus is narrower and tighter than in rabbits, for example (see **Fig. 42**). Some ovarian and mesometrial vessels are visible, but they tend to be small and hemorrhage is seldom a problem if using Hemoclips or a LigaSure device. In some of these cases, however, there can be excessive hemorrhage, and perioperative or postoperative death is possible due to blood loss. The uterus can be transfixed using 3-0 or 4-0 monofilament, absorbable suture material, and transected at the cervix or vagina. The muscle layer is closed using 4-0 monofilament, absorbable suture material in a simple continuous patter, and a subcuticular pattern can be used to close the skin or skin sutures or staples used.

Additional Ferret Surgical Procedures

The prevalence of neoplastic diseases in ferrets has changed over the past several decades with respect to primary organ system involved. Reproductive system neoplastic diseases were most common in the 1970s and 1980s or second only to

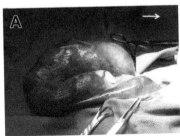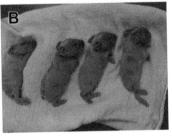

Fig. 40. Caesarian section in a female guinea pig. (*A*) Intraoperative appearance of the pregnant uterus. (*B*) New-born infants delivered by Caesarian section. *Arrow* indicates craniad.

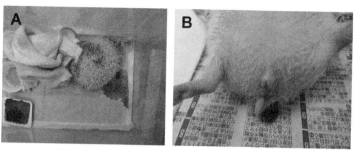

Fig. 41. Hematuria (*A*) and/or vulvar hemorrhage (*B*) in a female hedgehog with reproductive disease.

lymphoma.[32–34] The prevalence of reproductive system tumors has significantly decreased, however, whereas the prevalence of endocrine neoplasia, including adrenal adenoma/adenocarcinoma and pancreatic beta cell tumors (ie, insulinoma), has increased.[35–39] This changing prevalence of neoplastic diseases in ferrets can be attributed to the fact that most pet ferrets sold in North America and Japan are neutered and descented at an early age. Both authors have performed multiple ovariohysterectomies and anal sacculectomies on retired breeding ferrets (**Fig. 43**). The ovariohysterectomy procedure in a ferret is identical to that in a small cat. Both authors have experienced cases in which stump pyometra is diagnosed, and surgical excision of the distended uterine stump was completed. Castration of male ferrets is similar to the procedure used in a small dog (see **Fig. 35**).

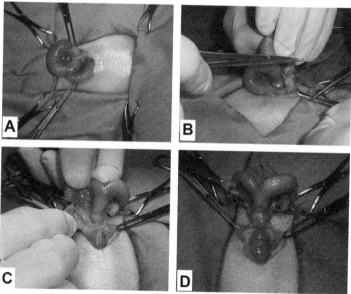

Fig. 42. Female hedgehog undergoing an ovariohysterectomy of diseased uterus. Female hedgehog uterine horns are coiled and the broad ligament of the uterus is narrower and tighter compared with the reproductive tract of other female small mammals. (*A*) Uterine horns exposed peri-operatively in a female hedgehog. (*B*) Ligature transfixation of uterine body of female hedgehog. (*C, D*) Excision of uterus and ovaries from the female hedgehog.

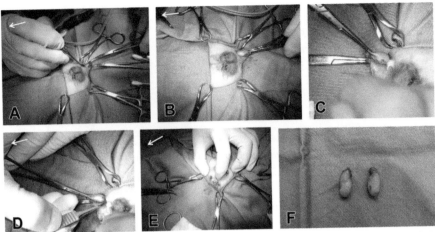

Fig. 43. Anal sacculectomy of a ferret. The perianal gland ducts are identified and os of the gland is clamped using a small hemostat (*A*). A circumferential incision is made (*B*) closely associated with the duct and the gland is slowly and carefully, bluntly dissected from the surrounding muscle (*C*). A scalpel blade and bipolar cautery are used to scrape the muscle from the serosal surface of each gland, being careful not to rupture the gland (*D*). Both glands are excised and the surgical wounds left open to heal by second intention (*E*). Excised anal glands are shown (*F*). *Arrows* indicates craniad.

Although uncommon, mammary gland neoplasia is observed in ferrets and is most commonly associated with concurrent adrenal disease and increased reproductive hormones. In cases of mild enlargement of mammary gland or enlargement of the nipples only (**Fig. 44**), these symptoms may resolves with surgical removal of the diseased adrenal gland or medical management by using deslorelin implants. On the other hand, in cases in which a solid mammary tumor is observed, the diseased mammary tissue should be surgically excised (see **Fig. 44**).

Endocrine Surgery

Adrenal adenoma/adenocarcinoma and pancreatic beta cell tumors are the 2 most common endocrine diseases in domestic ferrets, and both diseases can be managed either medically or surgically. The surgical techniques for adrenalectomy and excision of pancreatic beta cell tumors in ferrets are described.

Adrenalectomy

Many cases of adrenal adenoma/adenocarcinoma in ferrets are now managed using deslorelin implants to control the clinical signs. This medical management does not affect the disease progression, only the signs associated with increased androgens and estrogens. Surgical removal of the adrenal gland is an option, and can provide increased time to recurrence. Typical clinical signs associated with adrenal disease in ferrets include alopecia, pruritus, skin excoriations, lethargy, swollen vulva in females, stranguria in males due to prostatic enlargement and urethral compression, and thin skin. Diagnosis is based on endocrine panels and/or ultrasonographic evidence of an enlarged or misshapen adrenal gland or glands. The adrenal glands are located near the craniomedial pole of the kidneys and surrounded by large amount of fat within the retroperitoneal cavity. The right adrenal, like the kidney, is located more cranially and closely associated with the dorsomedial aspect of the caudal

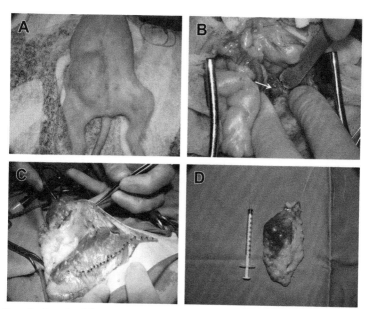

Fig. 44. Female ferret with mammary duct ectasia accompanied by adrenocortical carcinoma. (*A*) Appearance of the lesion (*B*) Note the enlarged left side adrenal gland (adenocortical carcinoma) (*arrow*). (*C*) Enlarged mammary gland was surgically resected. (*D*) The affected mammary gland was diagnosed as mammary duct ectasia.

vena cava. Therefore, surgical removal of the right adrenal gland is technically more challenging than surgical removal of the left adrenal gland. The surgical approach to the abdomen is routinely performed via a ventral midline approach and the retraction of the spleen and intestines from the surgical field to visualize the adrenal glands. Although both adrenals are located within the retroperitoneal fat (**Fig. 45**), the affected adrenal gland(s) is enlarged, irregularly shaped, discolored, and readily visible (**Fig. 46**). Although 1 gland may have an abnormal appearance on ultrasound images, both adrenal glands may be affected, and a subtotal, bilateral adrenalectomy is warranted. The authors usually attempt to remove the affected adrenal gland and debulk the other, leaving some of the capsule behind. The authors have not observed any

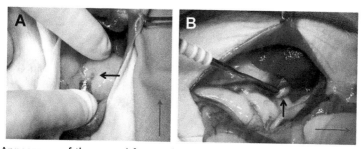

Fig. 45. Appearance of the normal ferret adrenal gland (*A*) left adrenal and (*B*) right adrenal. *Red arrow* indicates cranial. The adrenal glands (*black arrows*) are located within the retroperitoneal cavity and surrounded by a large amount of fat. (*B*) The right adrenal is located under the caudate liver lobe and adhered to the caudal vena cava.

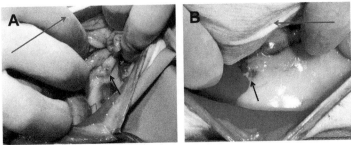

Fig. 46. Appearance of an abnormal ferret adrenal gland: (*A*) left adrenal and (*B*) right adrenal. Red arrow indicates cranial. Although both adrenals (*black arrows*) are located within the retroperitoneal fat, most of the affected adrenal is irregularly shaped, discolored, and readily visible.

ferret developing long-term hypoadrenocorticism crisis postbilateral adrenalectomy, but immediate postsurgical treatment with corticosteroids may be beneficial.[39] Accessory adrenal glands are occasionally observed and these tissues may compensate after the bilateral adrenalectomy in ferrets. The procedures associated with left adrenectomy (**Fig. 47**) and right adrenalectomy (**Fig. 48**) in ferrets are shown. Use of a CO_2 laser (**Fig. 49**) and cryosurgical probes has been described for right-sided

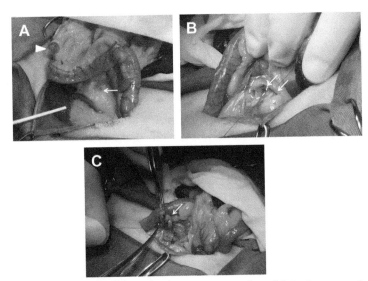

Fig. 47. Left adrenalectomy in a ferret. (*A*) The spleen and small intestines are retracted toward the right side in the body or exteriorized through the incision line. Confirm the left adrenal gland (*arrow*), which is located cranial to the cranial pole of the left kidney. A swollen lymph node (*arrowhead*) was observed, and the final diagnosis in this case was lymphoma. (*B*) Confirm the adrenolumbar vein (*arrows*), which runs from lateral to medial over the ventral surface of the left adrenal (*dotted line*), and ligate this vessel at the distal aspect using 4-0 absorbable suture or Hemoclips. (*C*) Separate the affected adrenal gland completely from the surrounding tissue, ligate the proximal part of the adrenolumber vein, and remove the affected gland (*arrow*).

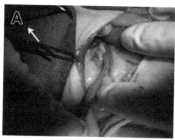
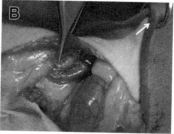

Fig. 48. Right adrenalectomy in a ferret. (*A*) Retract the spleen and intestines toward the left side in the body or exteriorize through the ventral midline incision. Confirm the right adrenal gland, which is located cranial to the cranial pole of the right kidney. The right adrenal gland is usually directly adhered to the vena cava and care must be taken to not lacerate this vessel during the procedure. (*B*) Hemoclips are useful for hemostatsis and ligation of vessels. Continue the same procedure as the left adrenalectomy, and detach the adrenal from the vena cava. *Arrow* indicates craniad.

adrenalectomy. A complete abdominal exploratory is important to evaluate the abdominal organs, especially to check the pancreas for nodules.

Insulinoma

Surgical treatment of insulinoma in ferrets

Insulinomas are functional tumors of the beta cells of the islands of Langerhans, which secrete insulin despite the presence of hypoglycemia, and insulinoma is the most common neoplastic diseases of ferrets.[39] A tentative diagnosis of insulinoma is based on clinical signs associated with hypoglycemia and confirmation of the low blood glucose concentration lower than 60 mg/dL.[39] Because most pancreatic beta cell tumors are not discrete nodules and, therefore, difficult to diagnose using imaging modalities, medical management is frequently the treatment of choice. Medical management includes corticosteroids, such as prednisolone or prednisone, administered orally. Treatment may alleviate clinical signs associated with hypoglycemia but does not alter the progression of the disease process. Surgical excision of discrete pancreatic nodules is the recommended treatment of insulinoma in ferrets (**Fig. 50**).

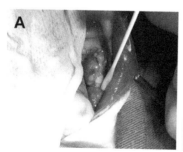
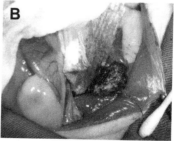

Fig. 49. Right side partial adrenalectomy in a ferret using a CO_2 laser. The affected adrenal infiltrated into caudal vena cava, and the owner denied aggressive surgery. After partial resection of the affected adrenal for histopathological evaluation, residual tissues were vaporized by CO_2 laser. (*A*) Appearance of the affected adrenal. (*B*) Appearance of the dorsal aspect of the adrenal gland after CO_2 laser vaporization.

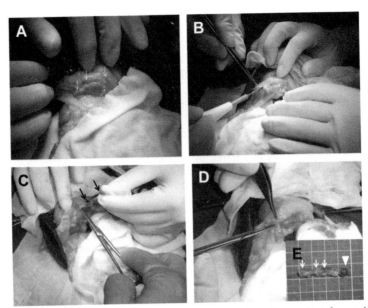

Fig. 50. Partial pancreatectomy as a surgical treatment of insulinoma in a ferret. (*A*) Multiple nodules (*arrows*) are confirmed in the left pancreatic lobe. (*B*) Incision of surrounding tissue associated with the affected pancreas lesion. Surgically removing any tumor nodules with a wide margin is important. (*C*) Isolate the affected nodule (*arrow*) and place a loop of suture around the lesion. Tighten the suture and allow it to crush through the pancreatic parenchyma. (*D*) Excise the specimen, distal to the ligature. (*E*) In the excised pancreas, there is 1 large nodule (*arrowhead*) and multiple small nodules (*arrows*).

REFERENCES

1. Lichtenberger M, Ko J. Anaesthesia and analgesia for small mammals and birds. Vet Clin North Am Exot Anim Pract 2007;10:293–315.
2. Flecknell PA, Richardson CA, Popovic A, et al. Anesthesia and immobilization of small mammals. In: Grimm KA, Tranquilli WJ, Lamont LA, editors. Essentials of small animal anesthesia and analgesia. 2nd edition. Ames (IA): Wiley-Blackwell; 2011. p. 300–25.
3. Johnson DH. Endoscopic intubation of exotic companion mammals. Vet Clin North Am Exot Anim Pract 2010;13:273–89.
4. Miller AL, Richardson CA. Rodent analgesia. Vet Clin North Am Exot Anim Pract 2011;14:81–92.
5. Van Oostrom H, Schoemacker NJ, Uilenreef JJ. Pain management in ferrets. Vet Clin North Am Exot Anim Pract 2011;14:105–16.
6. Souza MJ, Cox SK. Tramadol use in zoological medicine. Vet Clin North Am Exot Anim Pract 2011;14:117–30.
7. Capello V. Common surgical procedures in pet rodents. J Exotic Pet Med 2011; 20:294–307.
8. Johnson DH. Emergency presentations of the exotic small mammalian herbivore trauma patient. J Exotic Pet Med 2012;21:300–15.
9. Bennett RA. Surgery. In: Quesenberry KA, Carpenter JW, editors. Ferrets, rabbits and rodents: clinical medicine and surgery. 3rd edition. St Louis (MO): Saunders-Elsevier; 2012. p. 316–28.

10. Tynes V. Behavioral dermatopathies in small mammals. Vet Clin North Am Exot Anim Pract 2014;43:801–20.
11. Heatley JJ, Harris MC. Hamsters and gerbils. In: Mitchell MA, Tully TN, editors. Manual of exotic pet practice. St Louis (MO): Saunders-Elsevier; 2009. p. 406–32.
12. Riggs SM, Mitchell MA. Chinchillas. In: Mitchell MA, Tully TN, editors. Manual of exotic pet practice. St Louis (MO): Saunders-Elsevier; 2009. p. 474–92.
13. Greenacre CB. Spontaneous tumors of small mammals. Vet Clin North Am Exot Anim Pract 2004;7:627–51.
14. Campbell TW. Exotic animal hematology and cytology. 4th edition. Ames (IA): Wiley-Blackwell; 2015. p. 267–308.
15. Kondo H, Onuma M, Shibuya H, et al. Spontaneous tumors in domestic hamsters. Vet Pathol 2008;45:674–80.
16. Jenkins JR. Diseases of geriatric Guinea pigs and chinchillas. Vet Clin North Am Exot Anim Pract 2010;13:85–93.
17. Hoefer HL, Bell JA. Gastrointestinal diseases. In: Quesenberry KA, Carpenter JW, editors. Ferrets, rabbits and rodents: clinical medicine and surgery. 3rd edition. St Louis (MO): Saunders-Elsevier; 2012. p. 25–40.
18. Mehler SJ. Surgery. In: Fox JG, Marini RP, editors. Biology and diseases of the ferret. 3rd edition. Ames (IA): Wiley-Blackwell; 2014. p. 285–310.
19. Lennox AM. Gastrointestinal diseases of the ferret. Vet Clin North Am Exot Anim Pract 2005;8:213–25.
20. Fossum TW. Surgery of the liver. In: Fossum TW, Hedlund CS, Johnson AL, et al, editors. Small animal surgery. 3rd Edition. St Louis (MO): Elsevier; 2007. p. 531–59.
21. Rothuizen J, Twedt DC. Liver biopsy techniques. Vet Clin North Am Small Anim Pract 2009;39:469–80.
22. Ludwig L, Aiken S. Soft tissue surgery. In: Quesenberry KA, Carpenter JW, editors. Ferrets, rabbits and rodents: clinical medicine and surgery. 3rd edition. St Louis (MO): Saunders-Elsevier; 2012. p. 121–35.
23. Marini RP, Callahan RJ, Jackson LR, et al. Distribution of technetium 99m-labeled red blood cells during isoflurane anesthesia in ferrets. Am J Vet Res 1997;58:781–5.
24. Nwaokorie EE, Osborne CA, Lulich JP, et al. Epidemiology of struvite uroliths in ferrets: 272 cases (1981-2007). J Am Vet Med Assoc 2011;15:1319–24.
25. Nwaokorie EE, Osborne CA, Lulich JP, et al. Epidemiological evaluation of cystine urolithiasis in domestic ferrets (Mustela putorius furo): 70 cases (1992-2009). J Am Vet Med Assoc 2013;242:1099–103.
26. Hawkins MG, Bishop CR. Disease problems of guinea pigs. In: Quesenberry KE, Carpenter JW, editors. Ferrets, rabbits, and rodents: clinical medicine and surgery. 3rd edition. St Louis (MO): Elsevier; 2012. p. 295–310.
27. Morges MA, Grant KR, MacPhail CM, et al. A novel technique for orchiectomy and scrotal ablation in the sugar glider (Petaurus breviceps). J Zoo Wildl Med 2009;40:204–6.
28. Nielsen TD, Holt S, Ruelokke ML, et al. Ovarian cysts in guinea pigs: influence of age and reproductive status on prevalence and size. J Small Anim Pract 2003;44:257–60.
29. Pilny A. Ovarian cystic disease in guinea pigs. Veterinary Clin North Am Exot Anim Pract 2014;17:69–75.
30. Bean AD. Ovarian cysts in the guinea pig (Cavia porcellus). Veterinary Clin North Am Exot Anim Pract 2013;16:757–76.
31. Raymond JT, Garner MM. Spontaneous tumors in captive African hedgehogs (Atelerix albiventris): a retrospective study. J Comp Pathol 2001;124:128–33.

32. Li X, Fox JG, Padrid PA. Neoplastic diseases in ferrets: 574 cases (1968-1997). J Am Vet Med Assoc 1998;212:1402–6.
33. Dillberger JE, Altman NH. Neoplasia in ferrets: eleven cases with a review. J Comp Pathol 1989;100:161–76.
34. Beach JE, Greenwood B. Spontaneous neoplasia in the ferret (Mustela putorius furo). J Comp Pathol 1993;108:133–47.
35. Brown SA. Neoplasia. In: Hillyer EV, Quesenberry KE, editors. Ferrets, rabbits, and rodents: clinical medicine and surgery. Philadelphia: Saunders; 1997. p. 99–114.
36. Li X, Fox JG. Neoplastic disease. In: Fox JG, editor. Biology and diseases of the ferret. 2nd edition. Baltimore (MD): Williams & Wilkins; 1998. p. 405–47.
37. Williams BH, Weiss CA. Neoplasia. In: Quesenberry KE, Carpenter JW, editors. Ferrets, rabbits, and rodents: clinical medicine and surgery. 2nd edition. Philadelphia: Saunders; 2003. p. 91–106.
38. Miwa Y, Kurosawa A, Ogawa H, et al. Neoplasitic diseases in ferrets in Japan: a questionnaire study for 2000 to 2005. J Vet Med Sci 2009;71:397–402.
39. Beeber NL. Surgical management of adrenal tumors and insulinomas in ferrets. J Exotic Pet Med 2011;20:206–16.

Eye Removal Surgeries in Exotic Pets

Kathryn A. Diehl, MS, DVM, DACVO[a],*, Jo-Ann McKinnon, DVM, DACVO[b]

KEYWORDS

- Enucleation • Exenteration • Evisceration • Exotic pets • Rabbits • Birds • Snakes

KEY POINTS

- Considering the anatomic variation of exotic pets and how this affects surgical considerations, approach, and risks is key to a successful surgical outcome.
- Proper equipment and preparedness are important to a successful surgical outcome.
- The orbital venous plexus is well developed in rabbits and several other small mammal species.
- To reduce risk of disrupting the orbital venous plexus and possibly causing severe hemorrhage during enucleation, a subconjunctival approach is preferred over transpalpebral.
- Evisceration offers an alternative to enucleation in birds with ocular disease not involving the orbit or sclera.

GENERAL CONSIDERATIONS FOR OPHTHALMIC SURGERY IN EXOTIC PETS

Ophthalmic examination and diagnosis in exotic pets may be more challenging by nature of issues with stress on the animal and restraint, frequently small size of ophthalmic structures, and often less familiar differential list for the practitioner.[1] Once a diagnosis is made, therapeutic options may be limited by the morbidity associated with frequent administration of medication (capture, restraint) or the its side effects, especially with the small size of many of these patients and the risk of systemic absorption,[1,2] as well as possible underlying systemic disease with broader implications.[3]

Surgical management of ophthalmic disorders when possible may alleviate some of these concerns but comes with its own,[1] including patient and client, considerations such as anesthetic candidacy, safety, and cost. Furthermore, anatomic factors dictate that surgical options are often more limited and riskier than in traditional pet species. Finally, surgery may not eliminate the need for postoperative medical treatment and associated morbidity and mortality. The decision to pursue surgery should thus

The authors have nothing to disclose.
[a] Department of Small Animal Medicine and Surgery, University of Georgia – College of Veterinary Medicine, 2200 College Station Road, Athens, GA 30602, USA; [b] Loudon, TN, USA
* Corresponding author.
E-mail address: kadiehl@uga.edu

Vet Clin Exot Anim 19 (2016) 245–267
http://dx.doi.org/10.1016/j.cvex.2015.08.003   vetexotic.theclinics.com

come after thorough regard for both the short- and long-term outcome goals and prognosis. Ophthalmic surgical intervention may thus be indicated for pain relief, quality of life (alleviating or reducing medical treatment), restoration of function, biopsy, or cosmesis. Despite these indications, potential drawbacks of surgery may include continued need to treat, some loss of function and associated impact, healing issues and other complication risks, and poor cosmesis.

Anesthesia

For eye removal surgeries requiring general anesthesia, considerations and protocols are the same as for other surgeries, with nuances in terms of preanesthetic management, including variations in fasting, which may be limited or not performed in exotic pet species with generally high metabolic rates and uncommon or impossible (rabbits and rodents) emesis[4,5]; moisturization in amphibians[6] and fish[7]; drug doses and administration; patient size; difficult or impossible endotracheal intubation; adequate monitoring; thermoregulation[8]; and recovery, as expected for exotic pets. In addition, because the head is draped in for these procedures, there may be extra challenges in patient observation, and it is essential that appropriate capability and equipment for assessing cardiac, vascular, and respiratory status, as well as depth of anesthesia, are available and functioning.

In patients undergoing anesthesia, there is an increased risk of exposure-related corneal damage due to altered palpebral reflexes with frequent lagophthalmia and decreased tear production.[9] Unoperated eyes should be generously lubricated with an artificial tear ointment.

Retrobulbar local nerve blocks are commonly used in canine,[10] feline, and large-animal[11,12] ocular surgeries, particularly enucleations, to help manage intraoperative and postoperative pain and allow decreased depth of and safer general anesthesia, as well as improve ocular position (with slight exophthalmos and central rotation) and exposure. Owing to the small size of exotic pet species and, in some, an orbital venous plexus and risk of hemorrhage, these blocks are infrequently used, although they may be used with caution in rabbits[13] and other species. A gently curved 23- to 30-gauge needle is inserted at the lateral canthus, through the conjunctiva and along the globe posteronasally. After aspiration to ensure the needle is not in a vascular structure, an appropriate small volume of local anesthetic (eg, lidocaine, bupivicaine) is deposited extraconally. The needle is carefully removed. Potential complications include hemorrhage, laceration of and/or injection into the globe, and injection within the optic nerve sheath with possible effect on the contralateral eye.[14]

Traction on the extraocular muscles and optic nerve or pressure on the globe during surgery can result in bradycardia and even cardiac arrest because of the oculocardiac reflex.[15,16] Both the surgeon and anesthetist should be aware of and prepared for this potential event, which is best avoided altogether or possibly corrected when it does occur, by more gentle manipulation of the globe.

PATIENT PREPARATION

Preparation of the patient's eye and surgical field vary with the surgery to be performed as well as the species. Generally, where applicable, eyelashes are trimmed with small scissors with artificial tear ointment along the blade away from the cornea to catch cut lashes and reduce risk of them entering the surgical field.

In mammals with haired skin, for eyelid and eye removal procedures, an appropriate sized (1–2 in depending on patient size) border from the eyelid margins is clipped with scissors or electric clippers with a small blade (#40 or #50). Loose hairs are removed by gently blotting with tape. Some veterinary ophthalmologists advocate lubricating the ocular surface before clipping to protect it from stray hairs. Others recommend cleaning and rinsing the conjunctiva, including the fornices, after clipping to remove any hairs, then applying a lubricant so the hairs are not caught in it. In birds, the periocular feathers may be gently manually plucked in the direction of their growth, around the surgical site.[17,18] Reptiles, amphibians, and fish do not require preoperative trimming or descaling.

Presurgical disinfection can be extrapolated from ophthalmic surgical preparation of other veterinary patients. The eyelids and adjacent periocular skin and conjunctiva/ocular surface may be cleaned with dilute (half-strength aqueous) povidone-iodine solution and rinsing with sterile saline without damaging the cornea or causing periocular irritation,[19] although care must be taken in amphibians with their semipermeable skin and potential iodine toxicity.[6] Povidone-iodine has broad-spectrum antimicrobial and bactericidal effects, including against common bacterial and fungal species as well as viruses.[20] Povidone-iodine scrub, chlorhexidine scrub, and alcohol should not be used even if the prepared eye is being removed, as they could inadvertently damage the other eye/cornea.[21]

Gentle conjunctival cul-de-sac cleaning with dilute povidone-iodine solution–wetted sterile cotton tipped applicators, with care to avoid the cornea, and saline eye wash rinsing may remove debris and hairs.

POSITIONING

Depending on the species and surgery to be performed, the patient may be placed in dorsal, lateral, or ventral recumbency with the head close to the head end of the table and rotated such that the palpebral fissure of the operated eye is in a plane parallel to the floor/table (**Figs. 1–4**). This position allows improved ease of focus, especially if magnification is used for surgery. Vacuum or other moldable beanbags or other padding or supports, as well as adhesive tape, to maintain this head position are particularly helpful for ophthalmic procedures, again especially those requiring use of magnification. It is important to ensure that this arrangement, often with unnatural manipulation of the neck, does not interfere with patient ventilation.

Generally in ophthalmic surgical procedures, the surgeon is positioned at the head of the table and rests his or her forearms for stabilization. Care must be taken to not put pressure on the patient or anesthetic equipment.

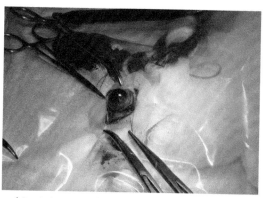

Fig. 1. Positioning and Steri-draping of a rabbit during enucleation. Note the use of retracting eyelid stay sutures manipulated by hemostats, as an alternative to an eyelid speculum.

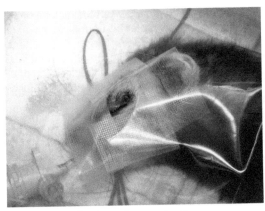

Fig. 2. Positioning and draping of a ferret for enucleation.

EQUIPMENT

Adequate lighting, appropriate magnification, good ophthalmic surgical instruments, and proper suture optimize surgical results and thus quality of care, especially with the small size of the tissues being manipulated in exotic pet ophthalmic surgery.

There are many excellent manufacturers of surgical loupes, with customizable working distance and degree of magnification. Less expensive, more universal, but adjustable jeweler's loupes or binocular head loupes (OptiVISOR, Donegan Optical Company, Inc, Lenexa, KS, USA) are also reasonable options to provide adequate magnification for many external ocular ophthalmic examination and surgical procedures.

Surgical instrumentation specifically designed for ophthalmic procedures tend to be small, sharp, and precise. Such instruments are easily damaged if not handled properly; thus, no discussion of ophthalmic surgical equipment is complete without covering care.

Instruments should be kept in a separate ophthalmic pack (various specialized trays are available) where they cannot rub against each other or be individually wrapped. Regardless, pieces of silicone tubing may be slipped over instrument tips to reduce risk of damage.

After use, instruments should be rinsed with distilled water and gently brushed, with great care along blades and tips, as needed to remove dried blood and tissue. They should then be sonicated in an ultrasonic cleaner with appropriate mild detergent, thoroughly rinsed with distilled water, and air dried before packing and sterilization. Gas sterilization is best, as steam may cause corrosion and dull instruments.[22]

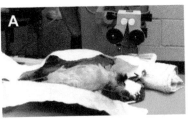
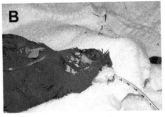

Fig. 3. Positioning of avian patients for ocular surgery. (*A*) Blue-and-yellow macaw (*Ara ararauna*) positioned under an operating microscope. (*B*) Red lori (*Eos bornea*) positioned for enucleation of the right globe.

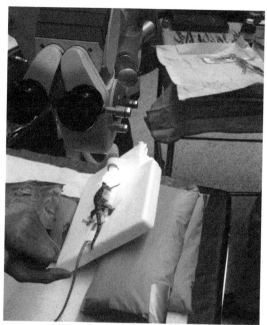

Fig. 4. Gargoyle gecko (*Rhacodactylus auriculatus*) positioned for ocular surgery under an operating microscope. Note the inclined styroform board used to aid in positioning of this small patient with the palpebral fissure parallel to the floor.

Instruments for Exposing or Stabilizing Tissues

Eyelid specula

Barraquer wire eyelid speculum (small or pediatric) provides invaluable exposure of the ocular surface and globe (**Figs. 5** and **6**). The degree of opening can be adjusted manually before placement. The hinge is placed temporally.

Tissue forceps

Forceps used for exotic animal eyelid skin, conjunctiva, and periocular dissection, most commonly during enucleation, should be light enough to stabilize the tissues without causing excessive trauma but not so delicate that they are bent by the tissues. Typically, these forceps have teeth in a 1×2 intermeshing box tooth pattern. Examples include delicate Adson rat tooth forceps or ideally 0.5- or 0.3-mm (across the tips) Bishop-Harmon forceps for eyelids and conjunctiva and 0.3-mm Colibri-style forceps with an angled shaft to allow visualization while grasping, for conjunctiva.[23]

Instruments for Separating, Incising, or Excising Tissues

Scalpels and blades

A #3 Bard-Parker scalpel handle with #15 blade can provide adequate depth control and incision direction for eyelids (**Fig. 7**). Alternatively, a Beaver handle/chuck with a #6400 or #6500 blade is smaller and lighter and may provide improved tactile feedback to the surgeon, thus improving precision.

Scissors

There are a variety of blunt-tipped scissors useful for eyelid, conjunctival, and periocular surgery cutting and dissection regardless of species. Steven tenotomy scissors

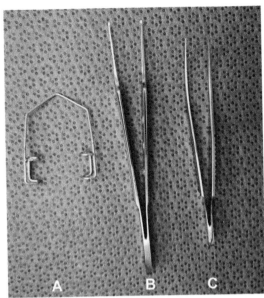

Fig. 5. Instruments for exposing or stabilizing tissues. (*A*) Barraquer wire eyelid speculum; (*B*) delicate Bishop-Harmon forceps; (*C*) Colibri-style forceps.

are general-purpose small scissors with curved or straight blades and variable tong lengths. Westcott tenotomy scissors with spring action handles also come in a variety of types and sizes but are more suitable for delicate incisions of conjunctiva and periocular tissue, as well as for cutting fine suture.

Lens loupes
A lens loupe has a blunt edge and open oval end and may be used to remove the lens and dissect free the uveal tract without damage to the sclera during evisceration. Several types, with variable shapes and sizes, exist.

Cyclodialysis spatulas
These slightly arching, thin, blunt-tipped blades may be used to dissect free the uveal tract without damage to the sclera during evisceration. They may be single or double ended.

Instruments and Material for Uniting Tissues (Suturing)

Needle holders
There are 2 categories for ophthalmic needle holders based on the size of the needle they are intended to grasp: Derf, for 5-0 to 4-0 suture material/needles, and fingertip-controlled, spring action–handled, microsurgical needle holders, with many suitable varieties (locking, nonlocking, straight, or curved tips), for 6-0 and smaller suture material/needles (**Fig. 8**).[24]

Suture needles
Each of the common point designs (taper, cutting, reverse cutting, and spatula) produces a different tissue tract and results in differing tissue damage. For eyelid skin, 4-0 to 6-0 reverse cutting swaged needles are most appropriate. Subcutaneous and periocular tissues may be apposed with 4-0 to 6-0 taper needles.[25]

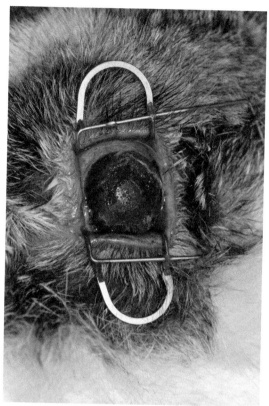

Fig. 6. Winged Barraquer eyelid speculum used on a rabbit for cyanoacrylate glue placement for a superficial nonhealing corneal ulcer.

Suture materials

Considerations for suture material choice include the type of tissue being repaired, as different tissues heal at variable rates and need different durations of effect and support. Different tissues also tolerate suture drag–induced trauma and inflammatory response differently. With irritation risk comes the likelihood of and concern for patient attempts at suture disruption. The likelihood of and concern for capillarity (wicking) by the suture material dictate the need for or acceptability of monofilament versus braided suture. Other factors in suture material choice are its ease of use and suture removal indication (skin) and logistics: can the patient be re-presented and compliant/tolerant?[26] Ideally, the smallest possible suture size that provides adequate and uniform tensile strength across the wound during or until healing, with the least amount of tissue reactivity and wicking tendency, should be used.

Absorbable sutures, commonly used in subcutaneous, conjunctival, and episcleral tissues, include polyglactin 910 (eg, Vicryl, generally braided except very small sizes) with good tensile strength for about 20 days[27] but fairly reactive, poliglecaprone 25 (Monocryl, monofilament), and polydioxanone (PDS II, monofilament). Nonabsorbable sutures, commonly used in skin, include nylon (monofilament, chronically strong and inert, or braided, strong and still inert with softer tags), polypropylene (Prolene, monofilament), and silk (braided). Braided options can wick, but this is uncommonly a problem if sutures are removed in a timely manner ($\sim$10 days).[28]

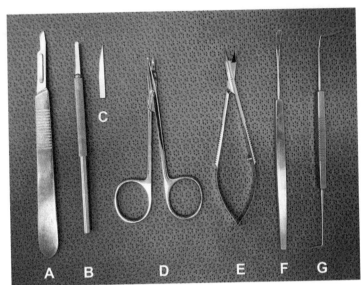

Fig. 7. Instruments for separating, incising, or excising tissues. (*A*) #3 Bard-Parker scalpel blade handle with #15 blade; (*B*) Beaver blade handle with #6400 Beaver blade; (*C*) #6500 Beaver blade; (*D*) Steven tenotomy scissors; (*E*) Westcott tenotomy scissors; (*F*) lens loupe; (*G*) cyclodialysis spatula.

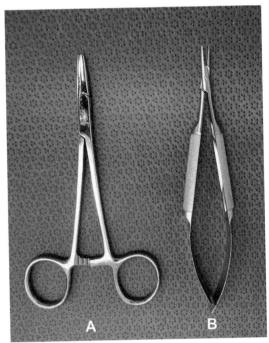

Fig. 8. Instruments for uniting tissues. (*A*) Derf needle holder; (*B*) nonlocking Barraquer microsurgical needle holder.

Miscellaneous Instruments and Accessories

Clear plastic, adhesive drapes (Steri-Drape, St Paul, MN, USA) and patient drapes; Schaedel cross-action towel clamps; sterile gauze, cotton-tipped applicators, and cellulose sponge spears (Weck-Cel cellulose sponges, Beaver-Visitec, Waltham, MA, USA), which avoid cotton fibers remaining in the wound, for hemostasis and visualization; irrigation cannulas for accurate and least disruptive moisturization of the operated ocular surface thus improving visualization and reducing risk of exposure damage; Jameson muscle hook for tissue and globe manipulation; and absorbable gelatin compressed sponge material (Gelfoam, Pfizer, New York, NY, USA), cautery, topical phenylephrine, and even thrombin 1000 IU/mL for hemostasis; may facilitate ophthalmic surgery.

ANATOMIC FACTORS

Although some of the more practically applicable nuances are discussed in the specific procedures and species, the reader is also referred to several texts[5,6,9,29–36] for further elaboration of anatomic variations as they relate to ophthalmic surgery in exotic pets. Generally, the surgeon should be aware and mindful of some important orbital vascular structures in some small mammal species that, especially given the small nature of these patients, increase the risk of significant blood loss and associated complications. In addition, variations in periocular/orbital glandular structures and their blood supplies may have implications in surgical procedures. Finally, for eyelid, ocular surface, and eye removal surgeries, the thin and usually less mobile nature of most exotic pets' skin, conjunctiva, and third eyelids, as well as the presence of less actual tissue, must be factored in to appropriate surgical planning for adequate wound closure.

POSTOPERATIVE MANAGEMENT

For best outcome after surgery, (self-inflicted) trauma to the site, which may delay or otherwise complicate healing, should be avoided. This is accomplished by ensuring a smooth recovery and placement of an Elizabethan collar if needed.

Discomfort should also be managed with appropriate (nonsteroidal) anti-inflammatory or opioid medications.[1]

Finally, any indicated medical therapy, monitoring, or follow-up should be pursued after surgery.

EYE REMOVAL SURGERY

Eye removal is the most common ophthalmic surgical procedure performed in exotic pets. Indications for this salvage procedure include irreversibly blind, painful eyes refractory to treatment or unable to be treated by reasonable or tolerated medical management. In exotic pets, this is often due to exophthalmos from orbital or retrobulbar disease (**Fig. 9**), especially associated with dental disease[5,34,35,37] or neoplasia,[38] both with secondary exposure corneal disease, or trauma. Other possible causes include corneal disease (**Fig. 10**A–C), especially perforated ulcers; full-thickness globe lacerations with extrusion of intraocular contents; chronic uveitis (**Fig. 10**D)[1]; otherwise inoperable eyelid[39] and intraocular[3,37,40–42] tumors; and primary or usually secondary glaucoma,[1,2,37] with buphthalmos and corneal disease.

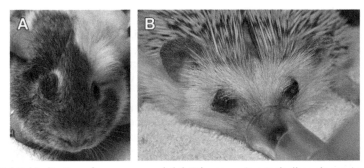

Fig. 9. Orbital indications for eye removal. (*A*) Odontogenic retrobulbar abscess in a guinea pig causing exophthalmos and exposure corneal dessication. (*B*) Bilateral corneal dessication due to exophthalmos of undetermined cause in a hedgehog.

ENUCLEATION

Enucleation is performed when disease is confined to the globe. Only the globe with short piece of optic nerve, third eyelid and associated glands, lid margins with meibomian glands as applicable, and conjunctiva with goblet cells are removed (remaining orbital contents are not). This procedure generally provides adequate tissue for appropriate histopathologic analysis. A space-filling orbital implant may be placed, and the cut eyelid margins are closed over the orbit, or rarely the eyelids are retained and an ocular prosthesis is designed and fitted.

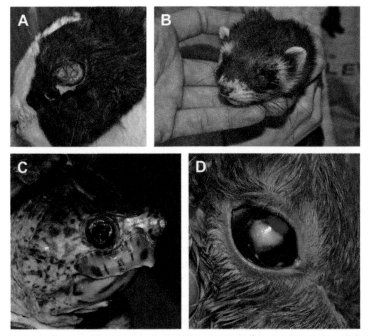

Fig. 10. Ocular indications for eye removal. (*A*) Corneal perforation and panophthalmitis in a rabbit. (*B*) Globe trauma with severe ocular surface damage in a ferret. (*C*) Corneal perforation in a razor-backed musk turtle (*Sternotherus carinatus*). (*D*) Phacoclastic uveitis secondary to infection with *Encephalitozoon cuniculi* in a rabbit.

EXENTERATION

Exenteration, which is removal of the globe and all orbital contents, is performed when there is extension of disease into the orbit or the orbital disease is the primary ophthalmic issue (retrobulbar abscess or severe infection, neoplasia). It is seldom safely possible in species with a prominent orbital venous plexus because of hemorrhage. As with enucleation, exenteration generally provides adequate tissue for appropriate histopathologic analysis. Orbital implants are usually contraindicated in these instances, although exceptions are possible.

EVISCERATION

Evisceration with intraocular implant placement is the removal of the intraocular contents (lens, vitreous, uveal tract, and retina) via a limbal or scleral incision and replacement inside the retained corneoscleral shell with a sterile silicone sphere. This procedure is usually performed on referral to improve cosmesis, in exotic species, particularly for exhibit or display animals,[1,2,43] by retaining a globe with normal eyelid function and ocular movement. Drawbacks to this surgery include reliance on a healthy ocular surface for success and minimizing risk of complication, incomplete removal of diseased tissue, providing less ideal tissue for histopathologic analysis and thus potentially impairing diagnosis, less immediate pain relief, greater risk with patient self-trauma in the postoperative healing period, and continued, possibly long-term, need for medical therapy. With these issues, this surgery is not indicated for common reasons for pursuit of eye removal in exotic pets, including orbital disease, infection, severe corneal disease, and intraocular or orbital neoplasia, although modified evisceration, leaving just the rigid scleral shell, may be appropriate particularly for birds and reptiles, as discussed later.

CONSIDERATIONS IN EXOTIC PETS

- Anatomic variations: Discussed generally earlier and more specifically later in discussion
- Infection: Infection is often the reason for damage and surgery in the first place. It can be difficult to manage medically and even surgically. If there is gross or other evidence of or concern for orbital or other residual infection, appropriate perioperative antibiotics should be administered and continued postoperatively as indicated by the surgical findings, culture and histopathology results, and patient response and complications.
- Blood loss: The small size of these patients and, in some, the presence of an orbital venous plexus/sinus make informed and careful surgery to best limit hemorrhage and achieve hemostasis a significant priority.
- Wound closure: With anesthesia more risky in exotic pets and a goal of most efficient surgery shortening anesthetic duration, as well as tissue limitations, the orbit is usually closed in only 1[38,42] to 2 layers.

ENUCLEATION PROCEDURE IN SMALL MAMMALS

Owing to concern for blood loss, subconjunctival enucleation, which prompts dissection closer to the globe, more likely avoiding larger vascular structures, is advocated instead of transpalpebral eye removal.[5]

Technique

- Administering anesthesia, patient preparation, and draping are done as described earlier. Place eyelid speculum and perform lateral canthotomy to facilitate maximal exposure (**Fig. 11**A): clamp the lateral canthus with a hemostat to aid in hemostasis, then cut up to ~5 mm of the preclamped canthus with Steven tenotomy scissors.

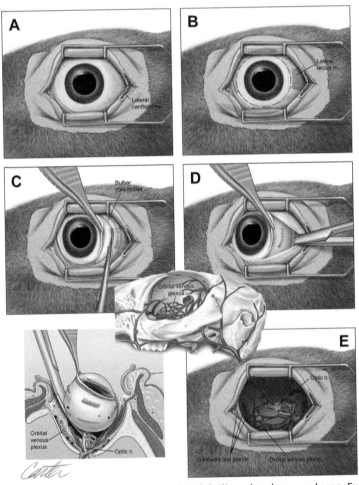

Fig. 11. Subconjunctival enucleation in a rabbit. (*A*) Clipped and prepped area. Eyelid speculum placed. Lateral canthotomy performed. (*B*) Bulbar conjunctival (peritomy) incision (*dashed line*) and underlying extraocular muscles. (*C*) Forceps grasp perilimbal bulbar conjunctiva and rotate globe to facilitate dissection and transection of extraocular muscles. (*D*) Surface and inset cross-sectional views showing optic nerve transection and proximity to the orbital venous plexus, which is not visualized intraoperatively but which the surgeon must be respect. Additional inset view of bony skull and orbit with venous vascular structures, most notably, the orbital venous plexus. (*E*) Orbit after globe removal with the eyelid margins and third eyelid still in place, showing the location and extent of the orbital venous plexus and its relationship with the third eyelid. (*Courtesy of* University of Georgia, Athens, GA. All rights reserved; with permission.)

- Grasping the bulbar conjunctiva a few millimeters posterior to the limbus with delicate Bishop-Harmon forceps, incise it (**Fig. 11B**) and sharply and bluntly deepen this dissection through the Tenon capsule to the level of the sclera with tenotomy scissors. Extend this dissection 360° around the globe with care to avoid undue traction on the globe and possible oculocardiac reflex or damage to the optic chiasm and contralateral optic nerve fibers, potentially blinding the other eye.
- Transect extraocular muscle attachments at their insertions on the globe (**Fig. 11C**). These attachments may not be identified or visualized in many small exotic pets because of their small size, but the globe should be freed from all significant attachments circumferentially.
- Clamp the optic nerve and associated vasculature first with a mosquito hemostat a few millimeters posterior to the globe if there is room in the orbit without excessive tension on the globe and nerve, then carefully transect above/superficial to this clamp or simply transect without clamping first, in this same location (**Fig. 11D; Fig. 12**). Do not incise the posterior eye wall, and remove the globe whole from the orbit, without leakage of ocular contents. As the globe is lifted from the orbit, transect any remaining tissue attachments.
- Hemostasis is generally achievable with several minutes of digital pressure through gauze sponges and, often, with placement of an absorbable gelatin sponge, which may be left in the orbit at closure.[42] Occasional suture ligation or cautery (although these are not possible and are ineffective for vascular plexuses/sinuses) or application of topical thrombin, rarely direct drip[44] or indirect via a soaked gelatin sponge, is indicated. If the orbital venous plexus/sinus is compromised, exsanguination may occur quickly, and prompt intervention, including direct pressure application for at least 5 minutes, is imperative.
- Remove the eyelid speculum, and excise full thickness the eyelid margins (~3 mm back), including canthal tissue, associated meibomian glands, and palpebral conjunctiva with Steven tenotomy scissors. Preclamping the planned incision line with hemostats may aid in hemostasis as will avoiding the angularis oculi vein near the superior medial canthus.[17,29]
- Owing to the secretory nature and potential for complications, including chronic discharge or drainage and/or cyst formation if left in the orbit, it is generally

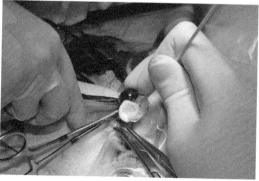

Fig. 12. Optic nerve transection on a rabbit during enucleation. Neither the optic nerve nor the very close underlying orbital venous plexus are visible.

recommended to remove the third eyelid and associated glands (which vary with species[5,34,37]) and conjunctiva. Before excision, clamp the third eyelid with mosquito hemostats across its base below the glands for improved exposure, more thorough removal, and reduced hemorrhage, as in rabbits, for example, the glands are intimately associated with and surrounded by the orbital venous plexus.[5,35] This procedure may be performed after partial wound closure to allow more rapid completion of surgery and hemostasis,[17] but bleeding may still be an issue difficult to control, and some surgeons admit likely incompletely removing the third eyelid and glands without known issues.

- If it can be identified and blood loss controlled, remove any remaining conjunctival fornix ring with tenotomy scissors.
- Hemostasis status, concern for infection, and surgeon preference dictate whether orbital flushing with saline pulsed from a syringe with or without suction is then used.
- Closure: In traditional larger veterinary patients, closure is usually in 3 layers: deep orbital, subcutaneous, and skin. In the interest of minimizing anesthesia time and risk, as well as because of less available tissue for closure, and some risk of reinciting hemorrhage, for enucleation/exenteration in small exotic pets, closure should be in 2 layers if possible:
  - Periorbital/deep fascial or usually the deepest subcutaneous tissue apposable without undue tension or gaps, with absorbable 4-0 to 6-0 simple continuous suture
  - Skin with nonabsorbable 4-0 to 6-0 simple interrupted, cruciate, or simple continuous suture (**Fig. 13**). If sutures are likely to be disturbed or disrupted by self-trauma, more common in mammals and especially rabbits,[5,17] and often difficult to limit or avoid, or sutures will not be able to be removed, absorbable 5-0 to 6-0 buried subcuticular sutures are indicated.[5]
- Always submit excised tissue for histopathology and culture and sensitivity if warranted.

Postoperative Care

Use of an Elizabethan collar is generally unnecessary but should be used as needed to prevent self-trauma to the orbit or surgical wound. If used, impact on patient stress, possibly with delayed healing, and impaired cecotrophy, important to digestive health in some species, should be monitored.

Pain management is critical, and systemic antibiotic therapy is indicated if there is evidence of or concern for orbital infection. Skin sutures, if placed, should be removed approximately 10 days postoperatively.

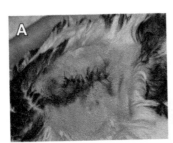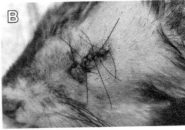

Fig. 13. Wound closure following enucleation in mammals. (A) Rabbit and (B) ferret, with simple interrupted skin sutures.

Postoperative Complications

Eyelid bruising and orbital swelling tends to peak at about 24 hours postoperatively. Over a couple of weeks postoperatively, overlying skin sinks into the orbit unless a space-filling orbital implant was placed (generally not performed in exotic pets, as it is purely cosmetic and increases risk of complication) before closure.

Potential complications include hemorrhage, infection, and wound healing issues or dehiscence. Persistence of underlying orbital, dental, or systemic disease may be encountered, if incomplete tissue removal was performed or the ophthalmic issue was just a symptom of another disease process that has not been addressed or resolved. If there is a return of swelling or drainage once postoperative changes have subsided, infection, suture reaction, retained secretory tissue possibly with cyst formation, retained neoplastic tissue, or seroma should be suspected and addressed as indicated. Other less common complications include orbital emphysema via persistently patent nasolacrimal duct and contralateral blindness.

Mammalian Enucleation: Species-Specific Nuances

A retrobulbar or posterior orbital venous plexus/sinus and associated risk of significant hemorrhage at surgery is present in rabbits (see **Fig. 11**D [inset]), extending from the globe equator to the posterior pole and intimately associated with the deep (harderian) gland of the third eyelid[5,17,29,34,35] (**Fig. 11**E); ferrets[9,34,44,45]; mice[9,29,46,47]; rats, although some texts show none,[29] others claim its smaller[9] presence in this species,[34,46,47] and regardless, with small patient size, blood loss is a concern; hamsters and chinchillas[9,46]; gerbils[9]; and guinea pigs.[46,48]

AVIAN EYE REMOVAL
Additional Considerations in Avian Patients

- Globe volume and weight: The relative proportion of the eye volume and weight within the skull to that of the head and even body of birds is high, so implications (eg, imbalance and effect on flying, catching food) of surgery to remove the eye may affect surgical technique.[18,30,34,49]
- Globe rigidity: Owing to the presence of scleral ossicles in a ring just posterior to the limbus, as well as more posterior scleral cartilage, the avian eye is inflexible. The tight fit of this unyielding globe in the orbit makes extraocular dissection while avoiding traction on the optic nerve and chiasm even more challenging in birds than in small mammals.[30,31,49]
- Proximity to the thin interorbital bony septum and thus the other eye: Care must be taken during any medial dissection.[17]
- Proximity to infraorbital diverticulum of the infraorbital sinus: The closeness of the globe to this structure mainly results in clinical signs of ophthalmic disease with sinus issues, but the surgeon should also be cognizant of and cautious because of this anatomy.[30,34]
- Blood loss: Even in the general category of exotic pets, low-volume blood loss is tolerated in birds. Careful surgery and prompt and effective hemostasis with the various options previously discussed as readily available are recommended.

The shape of the avian globe varies across species prompting different eye removal techniques. Owls have tubular eyes,[30] and transaural enucleation is an option recommended to remove the globe intact in these species.[34,50] Because they are generally not kept as pets, and this surgery is uncommonly performed in lieu of the other options discussed later, the reader is referred elsewhere for discussion of this surgery. Hawks and eagles have globular eyes. Commonly, the avian eye is flattened anteroposteriorly with a hemispherical posterior segment, as seen in psittaciformes and passerines.[30] The following 2 eye removal techniques are reasonable for any avian species.

ENUCLEATION: GLOBE COLLAPSING PROCEDURE

Globe collapsing enucleation removes the entire globe via enhanced visualization but distorts it in a manner that may affect histopathologic analysis.[17,31,50]

Technique

- Administration of anesthesia, patient preparation, and draping are done as described earlier.
- Place eyelid speculum and perform extended lateral canthotomy to facilitate maximal exposure (**Fig. 14**A): clamp the lateral canthus with a hemostat to aid in hemostasis; then, with tenotomy scissors or a scalpel, incise the preclamped

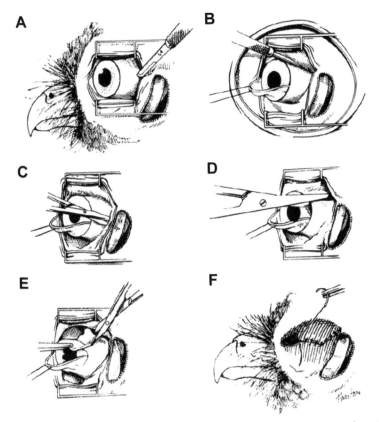

Fig. 14. Avian globe collapsing enucleation. (*A*) Eyelid speculum placed. Lateral canthotomy performed. (*B*) The peripheral cornea has been incised and is retracted inferiorly by a stay suture. Bulbar conjunctiva is incised down to the sclera circumferentially. (*C*) Extraocular muscles are transected during dissection. (*D*) The sclera is incised full thickness perpendicular to the limbus. (*E*) The cut edges of the sclera are folded in on each other. The optic nerve is transected. (*F*) Wound closure is routine. (*From* Murphy CJ, Brooks DE, Kern TJ, et al. Enucleation in birds of prey. J Am Vet Med Assoc 1983;183:1236; with permission.)

canthus and extend the incision superior-temporally up to as far as the anterior auricular margin.
- Incise full thickness approximately 180° of the superior-temporal peripheral cornea with scalpel and Westcott tenotomy scissors.
- Place a full-thickness corneal stay suture with 5-0 or 6-0 suture to improve ability to manipulate the globe and this corneal flap during surgery (**Fig. 14B**).
- Incise the thin bulbar conjunctiva and periorbital fascia a few millimeters back from the limbus down to the external sclera and extend this incision 360° with tenotomy scissors. Transect extraocular muscles at their insertions on the globe if and as they are encountered (**Fig. 14C**).
- Undermine the area deep to the anterior auricular skin incision to increase lateral and posterior globe exposure if and as needed.
- Superior-temporally, in a radial direction/perpendicular to the limbus and sparing/external to the uveal tract, cut the sclera/scleral ossicles full thickness with tenotomy or Metzenbaum scissors (**Fig. 14D**). With forceps facilitating it, this allows the now freed edges of sclera to be folded in on each other, collapsing the globe and improving exposure of its posterior aspect laterally (**Fig. 14E**) without undue traction on the globe and optic nerve. This approach also limits dissection medial to the globe whereby the fragile interorbital bony septum may be damaged.
- With improved visualization through globe collapse, clamp or ligate then transect the optic nerve and associated vasculature, along with any remaining tissue attachments, as described earlier, with particular preparedness for the potential for oculocardiac reflex bradycardia.
- Hemostasis is achieved as described earlier in mammals.
- Remove the speculum and excise the eyelid margins (without concern for meibomian glands, which are lacking in birds[30]), third eyelid, and conjunctiva as described earlier in subconjunctival enucleation in mammals.
- Wound closure (**Fig. 14F**) is accomplished in 2 layers with 4-0 to 7-0 suture varying with the patient size, but otherwise as described earlier, with birds less likely to disturb skin sutures than mammals.[17]
- Postoperative management and potential complications are as described earlier in mammals.

OCULAR EVISCERATION

The modified evisceration procedure for eye removal reduces the disfigurement and imbalance issues, which occur after removal of the entire globe in birds.[18,34,51,52] The sclera and its ossicles and cartilage and, in some cases, the third eyelid[18] remain. By definition, this procedure does not remove all ocular tissues and thus is not recommended in cases of known or suspected ocular/orbital infection or neoplasia and regardless has negative implications for most thorough histologic analysis of excised tissue. Owing to limited extraocular dissection, it protects the optic nerve and chiasm, interorbital bony septum, and infraorbital sinus, and reduces risk of hemorrhage, as well as is easier, shortening anesthesia time and decreasing risk, and possibly less painful.[51]

Technique

- Administration of anesthesia, patient preparation, and draping are done as described earlier.
- Place eyelid speculum (**Fig. 15A**).

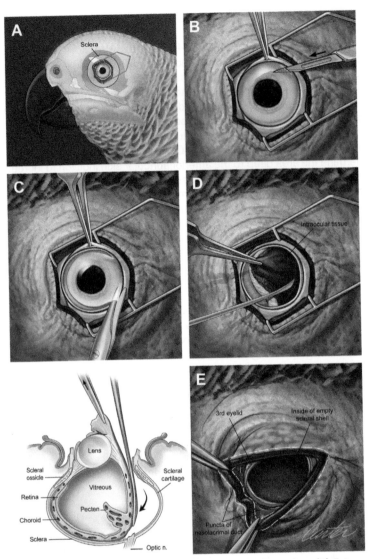

Fig. 15. African gray parrot (*Psittacus erithacus*) modified evisceration. (*A*) External surface overlying anatomic view of bony skull for orientation. Eyelid speculum placed. (*B*) Globe stabilized by forceps. Peripheral cornea penetrated full thickness with #6500 Beaver blade. (*C*) Incision extended circumferentially and cornea removed. (*D*) Surface and inset cross-sectional views: The intraocular contents are eviscerated from the sclera with forceps and lens loupe. (*E*) Speculum removed and eyelid margins excised (*dashed white line*) with care to preserve the nasolacrimal puncta. (*Courtesy of* University of Georgia, Athens, GA. All rights reserved; with permission.)

- Incise full thickness the peripheral cornea circumferentially with scalpel and Westcott tenotomy scissors (**Fig. 15**B, C) and remove it to de-roof the eye.
- Remove the iris, lens, vitreous, posterior uveal tract including pectin, and retina (via gentle traction and peeling with delicate forceps and a lens loupe or

cyclodialysis spatula) from the scleral shell (**Fig. 15D**), which along with the optic nerve, is left in the orbit.

- Use direct pressure with cotton-tipped applicators or cellulose spears for hemostasis and visualization to ensure all intraocular tissue is removed, leaving just the whitish sclera. Absorbable gelatin sponge material may then also be used to pack and remain in the scleral shell cup for continued hemostasis during and after surgery.
- Remove the speculum and excise the eyelid margins (**Fig. 15E**), third eyelid, and conjunctiva as described earlier. Alternatively, leave the third eyelid and conjunctiva in place and excise just the eyelid margins, with care taken to retain their superior and inferior nasolacrimal puncta near the medial canthus, to allow drainage of continued lacrimal secretions.[18]
- Close the incision wound in 1 to 2 layers as described earlier (**Fig. 16**).
- Postoperative management and potential complications are as described earlier.

REPTILE EYE REMOVAL

In reptiles with some eyelid structure, including chelonians, crocodilians, and most lizards, enucleation may be performed in a manner similar to that in exotic pet

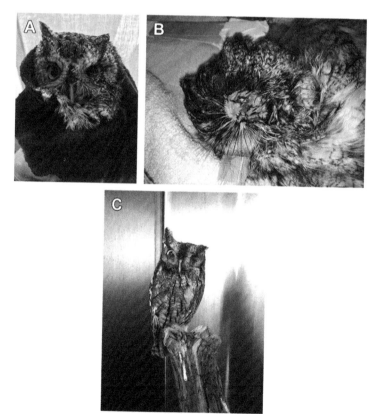

Fig. 16. Eastern screech owl (*Megascops asio*) presented for left eye removal for refractory traumatic uveitis. (*A*) Preoperative photograph with blepharospasm indicating ocular pain. (*B*) Intraoperative photograph of skin wound closure. (*C*) Postoperative photograph of the owl perching normally with no signs of discomfort or distress and good cosmetic outcome after modified evisceration. (*Courtesy of* Four Lakes Wildlife Center, Madison, WI.)

mammals or via the globe collapsing procedure. The modified evisceration technique as described in birds is also reasonable for eye removal surgery in reptiles. This procedure leaves behind a rigid sclera because of the presence of posterior cartilage and therefore somewhat decreases orbital sinking postoperatively, as compared with that with enucleation. Because of tissue limitations, closure with 4-0 to 7-0 suture varying with the patient size is generally in 1 layer, with skin apposed to slightly everted, as it may invert with healing, and this compensation reduces risk of dysecdysis complications in the future.[4,8,38] As with birds, reptiles are less likely to disturb skin sutures than mammals.[4]

In other reptiles, including snakes, with fused eyelids forming the precorneal spectacle, the entire globe with the spectacle is removed in a manner similar to that in mammals, but the wound is not closed. Instead, with topical antibiotic administration, it is allowed to granulate over 4 to 6 weeks.[8,32] Given this, the surgeon needs to thoroughly consider the indications for eye removal, as if there is no infection, drainage, or otherwise bother to the patient or client, the ultimate outcome may be as good as surgery with less morbidity (**Fig. 17**).

AMPHIBIAN EYE REMOVAL

Careful consideration before enucleation in amphibians is warranted because of the importance of the globe in swallowing, and some veterinarians advocate against this surgery.[34] In these species, a powerful retractor bulbi muscle pulls the globe back in the orbit and into the pharynx, which is separated from the eye by only a thin membrane.[33] This process helps to generate intraoral pressure and facilitate swallowing. If enucleation is pursued as in mammals or via a globe-collapsing procedure as in birds, care must be taken to avoid damage to this thin buccal-orbital membrane. Eyelid margins may be removed and the wound closed as described earlier; in species without eyelids, wound closure is not attempted, and the area is left to granulate, as in snakes. Topical and systemic antibiotics are administered during the healing process.[6] Modified evisceration and evisceration with intraocular implant placement have not been described in amphibians.

FISH EYE REMOVAL

Consideration of patient welfare and risk-benefit analysis dictates that enucleation is not commonly performed in fish.[3,7,34] When pursued, the periocular skin attaching the eye to the orbital rim is incised, allowing globe exposure. Muscles and the optic nerve

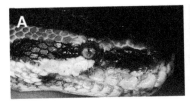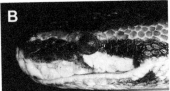

Fig. 17. Snake presented for bilateral enucleation 3 months after overzealous spectacle removal by the referring veterinarian left both eyes with exposed iris and lens. By that time, although the snake had experienced transient discomfort evident through behavior change, it had completed the healing process, granulating and scarring in both scleral cups, one with seeming, although opaque, spectacle regeneration and consistent light perception. (*A*) Phthisical right eye and (*B*) light perceiving left eye. Although ocular components generally removed at surgery were retained in this case, there were no complications, and further surgery was not indicated to try to improve on this outcome.

are transected with care to avoid cranial nerve VII (maxillary and buccal) and V (mandibular) branches that run along the inferior-lateral orbital margin. Hemostasis is achieved via direct pressure, application of a drop of phenylephrine or epinephrine or collagen powder, and/or cautery. The wound is then left open or may be packed with a waterproof methylcellulose, pectin, and gelatin paste. Parenteral antibiotic administration is recommended for about 10 days. Postoperative survival is often affected by blood loss and/or undetected underlying systemic disease, so again, risk and prognosis should be analyzed before pursuit of surgery. Although purely cosmetic, ocular prosthetic placement after exenteration in a display fish has been reported[53]; such is usually not indicated or elected in pets, especially given ultimately poor retention.

ACKNOWLEDGMENTS

The authors thank guest editor Dr Christoph Mans and Drs Kathern Myrna, Joerg Mayer, and David Williams for support, collaboration, and photographs; Drs Silvia Pryor and Isabelle Desprez for assistance with literature search and reference collection; and Kip Carter for design and creation of medical illustrations.

REFERENCES

1. Millichamp NJ. Ophthalmic disease in exotic species. Vet Clin North Am Exot Anim Pract 2002;5:223.
2. Millichamp NJ. Management of ocular disease in exotic species. Semin Avian Exot Pet 1997;6:152–9.
3. Wildgoose WH. Impress your fish clients: enucleation. North American Veterinary Conference: Small Animal and Exotics 2007;1448.
4. Mader DR, Bennett RA, Funk RS, et al. Surgery. In: Mader DR, editor. Reptile medicine and surgery. 2nd edition. St Louis (MO): Saunders Elsevier; 2006. p. 581–630.
5. Harcourt-Brown F. Textbook of rabbit medicine. Oxford (United Kingdom): Butterworth-Heinemann; 2002.
6. Wright KM. Surgical techniques. In: Whitaker BR, Wright KM, editors. Amphibian medicine and captive husbandry. 2nd edition. Malabar (FL): Krieger Pub. Co; 2001. p. 273–83.
7. Jurk I. Ophthalmic disease of fish. Vet Clin North Am Exot Anim Pract 2002;5: 243–60.
8. Alworth LC, Hernandez SM, Divers SJ. Laboratory reptile surgery: principles and techniques. J Am Assoc Lab Anim Sci 2011;50:11–26.
9. Williams DL, Gum GG. Laboratory animal ophthalmology. In: Gelatt KN, Gilger BC, Kern TJ, editors. Veterinary ophthalmology. 5th edition. Ames (IA): Wiley-Blackwell; 2013. p. 1692–724.
10. Myrna KE, Bentley E, Smith LJ. Effectiveness of injection of local anesthetic into the retrobulbar space for postoperative analgesia following eye enucleation in dogs. J Am Vet Med Assoc 2010;237:174–7.
11. Pollock PJ, Russell T, Hughes TK, et al. Transpalpebral eye enucleation in 40 standing horses. Vet Surg 2008;37:306–9.
12. Pollock PJ. How to perform a standing enucleation in the horse. Companion Animal 2012;17:4–7.
13. Hazra S, Palui H, Biswas B, et al. Anesthesia for intraocular surgery in rabbits. Scand J Lab Anim Sci 2011;38:81–7.

14. Regnier A. Clinical pharmacology and therapeutics. In: Gelatt KN, Gilger BC, Kern TJ, editors. Veterinary ophthalmology. 5th edition. Ames (IA): Wiley-Blackwell; 2013. p. 351–434.

15. Turner Giannico A, de Sampaio MOB, Lima L, et al. Characterization of the oculocardiac reflex during compression of the globe in Beagle dogs and rabbits. Vet Ophthalmol 2014;17:321–7.

16. Gum GG, MacKay EO. Physiology of the eye. In: Gelatt KN, Gilger BC, Kern TJ, editors. Veterinary ophthalmology. 5th edition. Ames (IA): Wiley-Blackwell; 2013. p. 171–207.

17. Holmberg BJ. Topics in medicine and surgery: enucleation of exotic pets. Journal of Exotic Pet Medicine Special Issue: Ophthalmology 2007;16:88–94.

18. Murray M, Pizzirani S, Tseng F. A technique for evisceration as an alternative to enucleation in birds of prey: 19 cases. J Avian Med Surg 2013;27:120–7.

19. Spiess BM, Pot SA. Diseases and surgery of the canine orbit. In: Gelatt KN, Gilger BC, Kern TJ, editors. Veterinary ophthalmology. 5th edition. Ames (IA): Wiley-Blackwell; 2013. p. 793–831.

20. Gelatt KN. The operating room. In: Gelatt KN, Gelatt JP, editors. Veterinary ophthalmic surgery. Oxford (United Kingdom): Elsevier/Saunders; 2011. p. 18–35.

21. Polak BCP. Drugs used in ocular treatment. Side Effects Drugs Annu 1985;9: 415–7.

22. Bistner SI, Batik G, Aguirre G. Atlas of veterinary ophthalmic surgery. Philadelphia: W. B. Saunders Co; 1977.

23. Klauss G. Topical review: ophthalmic surgical instruments. Clinical Techniques in Small Animal Practice Canine Ophthalmology 2008;23:3–9.

24. Troutman RC, Cantarella V. Microsurgery of the anterior segment of the eye: introduction and basic techniques. St Louis (MO): Mosby; 1974.

25. Schmiedt CW. Suture material, tissue staplers, ligation devices, and closure methods. In: Tobias KM, Johnston SA, editors. Veterinary surgery: small animal. St Louis (MO): Elsevier Saunders; 2012. p. 187–203.

26. Fossum TW. Biomaterials, suturing and hemostasis. In: Fossum TW, editor. Small animal surgery. 3rd edition. St Louis (MO): Mosby/Elsevier; 2007. p. 57–78.

27. Boothe HW. Suture material, tissue adhesives, staplers, and ligating clips. In: Slatter DH, editor. Textbook of small animal surgery. 3rd edition. Philadelphia: Saunders; 2003. p. 235–44.

28. Stades FC, van der Woerdt A. Diseases and surgery of the canine eyelid. In: Gelatt KN, Gilger BC, Kern TJ, editors. Veterinary ophthalmology. 5th edition. Ames (IA): Wiley-Blackwell; 2013. p. 832–93.

29. Popesko P, Rajtová V, Horák J. A colour atlas of the anatomy of small laboratory animals: volume one: rabbit, guinea pig; volume two: rat, mouse, hamster. London: Wolfe Pub; 1992.

30. Williams DL. Ophthalmology. In: Ritchie BW, Harrison GJ, Harrison LR, editors. Avian medicine: principles and application. Lake Worth (FL): Wingers Publishing, Inc; 1994. p. 673–94.

31. Bennett RA, Harrison GJ. Soft tissue surgery. In: Ritchie BW, Harrison GJ, Harrison LR, editors. Avian medicine: principles and application. Lake Worth (FL): Wingers Publishing, Inc; 1994. p. 1096–136.

32. Lawton MPC. Reptilian ophthalmology. In: Mader DR, editor. Reptile medicine and surgery. 2nd edition. St Louis (MO): Saunders Elsevier; 2006. p. 323–42.

33. Whitaker BR. The amphibian eye. In: Wright KM, Whitaker BR, editors. Amphibian medicine and captive husbandry. Malabar (FL): Krieger Pub. Co; 2001. p. 245–52. Original edition.

34. Williams DL. Ophthalmology of exotic pets. Chichester (United Kingdom): John Wiley & Sons; 2012.
35. Williams DL. The rabbit. In: Gelatt KN, Gilger BC, Kern TJ, editors. Veterinary ophthalmology. 5th edition. Ames (IA): Wiley-Blackwell; 2013. p. 1725–49.
36. Kern TJ, Colitz CMH. Exotic animal ophthalmology. In: Gelatt KN, Gilger BC, Kern TJ, editors. Veterinary ophthalmology. 5th edition. Ames (IA): Wiley-Blackwell; 2013. p. 1750–819.
37. van der Woerdt A. Ophthalmologic diseases in small pet mammals. In: Queensberry K, editor. Ferrets, rabbits and rodents: clinical medicine and surgery. 3rd edition. St Louis (MO): Elsevier Saunders; 2012. p. 523–31.
38. Darrow BG, Johnstone McLean NS, Russman SE, et al. Periorbital adenocarcinoma in a bearded dragon (Pogona vitticeps). Vet Ophthalmol 2013;16:177–82.
39. Hannon DE, Garner MM, Reavill DR. Squamous cell carcinoma in inland bearded dragons (Pogona vitticeps). J Herpetol Med Surg 2011;21:101–6.
40. McPherson L, Newman SJ, McLean N, et al. Intraocular sarcomas in two rabbits. J Vet Diagn Invest 2009;21:547–51.
41. Dickinson R, Bauer B, Gardhouse S, et al. Intraocular sarcoma associated with a rupture lens in a rabbit (Oryctolagus cuniculus). Vet Ophthalmol 2013;16:168–72.
42. Lima L, Montiani-Ferreira F, Sousa R, et al. Intraocular signet-ring cell melanoma in a hamster (Cricetulus griseus). Vet Ophthalmol 2012;15:53–8.
43. Sandemeyer LS, Breaux CB, McRuer DL, et al. Topics in medicine and surgery: case report: a new technique for intraocular prosthesis implantation in a great horned owl (Bubo virginianus). Journal of Exotic Pet Medicine Special Issue: Ophthalmology 2007;16:95–100.
44. Miller PE. Ferret ophthalmology. Semin Avian Exot Pet 1997;6:146.
45. Good KL. Ocular disorders of pet ferrets. Vet Clin North Am Exot Anim Pract 2002;5:325–39.
46. Washington IM, Van Hoosier G. Clinical biochemistry and hematology. In: Suckow MA, Stevens KA, Wilson RP, editors. The laboratory rabbit, guinea pig, hamster, and other rodents. Oxford (United Kingdom): Academic Press; 2012. p. 57–116.
47. Beaumont SL. Ocular disorders of pet mice and rats. Vet Clin North Am Exot Anim Pract 2002;5:311–24.
48. Clemons DJ, Seeman J, Terril LA. The laboratory guinea pig. 2nd edition. Boca Raton (FL): CRC Press; 2011.
49. Jones MP, Pierce KE, Ward D. Topics in medicine and surgery: avian vision: a review of form and function with special consideration to birds of prey. Journal of Exotic Pet Medicine Special Issue: Ophthalmology 2007;16:69–87.
50. Murphy CJ, Brooks DE, Kern TJ, et al. Enucleation in birds of prey. J Am Vet Med Assoc 1983;183:1234–7.
51. Dees DD, Knollinger AM, MacLaren NE. Modified evisceration technique in a golden eagle (Aquila chrysaetos). Vet Ophthalmol 2011;14:341–4.
52. Gelatt KN, Whitley RD. Surgery of the orbit. In: Gelatt KN, Gelatt JP, editors. Veterinary ophthalmic surgery. Oxford (United Kingdom): Elsevier/Saunders; 2011. p. 51–88.
53. Nadelstein B, Lewbart GA, Bakal R. Orbital exenteration and placement of a prosthesis in fish. J Am Vet Med Assoc 1997;211:603–6.

Exotic Mammal Laparoscopy

Izidora Sladakovic, BVSc (Hons I), MVS,
Stephen J. Divers, BVetMed, DZooMed, DECZM (Herpetology),
DECZM (Zoo Health Management), DACZM, FRCVS*

KEYWORDS

- Laparoscopy • Minimally invasive surgery • Endosurgery
- Laparoscopic instrumentation • Exotic mammal • Zoologic medicine

KEY POINTS

- Laparoscopy offers many advantages over traditional laparotomy and is considered a standard of care in human medicine.
- Laparoscopy is widely used in domestic animals and is a rapidly evolving field, but literature in exotic mammals is in the early stages.
- Organ biopsy and ovariectomy techniques have been described in exotic mammals.
- Advances in technology and instrumentation are creating opportunities to perform novel laparoscopic procedures in exotic mammals.

INTRODUCTION

Laparoscopy is considered a standard of care for many abdominal procedures in humans and is a rapidly evolving field in veterinary medicine, with advances in instrumentation and technology allowing increasing availability of laparoscopic procedures to veterinary patients. Indeed, minimally invasive surgery is now a required part of the American College of Veterinary Surgeons residency training programs. Laparoscopy offers many advantages over traditional laparotomy, including less tissue trauma, less pain, faster recovery times and return to normal function, and with experience, shorter surgery and anesthesia times. In contrast to elective surgical procedures of the abdomen performed using a traditional laparotomy approach through a small incision, a laparoscopic approach provides superior visualization of the abdominal cavity.

There is an increased interest in using laparoscopy in exotic mammals, zoo mammals, and free-ranging wildlife.[1] In zoo and free-ranging mammals, use of laparoscopy

The authors have nothing to disclose.
Department of Small Animal Medicine and Surgery (Zoological Medicine), University of Georgia College of Veterinary Medicine, 2200 College Station Road, Athens, GA 30602, USA
* Corresponding author.
E-mail address: sdivers@uga.edu

has been described in various species, most often performed for reproductive reasons.[2–12] Using minimally invasive laparoscopic techniques in zoo animals reduces the need for prolonged confinement, the possibility of wound dehiscence, and therefore, the need for repeat immobilizations. Likewise, in free-ranging wildlife, the option of confinement, monitoring, and repeat immobilization is often not available.

Exotic pet clinicians are increasingly required to provide the same level of high-quality care available for domestic pets, which includes minimally invasive surgery. Diagnostic endoscopy and endosurgery have already shown promise and are used widely by the authors in exotic mammals.[13,14] There is currently a paucity of published literature on the use of laparoscopy in exotic pet medicine. However, with the increasing availability of pediatric laparoscopic instruments, this will likely change in the future. In fact, rodents are used as models for development of surgical techniques in humans, including pediatric laparoscopic techniques.[15–18]

There is a steep learning curve in laparoscopy for inexperienced surgeons. Lack of tactile feedback from the long surgical instruments resulting in inappropriate tissue handling and altered depth perception displayed on a 2-dimensional monitor results in longer surgical times and more complications in inexperienced surgeons. For these reasons, it is important that appropriate training is sought for laparoscopic procedures.

The purpose of this article is to review instrumentation required for laparoscopy, patient selection and preparation, and laparoscopic approaches. This review is followed by a description of common laparoscopic techniques with a review of recent developments in exotic mammal laparoscopy. For a more extensive discussion on laparoscopic techniques in domestic animals, the reader is referred to dedicated laparoscopy resources.[19]

INDICATIONS AND CONTRAINDICATIONS

Indications for laparoscopy include organ biopsies under the magnification of a telescope, which can often provide a better view of pathologic abnormality, allowing for more accurate biopsies. Other indications of laparoscopy include laparoscopic surgeries, such as ovariectomy, adrenalectomy, splenectomy, liver lobectomy, and abdominal exploration.

Contraindications for laparoscopy include anesthetic contraindications, inability to intubate and ventilate (the exception to this may be when lift laparoscopy is used), lack of appropriate instrumentation, and presence of diaphragmatic defects. Obesity and abdominal adhesions can also create challenges. Lack of surgeon experience can be a contraindication. Using a predetermined time limit before conversion to traditional laparotomy and seeking appropriate training are strongly recommended and will reduce patient compromise.

INSTRUMENTATION

With a wide range of patient sizes and procedures that may be performed, there is a wide range of available instrumentation (**Table 1**), including

- Visualization and documentation devices
- Telescopes/endoscopes and operating sheaths
- Flexible instruments
- Trocars and cannulas
- Rigid instruments and handles
- Insufflation devices
- Coagulation devices

Table 1
Laparoscopic instrumentation for exotic mammals

Equipment Description	Primary Indications
Visualization & documentation	
Endovideo camera and monitor Xenon light source and light guide cable Digital capture device (eg, AIDA-Vet)	Required for all endoscopy procedures
Endoscopes	
1.9 mm × 18.5 cm telescope, 30° oblique, with integrated 3.3 mm operating sheath	Laparoscopy in animals <1 kg
2.7 mm × 18 cm telescope, 30° oblique 4.8 mm operating sheath	Laparoscopy in animals 1–10 kg
5 mm × 29 cm telescope 0°	Laparoscopy in animals >10 kg
Flexible instruments for use with operating sheaths	
Biopsy forceps Grasping forceps	1 mm instruments
34 cm biopsy forceps 34 cm single-action scissors Remote injection needle 34 cm grasping/retrieval forceps 60 cm wire basket retrieval Needle end radiosurgery electrode	1.7 mm instruments
Insufflation	
CO_2 insufflator with silicone tubing	Used for insufflation during laparoscopy
Rigid instruments, handles and cannulae for multiple-entry laparoscopy and thoracoscopy	
Cannulae	Available in 2.5, 3.5, 3.9 (graphite and plastic) and 6 mm (metal)
Reddick-Olsen dissecting forceps Metzenbaum scissors Babcock forceps	2 mm instruments
Fenestrated grasping forceps Metzenbaum scissors Reddick-Olsen dissecting and grasping forceps Short curved Kelly dissecting and grasping forceps Atraumatic dissecting and grasping forceps Babcock forceps Blakesley dissecting and biopsy forceps Scissors with serrated curved double action jaws Micro hook scissors, single action jaws Mahnes bipolar coagulation forceps Irrigation and suction cannula Palpation probe with cm markings Distendable palpation probe Ultramicro needle holder Knot-tier for extracorporeal suturing	3, 5 and 10 mm instruments
Handles (accept 2, 3 and 5 mm instruments)	Plastic or metal Mahnes-style or haemostat-style racket
Radiosurgery equipment	
3.8 or 4.0 MHz dual radiofrequency unit with foot pedal Monopolar lead to connect to plastic instrument handles Bipolar lead to connect to 3 mm Mahnes bipolar coagulation forceps	Enables endoscopic instruments to be used as monopolar devices and facilitates bipolar coagulation
LigaSure Atlas	Available in 5 mm and 10 mm

Telescopes are used to provide visualization within the abdominal cavity and come in a range of sizes. The most versatile telescope for exotic mammals less than 10 kg is the 2.7 mm × 18 cm, 0° or 30° oblique, which is a common device found in most exotic animal practices. For single-entry laparoscopy of animals less than 10 kg, this telescope can be housed within a 4.8-mm operating sheath, which includes ports for gas insufflation and an operating channel for introduction of 1.7-mm (5-Fr) flexible instruments. For multiple port laparoscopy of animals 1 to 10 kg, it can be housed within a 3.5-mm operating sheath, which can be introduced through a 3.9-mm cannula. A 1.9-mm integrated telescope is very useful for smaller species less than 1 kg and allows for the introduction of 1-mm flexible instruments; however, the range of 1-mm flexible instruments is limited. For larger animals of 10 to 300 kg, a 5-mm telescope is used, whereas telescopes 10 mm or larger may be preferred for even larger mammals.

Additional access ports are required for the introduction of instruments that are unable to be placed through the operating channel of a sheath and for the introduction of multiple instruments required for laparoscopic surgeries. Additional ports are created using a trocar within a cannula (**Fig. 1**). Cannulas come in different sizes, including 2.5 (for 2-mm rigid instruments), 3.5 (for 3-mm rigid instruments), 3.9 (for a 3.5-mm operating sheath), and 6 mm (for 5-mm instruments). In general, the larger the instrument size, the wider the instrument selection. Cannulas can be constructed of surgical steel

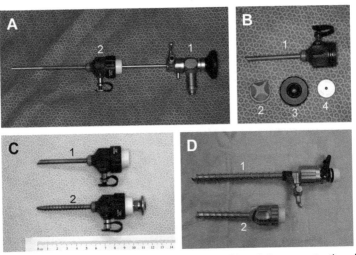

Fig. 1. Cannulas and trocars. (A) A 2.7-mm telescope within a 3.5-mm protection sheath (1) inserted through a 3.9 mm × 10 cm graphite/plastic cannula with insufflation side port (2). (B) A 3.9 mm × 10 cm graphite/plastic cannula disassembled to illustrate the graphite cannula (1), leaflet valve (2), screw cap (3), and instrument seal (4). (C) A 3.9 mm × 10 cm graphite/plastic cannula with insufflation side port (1), and 3.5 mm × 10 cm threaded cannula with insufflation side port and trocar inserted (2). The 3.9-mm cannula can accommodate the 2.7-mm telescope housed in a 3.5-mm protection sheath, while the 3.5-mm cannula can accommodate 3-mm instruments, and thanks to the threaded design, resists dislodgement in small exotic species. (D) Ternamian Endotip cannulas: 6 mm × 15 cm with insufflation side port and multifunctional valve (1), and 6 mm × 10.5 cm cannula with silicone leaflet valve (2). These metal cannulas are far heavier and best restricted to animals greater than 10 kg. (*Courtesy of* The University of Georgia; with permission. Copyright © 2015. All rights reserved.)

or graphite/plastic, with the latter being more suitable for smaller exotic pets because of their light weight.

The laparoscopic surgical pack will depend on the procedure planned and the size of the patient. In general, the authors recommend the following:

- A 1.9-mm telescope with 2.5-mm cannulas and 2-mm rigid instruments for animals weighing less than 1 kg;
- A 2.7-mm telescope system with 3.5-mm or 3.9-mm cannulas, and 3-mm rigid instruments (**Fig. 2**) for animals weighing between 1 and 10 kg;
- A 5-mm telescope with 6-mm cannulas and 5-mm rigid instruments for animals weighing more than 10 kg.

The rigid instruments have a standard attachment that can be used for a range of handles (**Fig. 3**). The handles are of plastic or metal construction and come with different features, including different styles of racket and a radiosurgical connection, allowing instruments to be used as monopolar devices.

When performing laparoscopic surgery, hemostasis is essential. In addition to the use of monopolar radiosurgery mentioned above, bipolar radiosurgery can be used with the use of 3-mm or 5-mm Mahnes bipolar coagulation forceps and is recommended for more vascular tissue. In larger patients wherein 6-mm cannulas or larger are used, the Ligasure Atlas system can be used for coagulation and cutting (**Fig. 4**).

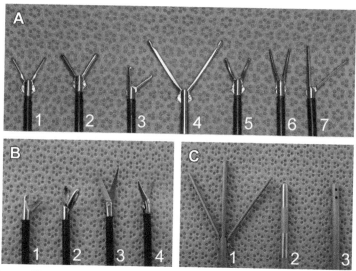

Fig. 2. Three-millimeter instruments. (*A*) Forceps: fenestrated atraumatic grasping forceps (*1*), Reddick-Olsen dissecting forceps (*2*), small Babcock forceps (*3*), large Babcock forceps (*4*), short curved Kelly dissecting and grasping forceps (*5*), long curved Kelly dissecting and grasping forceps (*6*), atraumatic dissecting and grasping forceps with single-action jaws (*7*). (*B*) Scissors and biopsy instruments: microhook scissors with single-action jaws (*1*), Blakesley dissecting and biopsy forceps (*2*), scissors with long sharp curved double action jaws (*3*), scissors with serrated curved double action jaws (*4*). (*C*) Probes: distendable palpation probe (*1*), palpation probe with centimeter markings (*2*), irrigation and suction cannula (*3*). These instruments are also available in 5 mm. (*Courtesy of* The University of Georgia; with permission. Copyright © 2015. All rights reserved.)

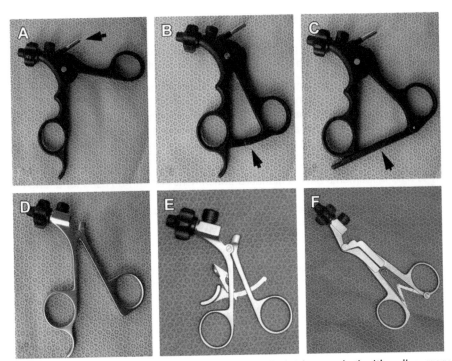

Fig. 3. Endoscopy instrument handles. (*A*) Plastic handle (without racket) with radiosurgery connector (*arrow*). (*B*) Plastic handle with hemostat-style racket (*arrow*). (*C*) Plastic handle with Mahnes-style racket (*arrow*). (*D*) Metal handle without racket or radiosurgery connection. (*E*) Metal handle with disengageable racket but no radiosurgical connection. (*F*) Metal Y-handle with spring action. (*Courtesy of* The University of Georgia; with permission. Copyright © 2015. All rights reserved.)

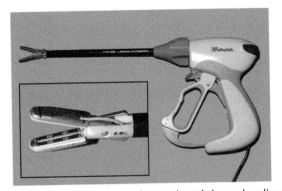

Fig. 4. The LigaSure Atlas (available in 20- and 37-cm lengths) vessel sealing/cutting system is a disposable human instrument but is frequently cleaned and resterilized for repeated veterinary use. (*Courtesy of* The University of Georgia; with permission. Copyright © 2015. All rights reserved.)

For visualization, the monitor should be placed in front of the surgeon with laparoscopic instruments and telescope facing away from the surgeon and toward the monitor. A second slave monitor on the opposite side of the operating room allows viewing from both sides of the table and avoids the need to move the endoscopy tower.

PATIENT PREPARATION AND POSITIONING

Assessment of husbandry, history, and physical examination findings is essential for appropriate risk assessment of the laparoscopic procedure. Hematology, biochemistry, a clotting profile, urinalysis, and diagnostic imaging can be useful. The reader is referred to dedicated references on general anesthetic management and drug protocols.[20,21]

- Patients undergoing laparoscopy must be intubated because ventilation is required. Insufflation of the abdomen results in restricted movement of the diaphragm and an increase in end-tidal CO_2 and acidosis, which is managed by positive-pressure ventilation (**Fig. 5**). As a result, monitoring of cardiopulmonary parameters, including end-tidal CO_2 and blood pressure, is vital for patients undergoing laparoscopy.
- The extent of fur clipping will depend on the type of laparoscopic procedure performed. Thermal support is vital, regardless of the extent of the clip, particularly in smaller patients.
- Position of the patient depends on the procedure to be performed; dorsal recumbency is used in most cases, at least to place the first port and the telescope.
- A tilting table allowing both side-to-side and front-to-back movement is ideal and provides greatest versatility, allowing displacement of organs by gravity to improve visualization (**Fig. 6**). When using a tilting table, it is important to secure the patient to the table to prevent slipping and falling. If a tilting table is not available, a variety of positioning aids can be used. Tabletop tilting platforms are also available.

APPROACH

The approach to laparoscopic techniques in exotic mammals is similar to that used in domestic dogs and cats, keeping in mind the differences in anatomy and size. The choice of location of cannula insertion and number of ports required depends on the procedure to be performed. A single-port technique is used most often for

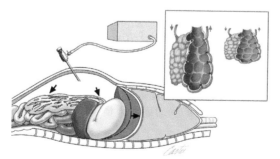

Fig. 5. The compressive effects of insufflation on abdominal viscera and lung alveoli. (*Courtesy of* The University of Georgia; with permission. Copyright © 2015. All rights reserved.)

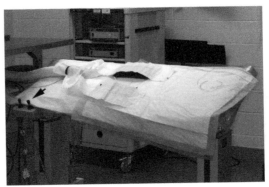

Fig. 6. Electronic tilting table with joy-stick control (*arrow*). (*Courtesy of* The University of Georgia; with permission. Copyright © 2015. All rights reserved.)

abdominal cavity exploration and collection of biopsies. Multiple-port techniques are used for a variety of surgical procedures, and larger or more complex biopsy collections.

SINGLE-PORT TECHNIQUE

Entry into the abdominal cavity can be achieved using a closed or an open approach. A closed approach is performed using a Veress needle, which has an outer sharp needle and an inner blunt spring-loaded obturator. The obturator advances beyond the sharp needle after entry into the abdominal cavity. The placement of the Veress needle is quicker than an open approach; however, there is increased risk of visceral damage including the spleen, and the voluminous and delicate gastrointestinal tract of herbivorous mammals. The authors prefer an open approach (Hasson technique). A small skin incision is made at a point along the linea alba. In general, this is made over or in the region of the umbilicus. The size of the incision depends on the size of the animal and the telescope-sheath to be used. In most exotic mammals less than 10 kg, this is 3 to 4 mm. The muscle layer is elevated and a stab incision is made through the linea alba. A 2.7-mm telescope, housed within a 4.8-mm sheath, is inserted through the incision into the peritoneal cavity, and entry into the peritoneal cavity is confirmed on the display monitor. Once the entry is confirmed, a mattress suture may need to be placed through the incision and around the sheath to create an airtight seal (**Fig. 7**). Carbon dioxide insufflation is then initiated (for example, at a rate of 0.5 L/min for a 2-kg mammal) to a pressure of 8 to 12 mm Hg. In very small mammals, air delivered manually by a syringe through the ingress port can also be used. A recent study in cats has shown no difference in working space comparing 8 and 15 mm Hg; however, there was a significant difference in cardiopulmonary parameters.[22] There are no such studies in exotic mammals, and anatomic differences must be taken into account. To reduce discomfort and cardiopulmonary derangements, the lowest pressure required to provide adequate visualization and working space is advised. After insufflation, the abdominal viscera can be viewed and appropriate documentation can be undertaken (**Fig. 8**). The telescope sheath instrument port can then be used for collection of biopsy samples.

MULTIPLE-PORT TECHNIQUES

Multiple ports are required for laparoscopic surgery, more extensive abdominal exploration, and larger biopsy collection (**Fig. 9**). The first port is created as

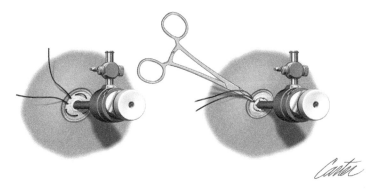

Fig. 7. The Hasson technique for the placement of the initial cannula. The mattress suture can either be secured using hemostats or tied. (*Courtesy of* The University of Georgia; with permission. Copyright © 2015. All rights reserved.)

described above for single-port technique using an appropriate-sized cannula. Following insufflation, additional ports are placed by making a small skin incision over the proposed port site. A cannula with a trocar is inserted through the abdominal wall, with the abdominal cavity insufflated, using the telescope to view the insertion site and avoiding accidental visceral trauma (**Fig. 10**A). Once the cannula is

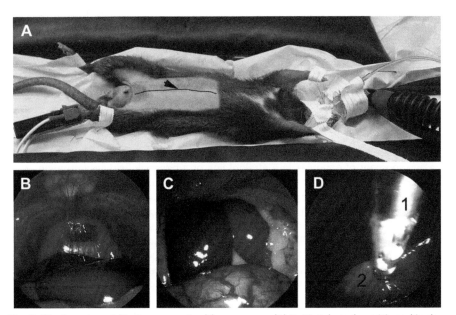

Fig. 8. Single-entry rat (*Rattus norvegicus*) laparoscopy. (*A*) Rat intubated, positioned in dorsal recumbency, and prepared for laparoscopy. The linea alba is indicated, and the preferred insertion point is the umbilicus (*arrow*). (*B, C*) Laparoscopic view of the rat's abdominal cavity. (*D*) Biopsy forceps (*1*) harvesting a liver (*2*) sample from a rat. (*Courtesy of* The University of Georgia; with permission. Copyright © 2015. All rights reserved.)

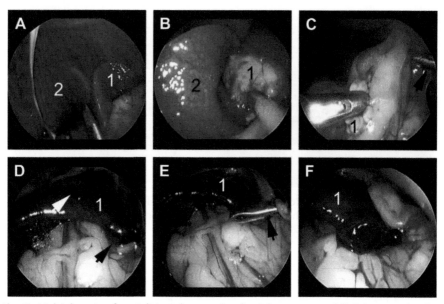

Fig. 9. Multiple-entry ferret (*Mustela putorius furo*) laparoscopy. (*A*) Using a palpation probe to examine between the left lateral (*1*) and left medial (*2*) lobes of the liver. (*B*) Identification of an abnormally thickened gallbladder (*1*) between the quadrate and right medial liver lobes (*2*). (*C*) Endoscopic biopsy of the pancreas (*1*) using 3-mm biopsy forceps that confirmed the presence of an insulinoma. Note the use of 3-mm atraumatic tissue forceps (*arrow*) to retract the mesentery. (*D*) View of the spleen (*1*) demonstrating a nodular abnormality (*black arrow*), and the previous site of attempted ultrasound-guided fine-needle aspiration (*white arrow*). (*E*) Biopsy of the spleen (*1*) using 3-mm biopsy forceps (*arrow*). (*F*) Postbiopsy view of the spleen (*1*); note the absence of severe hemorrhage. (*Courtesy of* The University of Georgia; with permission. Copyright © 2015. All rights reserved.)

inserted, the trocar is removed. An instrument, such as a biopsy forceps, can then be inserted (**Fig. 11**).

A 3-port technique is one of the most versatile and commonly used approaches. The arrangement of cannulas in a straight line or a baseball field configuration, with the instruments facing away from the surgeon and toward the monitor, creates triangulation and provides depth perception (**Fig. 12**). Cannulas are placed in a sagittal or transverse plane depending on the procedure planned or organ of interest. For access to dorsolateral structures, such as ovaries and kidneys, a sagittal arrangement of cannulas along the ventral midline is used (**Fig. 13**). For access to cranial (liver, gallbladder, pancreas, stomach) or caudal (bladder, large intestines) structures, a transverse arrangement is used, with the first port placed on the midline (**Fig. 14**). Some procedures require paramedian or paralumbar approaches, such as adrenalectomies (**Fig. 15**).

To ensure optimal port placement, the instrument and port angles are important. The manipulation angle is the angle created by the 2 working ports and should be 60°. The azimuth angle is the angle between one instrument and the axis of the telescope. The azimuth angles for the 2 instruments should be equal. The elevation angle is the angle between the instrument and the horizontal plane; the ideal is 60°.

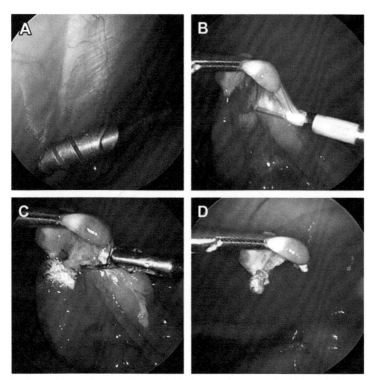

Fig. 10. Endoscopic ovariectomy in a rabbit (*Oryctolagus cuniculus*). (*A*) Placement of a 3.5-mm graphite/plastic-threaded cannula under endoscopic guidance. (*B*) View of the ovary elevated using atraumatic (fenestrated) grasping forceps to reveal the vasculature within the mesovarium. The bipolar forceps are advanced to coagulate the vessels before transection in this rabbit. (*C*) Monopolar scissors being used to coagulate and cut to dissect the ovary free from the mesovarium. (*D*) The cannula was slid up the shaft of the grasping forceps and is outside the abdominal cavity (not shown). The forceps and ovary are gently withdrawn through the hole in the body wall. (*Courtesy of* The University of Georgia; with permission. Copyright © 2015. All rights reserved.)

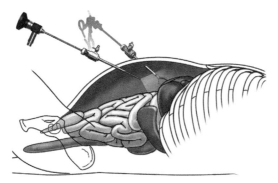

Fig. 11. A 2-port approach for a liver biopsy. (*Courtesy of* The University of Georgia; with permission. Copyright © 2015. All rights reserved.)

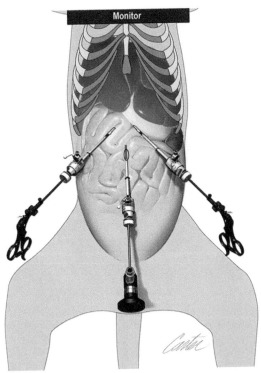

Fig. 12. A baseball-field configuration of a 3-port approach using a transverse arrangement. (*Courtesy of* The University of Georgia; with permission. Copyright © 2015. All rights reserved.)

PROCEDURES
Biopsy

Biopsies can be performed using a single-portal technique by introducing 1.7-mm biopsy forceps through the instrument channel of the operating sheath. A second port may be placed to allow insertion of larger biopsy forceps. Liver biopsy techniques have been described in rabbits and rats.[16,23] The study in rabbits compared 1.7-mm and 3-mm biopsy forceps for diagnostic quality of liver biopsy samples and found that the larger biopsy forceps provided samples with a higher number of portal triads and central veins, but had more severe artifactual changes.[23]

Ovariectomy

Ovariectomies have become the preferred method of sterilization in dogs and cats in Europe (and have also been recommended as the technique of choice in the United States). The technique has been used by the authors in both exotic and zoo animals. With the removal of an ovary inhibiting the development of uterine pathologic abnormality, ovariectomy seems protective against uterine neoplasia. However, because of the high risk of developing uterine adenocarcinoma, the authors recommend ovariectomy only in rabbits younger than 9 months of age. At the time of ovariectomy, the uterus should be evaluated, and if uterine pathologic abnormality is suspected, a complete ovariohysterectomy should be performed.

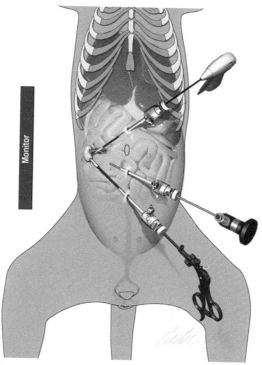

Fig. 13. The general position and orientation of the telescope and 2 instruments in a sagittal arrangement for access to the right dorsolateral ovary in a generic carnivore. (*Courtesy of The University of Georgia; with permission. Copyright © 2015. All rights reserved.*)

An ovariectomy can be performed using a 2-port or 3-port technique. A 2-port technique has been described in dogs and requires an extensive lateral fur clip and lateral recumbency to allow transfixation of the ovary to the abdominal wall. Although the technique reduces the number of ports placed, it may be undesirable in some animals to extend the fur clipping, particularly in zoo display animals.

A 3-port technique is most commonly used for performing an ovariectomy, especially in herbivores and omnivores wherein the voluminous gastrointestinal tract can make ovary location and manipulation more difficult. The first port is created through the umbilicus as described above. After insufflation of the abdomen, the abdominal cavity is examined with the telescope. Two additional cannulas are inserted 3 to 5 cm cranial and caudal to the first port, as described above for multiple-port entry (see **Fig. 10**A). Once the telescope and the cannulas are in position, the table is tilted approximately 30° laterally, causing the viscera to fall to the dependant side, revealing the contralateral ovary. Grasping forceps are inserted through a cannula (left cannula for a right-handed surgeon and right cannula for a left-handed surgeon) and the ovary is grasped. It is best to use handles with a racket to ensure the ovary is not dropped. The ovary is elevated, and the ovarian vessels are exposed. The vasculature is coagulated using radiosurgery or LigaSure, depending on the instrument size used and the size of the patient (**Fig. 10**B, C). Once the ovary is free, the cannula is removed from the abdominal wall up the shaft of the instrument, and the ovary is removed through the port site (**Fig. 10**D). After the surgical site is inspected for hemorrhage, the patient

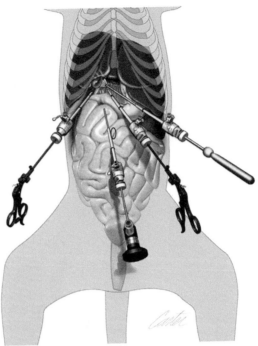

Fig. 14. A multiple-port approach for a laparoscopic cholecystectomy. (*Courtesy of* The University of Georgia; with permission. Copyright © 2015. All rights reserved.)

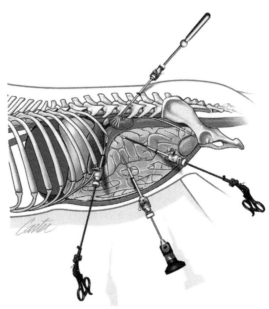

Fig. 15. A paralumbar approach for a laparoscopic adrenalectomy. (*Courtesy of* The University of Georgia; with permission. Copyright © 2015. All rights reserved.)

is tilted to the opposite side and the procedure is repeated from the other side of the table. Three-port ovariectomy technique has been described in rabbits[24]; however, the authors have used the technique in various species including large zoo animals (**Fig. 16**).

Endoscope-Assisted Laparotomy

Endoscopy can also be used for performing procedures through a smaller surgical incision, often an enlarged port entry site. Endoscope-assisted laparotomy is most useful when entering a viscus, such as the gastrointestinal tract or the bladder, because there is reduced risk of leakage of gastrointestinal tract content or urine into the abdominal cavity. The telescope is used to isolate an organ, such as a loop of bowel, which can then be exteriorized through the enlarged port entry site. A biopsy or enterotomy can then be performed traditionally, outside of the body cavity (**Fig. 17**).

Other Procedures

There is a paucity of published literature in exotic pet laparoscopic procedures; however, this is likely to change in the future. In domestic animals, laparoscopy is used for abdominal exploration, various organ biopsy, liver lobectomy, cholecystectomy and cholecystocentesis, splenectomy, gastrointestinal foreign body removal and feeding tube placement, urinary tract procedures (nephrectomy, cystotomy), reproductive tract procedures, including cryptorchid and abdominal castrations, and adrenalectomy.[19] There are numerous indications of these procedures in exotic animal medicine, because diseases requiring these procedures are commonly diagnosed.

Closure

On completion of a laparoscopic procedure, the insufflation gas is removed from the abdominal cavity by applying gentle external pressure on the abdomen or by the use

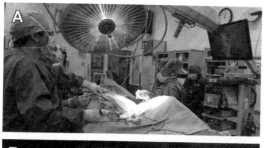
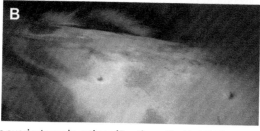

Fig. 16. Endoscopic ovariectomy in a tiger (*Panthera tigris*). (*A*) Three-port ovariectomy in a tiger using 5-mm instrumentation and Ligasure Atlas. (*B*) After closure view of the ventral abdomen. (*Courtesy of* The University of Georgia; with permission. Copyright © 2015. All rights reserved.)

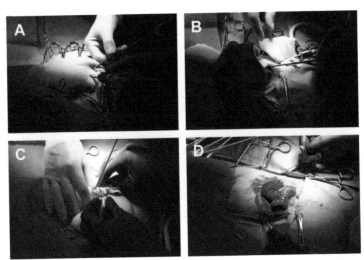

Fig. 17. Endoscope-assisted intestinal surgery in a ferret. (*A*) Ferret in dorsal recumbency, with a telescope in the midline cannula and a rigid instrument in the lateral cannula. (*B*) Lateral port being surgically enlarged. (*C*) A loop of small intestine being exteriorized through an enlarged port site. (*D*) A loop of small intestine exteriorized for surgical intervention through an enlarged port site. (*Courtesy of* The University of Georgia; with permission. Copyright © 2015. All rights reserved.)

of vacuum to one of the cannula side ports, reducing postoperative discomfort. The port sites are closed using a single skin suture or tissue adhesive; for the first port placed using Hasson technique, the linea alba is closed with a single suture, followed by routine skin closure.

Complications

Complications are often related to surgeon inexperience and include inadvertent organ trauma, hemorrhage, traumatic tissue handling, and initially prolonged anesthetic and surgical time. With experience, these complications decrease. To ensure laparoscopy caseload and increasing experience, it is recommended that the surgeon retain the option of converting to a traditional laparotomy if required. This recommendation should be communicated to the owner; a signed consent form stating this is advised.

Insufflation-related complications include impaired ventilation, acidosis, and reduced venous return to the heart. Leaving insufflation gas in the abdominal cavity causes increased discomfort on recovery.

Postoperative Care

In the absence of complications, the authors have observed rapid return to feeding and normal behavior in patients undergoing laparoscopy over traditional laparotomy. In rats, postoperative pain after liver biopsy obtained by laparoscopy was associated with fewer signs of pain compared with laparotomy.[16] Analgesia in the form of nonsteroidal anti-inflammatories and opioids should be administered as required. Supportive care, including fluid therapy and nutritional support, should also be provided as required.

Future Considerations

Some of the current areas of research in domestic animals include lift laparoscopy, single-incision laparoscopic surgery through specialized ports, and natural orifice laparoscopic surgeries. These current areas of research are beyond the scope of this article; however, lift laparoscopy is briefly mentioned. Lift laparoscopy relies on passive filling of the abdominal cavity with room air and creating an isobaric pneumoperitoneum by lifting the abdominal using a custom-made device. In humans, lift laparoscopy is associated with less cardiopulmonary changes and less shoulder pain and has been used in sedated patients under local anesthesia. Lift laparoscopy is being investigated in dogs and cats as an alternative to CO_2 insufflation. Studies comparing lift laparoscopy and capnoperitoneum laparoscopy have shown less frequency of hypercapnia and lower requirement for anesthetic gas. However, no difference in pain was noted and subjectively poorer visualization occurred with lift laparoscopy.[25,26] Lift laparoscopy may be a viable option in cases where CO_2 insufflation is undesirable or contraindicated, or in cases where endotracheal intubation is not possible.

SUMMARY

Ongoing development and application of laparoscopic techniques to exotic mammals is an exciting area of research. The ability to apply minimally invasive techniques to these patients will reduce morbidity and mortality, and many exotic pet clients recognize this.

ACKNOWLEDGMENTS

The authors are grateful to their endoscopy technicians, Ashley Schuller and Carole McElhannon, and to the numerous students, technicians, interns, residents, and faculty that assist with cases in the Veterinary Medical Learning Center at the University of Georgia. They are also grateful to Karl Storz Veterinary Endoscopy for their continued support of the research and development programs.

REFERENCES

1. Pizzi R. Minimally invasive surgery techniques. In: Miller RE, Fowler ME, editors. Fowler's zoo and wild animal medicine, vol. 8. St Louis (MO): Elsevier; Saunders; 2015. p. 688–98.
2. Portas TJ, Hermes R, Bryant BR, et al. Anesthesia and use of a sling system to facilitate transvaginal laparoscopy in a black rhinoceros (Diceros bicornis minor). J Zoo Wildl Med 2006;37:202–5.
3. Sweet J, Hendrickson DA, Stetter M, et al. Exploratory rigid laparoscopy in an African elephant (Loxodonta africana). J Zoo Wildl Med 2014;45:941–6.
4. Pizzi R, Cracknell J, David S, et al. Laparoscopic cholecystectomy under field conditions in Asiatic black bears (Ursus thibetanus) rescued from illegal bile farming in Vietnam. Vet Rec 2011;169:469.
5. Kolata RJ. Laparoscopic ovariohysterectomy and hysterectomy on African lions (Panthera leo) using the ultracision harmonic scalpel. J Zoo Wildl Med 2002;33: 280–2.
6. Steeil JC, Sura PA, Ramsay EC. Laparoscopic-assisted ovariectomy of tigers (Panthera tigris) with the use of the LigaSure device. J Zoo Wildl Med 2012;43: 566–72.
7. Hartman MJ, Monnet E, Kirberger RM, et al. Laparoscopic sterilization of the African lioness (Panthera leo). Vet Surg 2013;42:559–64.
8. Rubio-Martínez LM, Hendrickson DA, Stetter M, et al. Laparoscopic vasectomy in African elephants (Loxodonta africana). Vet Surg 2014;43:507–14.

9. Marais HJ, Hendrickson DA, Stetter M, et al. Laparoscopic vasectomy in African savannah elephant (Loxodonta africana); surgical technique and results. J Zoo Wildl Med 2013;44:S18–20.

10. Radcliffe RM, Hendrickson DA, Richardson GL, et al. Standing laparoscopic-guided uterine biopsy in a southern white rhinoceros (Ceratotherium simum simum). J Zoo Wildl Med 2000;31:201–7.

11. Lee SY, Jung DH, Park SJ, et al. Unilateral laparoscopic ovariectomy in a red fox (Vulpes vulpes) with an ovarian cyst. J Zoo Wildl Med 2013;45:678–81.

12. Higgins JL, Hendrickson DA. Surgical procedures in pinniped and cetacean species. J Zoo Wildl Med 2013;44:817–36.

13. Divers SJ. Exotic mammal diagnostic endoscopy and endosurgery. Vet Clin North Am Exot Anim Pract 2010;13:255–72.

14. Divers SJ. Exotic mammal diagnostic and surgical endoscopy. In: Quesenberry K, Carpenter JW, editors. Ferrets, rabbits and rodents: clinical medicine and surgery. 3rd edition. St Louis (MO): Elsevier; Saunders; 2012. p. 485–501.

15. Fernandez-Pineda I, Millan A, Morcillo J, et al. Laparoscopic surgery in a rat model. J Laparoendosc Adv Surg Tech A 2010;20:575–6.

16. Préfontaine L, Hélie P, Vachon P. Postoperative pain in Sprague Dawley rats after liver biopsy by laparotomy versus laparoscopy. Lab Anim 2015;44:174–8.

17. Targarona EM, Espert JJ, Bombuy E. Laparoscopic splenectomy in a rat model: developing an easy technique. J Laparoendosc Adv Surg Tech A 1999;9:503–6.

18. Van Velthoven RF, Hoffmann P. Methods for laparoscopic training using animal models. Curr Urol Rep 2006;7:114–9.

19. Rawlings CA. Laparoscopy. In: Tams TR, Rawlings CA, editors. Small animal endoscopy. 3rd edition. St Louis (MO): Elsevier; Mosby; 2011. p. 397–477.

20. Hawkins MG, Pascoe PJ. Anesthesia, analgesia, and sedation of small mammals. In: Quesenberry K, Carpenter JW, editors. Ferrets, rabbits and rodents: clinical medicine and surgery. 3rd edition. St Louis (MO): Elsevier; Saunders; 2012. p. 429–51.

21. West G, Heard DJ, Caulkett N. Zoo animal and wildlife immobilization and anesthesia. Ames (IA): Blackwell Publishing; 2007.

22. Mayhew PD, Pascoe PJ, Kass PH. Effects of pneumoperitoneum induced at various pressures on cardiorespiratory function and working space during laparoscopy in cats. Am J Vet Res 2013;74:1340–6.

23. Proença L, Camus M, Nemeth N, et al. Diagnostic quality of percutaneous fine-needle aspirates and laparoscopic biopsy specimens of the liver in rabbits (Oryctolagus cuniculus). J Am Vet Med Assoc 2015;246:313–20.

24. Divers SJ. Clinical technique: endoscopic oophorectomy in the rabbit (Oryctolagus cuniculus): the future of preventative sterilizations. J Exot Pet Med 2010;19:231–7.

25. Fransson BA, Ragle CA. Lift laparoscopy in dogs and cats: 12 cases (2008–2009). J Am Vet Med Assoc 2011;239:1574–9.

26. Fransson BA, Grubb TL, Perez TE, et al. Cardiorespiratory changes and pain response of lift laparoscopy compared to capnoperitoneum laparoscopy in dogs. Vet Surg 2014;9999:1–8.

Index

Note: Page numbers of article titles are in **boldface** type.

Vet Clin Exot Anim 19 (2016) 287–324
http://dx.doi.org/10.1016/S1094-9194(15)00096-1
1094-9194/16/$ – see front matter © 2016 Elsevier Inc. All rights reserved.

vetexotic.theclinics.com